PROGRESS IN CLINICAL AND BIOLOGICAL RESEARCH

Series Editors

RECENT TITLES

ﹾ the publisher for information about previous titles in this series

ETIOLOGY OF BREAST AND GYNECOLOGICAL CANCERS

ETIOLOGY OF BREAST AND GYNECOLOGICAL CANCERS

Proceedings of the Ninth International Conference on Carcinogenesis and Risk Assessment, Held in Austin, Texas, November 29 – December 2, 1995

Editors

C. Marcelo Aldaz
University of Texas
M.D. Anderson Cancer Center
Science Park – Research Division
Smithville, Texas

Michael N. Gould
Comprehensive Cancer Center
University of Wisconsin
Madison, Wisconsin

John McLachlan
Department of Pharmacology
Center for Bioenvironmental Research
Tulane University
New Orleans, Louisiana

Thomas J. Slaga
University of Texas
M.D. Anderson Cancer Center
Science Park – Research Division
Smithville, Texas

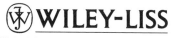

A JOHN WILEY & SONS, INC., PUBLICATION
New York • Chichester • Weinheim • Brisbane • Singapore • Toronto

The publication of this volume was facilitated by the authors and editors who submitted the text in a form suitable for direct reproduction without subsequent editing or proofreading by the publisher.

Library of Congress Cataloging-in-Publication Data

International Conference on Carcinogenesis and Risk Assessment (9th :
   1995 : Austin, Tex.)
      Etiology of breast and gynecological cancers : proceedings of the
   Ninth International Conference on Carcinogenesis and Risk
   Assessment, held in Austin, Texas, November 29–December 2, 1995 /
   editors, C. Marcelo Aldaz ... [et al.].
      p.   cm — (Progress in clinical and biological research :
   396)
      Includes bibliographical references and index.
      ISBN 0-471-16901-3 (alk. paper)
      1. Breast—Cancer—Etiology—Congresses. 2. Generative organs,
   Female—Cancer—Etiology—Congresses. 3. Carcinogenesis—
   Congresses. I. Aldaz, C. Marcelo, 1956–   . II. Title
   III. Series.
      [DNLM: 1. Breast Neoplasms—genetics—congresses. 2. Breast
   Neoplasms—chemically induced—congresses. 3. Genital Neoplasms,
   Female—genetics—congresses. 4. Genital Neoplasms, Female—
   chemically induced—congresses. 5. Environmental Exposure—adverse
   effects—congresses. 6. Risk Assessment—congresses. W1 PR668E
   v.396 1997 / WP 870 I58159e 1997]
   RC280.B8I5626 1997
   616.99'449071—dc21
   DNLM/DLC
   for Library of Congress   97-40180
                                                                  CIP

The text of this book is printed on acid-free paper.

10 9 8 7 6 5 4 3 2 1

Contents

Contributors

C. Marcelo Aldaz, Department of Carcinogenesis, University of Texas M.D. Anderson Cancer Center, Science Park - Research Division, Smithville, TX 78957 **[63]**

Christine B. Ambrosone, Division of Molecular Epidemiology, National Center for Toxicological Research, Jefferson, AR 72079 **[83]**

Christina A. Bandera, Division of Gynecologic Oncology, Department of Obstetrics and Gynecology, University of Pennsylvania Medical Center, Philadelphia, PA 19104 **[185]**

Charles W. Boone, Chemoprevention Branch, Division of Cancer Prevention and Control, National Cancer Institute, National Institutes of Health, Bethesda, MD 20892 **[159]**

Jeff Boyd, Division of Gynecologic Oncology, Department of Obstetrics and Gynecology, University of Pennsylvania Medical Center, Philadelphia, PA 19104 **[185]**

Andrew J. Brenner, Department of Carcinogenesis, University of Texas M.D. Anderson Cancer Center, Science Park - Research Division, Smithville, TX 78957 **[63]**

Kevin D. Brown, Laboratory of Gene Transfer, National Center for Human Genome Research, National Institutes of Health, Bethesda, MD 20892 **[101]**

Kenneth H. Buetow, Division of Population Science, Fox Chase Cancer Center, Philadelphia, PA 19111 **[53]**

Bill Bullock, Bowman Gray School of Medicine, Wake Forest University, Winston-Salem, NC 27709 **[217]**

Byron E. Butterworth, Chemical Industry Institute of Technology, Research Triangle Park, NC 21709 **[125]**

Phillip Carthew, MRC Toxicology Unit, University of Leicester, Leicester LE1 9HN, United Kingdom **[257]**

Tae-Ton Chun, Departments of Biochemistry and Meat and Animal Science, University of Wisconsin, Madison, WI 53706 **[233]**

Jeanne M. Connolly, Division of Nutrition and Endocrinology, American Health Foundation, Valhalla, NY 10595 **[147]**

James A Crowell, Chemoprevention Branch, Division of Cancer Prevention and Control, National Cancer Institute, National Institutes of Health, Bethesda, MD 20892 **[159]**

Robert Dickson, Department of Anatomy and Cell Biology, Georgetown University Medical Center, Lombardi Cancer Research Center, Washington, DC 20007 **[217]**

The numbers in brackets are the opening page numbers of the contributors' articles.

Susan R. Eldridge, Pathology Associates International, Frederick, MD 21701 **[125]**

Jeffrey L. Everitt, Department of Experimental Pathology and Toxicology, Chemical Industry Institute of Toxicology, Research Triangle Park, NC 27709 **[205]**

Leslie G. Ford, Community Oncology and Rehabilitation Branch, Division of Cancer Prevention and Control, National Cancer Institute, Bethesda, MD 20892 **[271]**

Judy E. Garber, Dana-Farber Cancer Institute, Boston, MA 02115 **[53]**

Andrew K. Godwin, Division of Population Science, Fox Chase Cancer Center, Philadelphia, PA 19111 **[53]**

Jack Gorski, Departments of Biochemistry and Meat and Animal Science, University of Wisconsin, Madison, WI 53706 **[233]**

Marco M. Gottardis, Department of Toxicology, Ligand Pharmaceuticals, La Jolla, CA 92037 **[205]**

Michael N. Gould, University of Wisconsin Comprehensive Cancer Center, Madison, WI 27511 **[125]**

Karen Gray, Laboratory of Reproductive and Developmental Toxicology, National Institute of Environmental Health Science, Research Triangle Park, NC 27709; present address: Department of Obstetrics and Gynecology, Uniformed Services University of Health Sciences, Bethesda, MD 20814 **[217]**

David Gregg, Departments of Biochemistry and Meat and Animal Science, University of Wisconsin, Madison, WI 53706 **[233]**

Ernest T. Hawk, Chemoprevention Branch, Division of Cancer Prevention and Control, National Cancer Institute, National Institutes of Health, Bethesda, MD 20892 **[159]**

Sue R. Howe, Department of Biochemistry, University of Texas Southwestern Medical Center, Dallas, TX 75235 **[205]**

Barbara Sorenson Hulka, Epidemiology Department, The University of North Carolina at Chapel Hill, Chapel Hill, NC 27599-7400 **[17]**

Karen A. Johnson, Community Oncology and Rehabilitation Branch, Division of Cancer Prevention and Control, National Cancer Institute, Bethesda, MD 20892 **[271]**

V. Craig Jordan, Robert H. Lurie Cancer Center, Northwestern University Medical School Chicago, IL 60611 **[245]**

Gary J. Kelloff, Chemoprevention Branch, Division of Cancer Prevention and Control, National Cancer Institute, National Institutes of Health, Bethesda, MD 20892 **[159]**

Johnathan M. Lancaster, Laboratory of Molecular Carcinogenesis, National Institute of Environmental

Health Sciences, National Institutes of Health, Research Triangle Park, NC 27709 [31]

Charles E. Land, Radiation Epidemiology Branch, Division of Cancer Epidemiology and Genetics, National Cancer Institute, Bethesda, MD 20892-7362 [115]

Chang-Kee Lim, MRC Toxicology Unit, University of Leicester, Leicester LE1 9HN, United Kingdom [257]

Xin-Hua Liu, Division of Nutrition and Endocrinology, American Health Foundation, Valhalla, NY 10595 [147]

Ronald A. Lubet, Chemoprevention Branch, Division of Cancer Prevention and Control, National Cancer Institute, National Institutes of Health, Bethesda, MD 20892 [159]

Elizabeth A. Martin, MRC Toxicology Unit, University of Leicester, Leicester LE1 9HN, United Kingdom [257]

John McLachlan, Laboratory of Reproductive and Developmental Toxicology, National Institute of Environmental Health Science, Research Triangle Park, NC 27709; present address: Department of Pharmacology, Center for Bioenvironmental Research, Tulane University, New Orleans, LA 70112 [217]

Glenn Merlino, Laboratory of Molecular Biology, National Cancer Institute, National Institutes of Health, Bethesda, MD 20892 [217]

Stephen A. Narod, Women's College Hospital, Toronto, Ontario M5G 1N9, Canada [53]

Susan G. Nayfield, Chemoprevention Branch, Division of Cancer Prevention and Control, National Cancer Institute, National Institutes of Health, Bethesda, MD 20892 [159]

Catherine M. Phelan, Department of Medical Genetics, Montreal General Hospital, Montreal, Quebec H3G 1A4, Canada [53]

Kimberly Raszmann, Laboratory of Reproductive and Developmental Toxicology, National Institute of Environmental Health Science, Research Triangle Park, NC 27709 [217]

Timothy R. Rebbeck, Departments of Biostatistics and Epidemiology, University of Pennsylvania School of Medicine, Philadelphia, PA 19104 [53]

David P. Rose, Division of Nutrition and Endocrinology, American Health Foundation, Valhalla, NY 10595 [147]

Irma H. Russo, Breast Cancer Research Laboratory, Fox Chase Cancer Center, Philadelphia, PA 19111 [1]

Jose Russo, Breast Cancer Research Laboratory, Fox Chase Cancer Center, Philadelphia, PA 19111 [1]

Stephen H. Safe, Department of Veterinary Physiology and Pharmacology, Texas A&M University, College Station, TX 77843-4466 [133]

Peter G. Shields, Laboratory of Human Carcinogenesis, National Cancer Institute, Bethesda, MD 20892 **[83]**

Caroline C. Sigman, CCS Associates, Mountain View, CA 94043 **[159]**

Lewis L. Smith, MRC Toxicology Unit, University of Leicester, Leicester LE1 9HN, United Kingdom **[257]**

Vernon E. Steele, Chemoprevention Branch, Division of Cancer Prevention and Control, National Cancer Institute, National Institutes of Health, Bethesda, MD 20892 **[159]**

Jerry Styles, MRC Toxicology Unit, University of Leicester, Leicester LE1 9HN, United Kingdom **[257]**

Danilo A. Tagle, Laboratory of Gene Transfer, National Center for Human Genome Research, National Institutes of Health, Bethesda, MD 20892 **[101]**

Debra A. Tonetti, Robert H. Lurie Cancer Center, Northwestern University Medical School, Chicago, IL 60611 **[245]**

Amy H. Walker, Departments of Biostatistics and Epidemiology, University of Pennsylvania School of Medicine, Philadelphia, PA 19104 **[53]**

Cheryl Walker, Department of Carcinogenesis, University of Texas M.D. Anderson Cancer Center, Science Park - Research Division, Smithville, TX 78957 **[205]**

Barbara L. Weber, Departments of Medicine and Genetics, University of Pennsylvania School of Medicine, Philadelphia, PA 19104 **[53]**

Douglas Wendell, Departments of Biochemistry and Meat and Animal Science, University of Wisconsin, Madison, WI 53706 **[233]**

Ian N.H. White, MRC Toxicology Unit, University of Leicester, Leicester LE1 9HN, United Kingdom **[257]**

Roger W. Wiseman, Laboratory of Molecular Carcinogenesis, National Institute of Environmental Health Sciences, National Institutes of Health, Research Triangle Park, NC 27709 **[31]**

Timothy Zacharewski, Department of Pharmacology and Toxicology, University of Western Ontario, London, Ontario N6A 5C1 **[133]**

Preface

This book presents a summary of the Ninth International Conference on Carcinogenesis and Risk Assessment, "Etiology of Breast and Gynecological Cancers." This conference was held from November 29 to December 2, 1995, at the Barton Creek Conference Resort in Austin, Texas. It was the ninth conference in a series covering research and contemporary issues on carcinogenesis and risk assessment.

Breast cancer together with gynecological cancer accounts for over 150 cancers per 100,000 persons at risk. While the incidence of breast cancer predominates, the total mortality from gynecological cancers is approximately 50% of that from breast cancer, making both cancer types a major public health concern. Not only do these cancers have a common target population, but many also have common etiological features. Both share a major hormonal component in their etiology. In addition, gynecological cancers such as ovarian cancer and breast cancer have elevated risk due to similar genetic changes in genes such as BRCA1. Furthermore, both gynecological and breast cancer have important environmental factors involved in their etiology. These factors include ionizing radiation, viruses, chemical xenobiotics, diet, and nutrition.

Based on these common etiological factors and target population, the organizers of this series of meetings chose to devote this conference to the interactions of environmental factors and host genetics in the etiology of breast and gynecological cancers. This volume contains outstanding chapters from those who presented papers at this meeting. This book reviews important environmental and genetic factors, including hormones, radiation, viruses, and predisposing genetics that are key to the induction of these cancers. These topics are presented by laboratory and clinical investigators as well as by epidemiologists, giving broad prospective to the causes and risk factors for the diseases. Emphasis was also placed on discussion of validation and extrapolation issues from animal models to man and their impact in risk assessment. Finally, intervention strategies are discussed in terms of chemoprevention, which has the potential to reduce the morbidity and mortality from these cancers of women.

C. Marcelo Aldaz
Michael N. Gould
John McLachlan
Thomas J. Slaga

Acknowledgments

The conference on which this volume is based, "Etiology of Breast and Gynecological Cancers," was supported in part by grants from the National Cancer Institute (R13 CA/HD 69052-01) and the National Institute of Environmental Health Sciences and by generous contributions from both academia and private industry. The conference organizers sincerely wish to thank the following sponsors: Hoffman LaRoche Inc.; the Procter and Gamble Company; the Rohm and Hass Company; The University of Texas M.D. Anderson Cancer Center, Science Park Division; the ILSI-Health and Environmental Sciences Institute; the American Industrial Health Council; Allied Signal Inc.; Chevron; Glaxo Wellcome; Dermigen Inc.; and Wyeth-Ayerst Research.

The Chairs of this meeting Drs. C. Marcelo Aldaz, Michael N. Gould, and John McLachlan, were assisted in the planning and organization of the conference by Program Committee members Drs. Byron E. Butterworth, R. Michael McClain, Denise Robinson, Thomas J. Slaga, Cheryl Walker, and Roger W. Wiseman.

The meeting organizers would like to thank the speakers who participated in this meeting and who contributed the outstanding chapters that make up this volume. We also want to thank Dr. Lea I. Sekely for her encouragement and helpful decisions. Special thanks go to the conference staff, Karen Engel, Mary Lou Fendley, Judy Ing, and LeNel Rice. Thanks for secretarial assistance in the preparation of this volume go to Mary Lou Fendley and Carrie McKinley.

Etiology of Breast and
Gynecological Cancers, pages 1–16
© 1997 Wiley-Liss, Inc.

TOWARD A UNIFIED CONCEPT OF MAMMARY CARCINOGENESIS

Jose Russo, M.D. and Irma H. Russo, M.D.

Breast Cancer Research Laboratory, Fox Chase Cancer Center,
Philadelphia, PA 19111.

INTRODUCTION

The study of human breast cancer reveals that the development of this disease, which is estimated will be diagnosed in 184,300 women in the United States in 1996 (Parker, et al., 1996), is associated with a combination of factors, either external, such as diet, socioeconomic status, or exposure to ionizing radiations, or internal, namely endocrinologic, familial or genetic factors. Among these factors, gender, age, genetic predisposition and reproductive history have been identified to play major roles, as evidenced by the fact that women are more prone to develop breast cancer than men, the disease is diagnosed more frequently in women over 40 years of age, and family history of breast or breast/ovarian cancer increases by nine fold cancer risk (Parker, et al., 1996). Reproductive history can influence positively or negatively the risk of developing breast cancer, since early first full-term pregnancy is associated with a lower incidence of breast cancer (Boring, et al.,1993; De Waard and Trichopoulos, 1988; Henderson, et al., 1993; John and Kelsey, 1993; MacMahon, et al., 1970; McGregor, et al., 1977; Rosner, et al., 1994), whereas nulliparity, late first full term or interrupted pregnancy are associated with a greater risk of disease development (Daling, et al., 1994, Newcomb, et al., 1996). Despite the wealth of information available on human breast cancer, neither the etiologic agent nor the mechanism(s) responsibles of its causation and initiation have been identified (Russo, J. and Ruso, I.H., 1994); this knowledge is indispensable for developing effective measures for the prevention and effective therapy of the disease. Its acquisition, however, is hindered by the lack of understanding of the the pathogenesis of the disease and the molecular basis of breast epithelial cell transformation (Russo, J., and Russo, I.H., 1994). Little is known on the pathogenesis of breast cancer, namely due to the long silent phase between initiation and tumor detection, the lack of identification of a specific site in which the initial event occurred, or the timing of its initiation (Russo, J.and Russo, I.H., 1987a; Russo, J., et al., 1990). More incomplete is our knowledege of the biological and molecular basis of the phenomena that lead a normal breast epithelial cell to malignancy (Russo, J., et al., 1988, 1989a, 1993; Soule, et al., 1990; Tait, et al., 1990; Basolo, et al., 1991; Russo, J. and Russo, I.H., 1993; Calaf and Russo, 1993). Many of the gaps in knowledge of the biology of the human disease have been bridged by extrapolations from experimental animal model data (Russo, I.H. and Russo, J., 1988; Russo, I.H., et al., 1989, 1991;

Russo, I.H., and Russo, J., 1989, 1993, 1994). Studies of the rat mammary carcinogenesis model have provided interesting insights on the origins of cancer. This model provides evidence that chemical carcinogens are causative agents of mammary cancer, that the initiation of the disease requires the interaction of the carcinogen with an undifferentiated and highly proliferating mammary gland, and that full term pregnancy protects the gland from neoplasia through the induction of differentiation. These findings have highlighted the importance of understanding the development of the breast, especially in its early phases, around puberty, in order to verify whether at this stage it exhibits characteristics indicative of a higher susceptibility to cancer initiation. This review covers some of the most relevant aspects of the developmental pattern of the postpubertal breast, new advances in the pathogenesis of breast cancer and *in vitro* cell transformation of human breast epithelial cells, in correlation with experimental data obtained in the rat mammary tumor model which has provided an understanding of the factors that modulate the susceptibility of this organ to carcinogenesis and their implications in the development of strategies for breast cancer prevention.

POSTPUBERTAL DEVELOPMENT OF THE HUMAN BREAST

The understanding of breast development requires to keep in mind that the human breast is one of the few organs of the body that is not completely developed at birth, and that only reaches its fully differentiated condition after a full term pregnancy, under the stimulus of new endocrine organs, the placenta and the developing fetus (Russo, J., and Russo, I.H., 1987a). The breast is composed of ducts The more branching the more differentiated the organ is. The branching pattern of the breast is manifested in the histological sections by the number of cross sectioned ductules per lobular unit. Each lobular structure has been morphologically characterized by their size, number of ductules per unit, and the number of cells per ductule, reflecting different stages of development (Figure 1). The earliest or more undifferentiated structure identified in the breast of postpubertal nulliparous women is the lobule type 1 (Lob 1), also called terminal ductal lobular unit (TDLU); it is composed of clusters of 6 to 11 ductules per lobule. They progress to lobules type 2 (Lob 2), which have a more complex morphology, being composed of a higher number of ductular structures per lobule. During pregnancy, Lob 1 and Lob 2 rapidly progress to lobules type 3 (Lob 3), which are characterized by having an average of 80 alveoli per lobule, and to actively secreting lobules type 4 (Lob 4), which have been observed only during the lactational period. After weaning, all the secretory units of the breast regress, reverting to Lob 3 and Lob 2. Further regression occurs after menopause, when Lob 1 increase in number at the expense of Lob 2 and Lob 3 (Russo, J., et al., 1992). Lob 1 comprise 50 to 60% of the total lobular component of the nulliparous women's breast at all ages, constituting the structure most frequently found. They are followed in frequency by the Lob 2, which represent 30-35% of the total, whereas only 5-10% are Lob 3, representing the least frequent ones. In the breast of parous women, on the other hand, Lob 3 predominate, comprising 80 to 100% of the total lobular component (Russo J, et al., 1992). In addition to variations in their morphological and functional characteristics, the Lob 1 and Lob 2 found in the breast of nulliparous women, and the Lob 3 present in the breast of parous women differ in their rate of cell proliferation (Russo, J. and Russo, I.H., 1987b; Russo, J. et al., 1992).

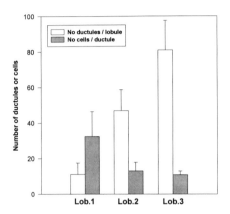

Figure 1. Profile of the human breast lobular structures

The determination of the proliferative activity of the mammary epithelium by measuring the uptake of ^{3}H-thymidine, reveals that the highest rate of cell proliferation, expressed as DNA labeling index (DNA-LI), or percentage of cells incorporating the radiolabeled precursor, occurs in the Lob 1, in which approximately 5 % of the cells are in the S phase of the cycle, decreasing five times in Lob 2 and 20 times in Lob 3 (Russo, J. and Russo, I.H., 1987b). The non-histone auxiliary protein for DNA polymerase delta proliferating cell nuclear antigen (PCNA), which detects a 36KD acidic nuclear protein essential for DNA synthesis, is expressed intensely in cells traversing the S phase and at lower levels in the M, G_1 and G_2 phases of the cell cycle. There is good correlation of these staining characteristics with data reported in the literature using ^{3}H-thymidine or 5-bromo-2'-deoxyuridine (BrdU) incorporation (Foley, et al., 1993). The nuclei of the cells in the S phase, that heavily reacted with PCNA antibody, represent the same cells incorporating ^{3}H-thymidine or BrdU; the nuclei with a granular stain are in G_1, the cells with cytoplasmic and nuclear mottled stain are in G_2, and those lacking the immunocytochemical stain are in G_0. Ki 67 is a protein expressed in the outer part of the nucleolus; it is known to be encoded by a gene located in the long arm of chromosome 10 (10q25), and especially in the granular component, appearing in late G_1, S, G_2, and M phases of the cell cycle. The use of this technique has allowed us to determine that Lob 1 in the breast of nulliparous women have a higher proliferative index than those present in the breast of age-matched parous women (Figure 2).

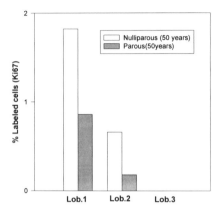

Figure 2. Proliferative activity in the Lob 1 of nulliparous and parous women's breasts.

More significant is the observation that both Lob 1 and Lob 3 in the parous woman's breast contain cells which are predominantly in the G_0 or resting phase of the cycle. The Lob 1 of the nulliparous woman breast, on the other hand, are composed of proliferating cells, with a very low percentage of them in the G_0 phase. The traditional method of counting those cells traversing the mitotic phase, or mitotic index, can be applied to tissues processed for any of the above mentioned procedures, since they are morphologically recognizable. The combination of these techniques has allowed us to determine that in addition to the morphological differences observed among lobular structures in different stages of development, there are differences in their cell kinetic characteristics. Among all the lobule types described, Lob 1 have a highest percentage of cells in G_1 and S phases. Their number decreases progressively as the structures become more differentiated. The fraction of cells in G_0 or resting phase, on the other hand, is minimal in Lob 1, progressively increasing in Lob 2, 3 and 4 (Figure 3).

PATHOGENESIS OF BREAST CANCER

One important concept that emerged from our study of breast development is that the TDLU, which had been originally identified by Wellings, et al. (1975) as the site of origin of the most common breast malignancy, the ductal carcinoma (Wellings, et al.,1975; Wellings, 1980), corresponds to a specific stage of development of the mammary parenchyma, the lobule type 1. This observation is supported by comparative studies of normal and cancer-bearing breasts obtained at autopsy. It was found that the non tumoral parenchyma in cancer associated breasts contained a significantly higher number of hyperplastic terminal ducts, atypical Lob 1 and ductal carcinomas *in situ* originated in Lob 1 than those breasts of women free of breast cancer, indicating that the Lob 1 is affected by preneoplastic as well as neoplastic processes.

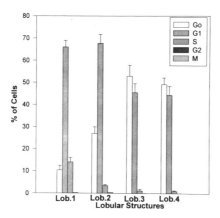

Figure 3. Percentage of cells in the various phases of the cell cycle.

More differentiated lobular structures have been found to be affected by neoplastic lesions as well, although they originate tumors whose malignancy is inversely related to the degree of differentiation of the parent structure, ie., Lob 2 originate lobular carcinomas *in situ*, whereas Lob 3 give rise to more benign breast lesions, such as hyperplastic lobules, cysts, fibroadenomas and adenomas, and Lob 4 to lactating adenomas.(Russo, J., et al., 1989b, 1994). We concluded from these observations that each specific compartment of the breast gives origin to a specific type of lesion. The finding that the most undifferentiated structures originate the most undifferentiated and aggresive neoplasms acquires relevance to the light that these structures are more numerous in the breast of nulliparous women, who are, in turn, at a higher risk of developing breast cancer. We concluded that the Lob 1 found in the breast of nulliparous women never went through the process of differentiation, whereas the same structures, when found in the breast of postmenopausal parous women did (Russo, J, et al., 1992). Genetic influences, which are responsible of at least 5% of the breast cancer cases (Russo, J. et al., 1996), seem to influence the pattern of breast development and differentiation, as evidenced by the study of prophylactic mastectomy specimens obtained from women with familial breasts and breast/ovarian cancer or carriers of the BRCA1 gene, as determined by linkage analysis (Figure 4).

The study of prophylactic mastectomy specimens obtained from both nulliparous and parous women revealed that the morphology and architecture of the breast were similar in these two groups of women. Their breasts were almost predominantly composed of

Lob 1, only a few specimens contained Lob 2 and Lob 3, in frank contrast to the predominance of Lob 3 found in parous women without family history of breast cancer (Russo, J., et al., 1996). Thus, the developmental pattern of the breast in parous women of the familial breast cancer group was similar to that of nulliparous women of the same group, and less developed than the breast of parous women without history of familial breast cancer. The breast of familial breast cancer group women presented differences in the branching pattern, and the Lob 1 present were frequently associated with ductal hyperplasia. These observations suggest that the genes that control the branching pattern of the breast during lobular development might have have been affected in those women belonging to families with a history of breast and breast/ovarian cancer (Marquis, et al., 1995; Russo J, et al., 1996), (Figure 4).

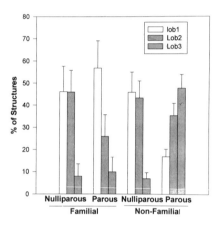

Figure 4. Developmental pattern of the breast in women with and without history of familial breast cancer.

TRANSFORMATION OF HUMAN BREAST EPITHELIAL CELLS

It is not known when in the lifetime of a woman the initiation of breast cancer takes place, or whether a specific agent causes it. The facts that late menarche and a full-term pregnancy completed before age 24, or early full-term pregnancy, reduces the risk of breast cancer development, whereas early menarche, nulliparity and exposure to ionizing radiations at ages younger than 19 (McGregor, et al., 1977) are associated with a higher breast cancer incidence (Russo, J. and Russo, I.H., 1987a), indicate that the period encompassed between menarche and first full-term pregnancy represents a window of high susceptibility for the initiation of breast cancer. In the previous section it has been indicated that ductal carcinomas originate in TDLU (Lob 1) and lobular carcinomas in Lob 2, whereas the Lob 3 is not associated with the development of malignancies (Russo, J. and Russo, I.H., 1987a, 1994; Wellings, et al., 1975). In order to ascertain whether Lob 1 and Lob 2 are more susceptible than Lob 3 to undergo neoplastic transformation, we have developed an *in vitro* system that reproduces the *in vivo* conditions of the breast epithelium. For these purposes, we utilize normal breast tissues from reduction mammoplasties which are obtained fresh and sterile. Upon digestion of the tissues with collagenase and hyaluronidase, epithelial cells in aggregates, or organoids, are separated by micromanipulation. Organoids are classified as Lob 1, Lob 2 or Lob 3 by applying the same criteria developed for classifying these structures in whole mount and histopathological preparations. Plating of each lobular type separately allows one to evaluate whether the behavior of cells in culture correlates with the specific type of lobule that originated them. Cells from Lob 1 and Lob 2, which in organ culture have shown to exhibit a higher DNA-LI, attach to the dishes promptly and start growing logarithmically, whereas cells from Lob 3, which have a lower DNA-LI, have a long lag phase before they attach to the dish and start growing. We determined that the number of doublings per unit of time was also higher in Lob 1 and Lob 2 than in Lob 3 (Russo, J., et al., 1989). For testing the susceptibility of the different lobule types to be transformed by chemical carcinogens *in vitro* a total of 52 human breast samples were processed. Organoids representing Lob 1, Lob 2 and Lob 3 were plated, and when the cells reached their logarithmic phase of growth they were treated with the chemical carcinogens N- methyl-N-nitrosourea (NMU), 7,12-dimethylbenz(a)anthracene (DMBA), methyl-N- nitro-nitroso-guanidine (MNNG) or benz(a)pyrene (BP) for 24 hours. The cells were followed up for several passages until they exhibited changes indicative of neoplastic transformation, such as variations in cell morphology, loss of contact inhibition, and anchorage independent growth. The changes in cell shape induced by the carcinogens was the result of increased number of surface microvilli and decreased cell-cell interaction. The property to form domes when plated in plastic flasks, which is characteristic of normal breast epithelial cells, was lost in carcinogen treated cells; this phenomenon was interpreted to be the result of an abnormal pattern of growth caused by altered contact inhibition. Treated cells showed increased ability to survive and to form colonies in agar methocel, and to exhibit multinucleation (Russo J, et al., 1993). These types of responses, however, were observed only in the epithelial cells derived from breast tissues containing Lob 1 and Lob 2. The phenomena were not observed in the breast cells derived from Lob 3 (Russo, J., et al., 1993).

These observations led us to conclude that primary cultures of human breast epithelial cells are susceptible to be transformed *in vitro* by chemical carcinogenes, however, the expression of phenotypes indicative of neoplastic transformation depends upon the stage of development of the breast and of the *in vivo* cell proliferation rate (Russo J, et al., 1989a; 1993). The finding that Lob 1 and Lob 2 express more readily changes indicative of neoplastic transformation *in vitro* indicates that these structures are more susceptible to the transforming effect of genotoxic agents, thus supporting the observations that they are the site of origin of mammary carcinomas; it also correlates with the lack of association of the Lob 3 with the development of malignant neoplasms

(Russo, J., et al., 1989b; 1990). Of greater relevance is the observation that the breast of nulliparous women contains more numerous Lob 1 and Lob 2 than the breast of parous women, in which predominates the Lob 3, further emphasizing the protective effect of gland differentiation, which modulates the response of breast epithelial cells to carcinogens under *in vitro* conditions.

EXPERIMENTALLY INDUCED MAMMARY TUMORS IN RATS

The elucidation of how host factors influence the initiation of the neoplastic process, and the determination of whether in women the susceptibility of the mammary gland varies with age and reproductive history require the availability of adequate experimental models. The induction of rat mammary carcinomas with chemical carcinogens, one of the most widely studied models more closely fulfills the above requirements. Many strains of rats develop spontaneous tumors, and respond to a variety of chemical carcinogens and radiation with development of either hormone-dependent or independent mammary tumors (Russo, J., et al., 1990). Two experimental systems have been preferentially utilized in the study of rat mammary tumorigenesis, Sprague-Dawley (S-D) rat inoculation with the polycyclic hydrocarbon DMBA (Huggins, et al., 1959; Huggins and Yang, 1962), and S-D or Fischer 344 rat injection of NMU. DMBA, given by gavage in a single dose of 2.5 to 20 mg induces tumors with latencies that generally range between 8 and 21 weeks, with final tumor incidences close to 100% if sufficient time elapses before necropsy. NMU, given by intravenous or subcutaneous injection in a single dose of 25 or 50 mg/kg body weight yields tumors with latency and incidence similar to those reported for DMBA (Rogers and Lee, 1986; Russo, J., et al., 1990).

These models of mammary carcinogenesis constitute useful tools for analyzing the interaction of the two major basic components of the neoplastic process, the etiologic agent, in this case the chemical carcinogen, and the target organ, obviously the mammary gland (Russo, J. and Russo, I.H., 1987). The mammary gland, however, does not respond as a unit to the carcinogenic insult. The mammary parenchyma develops from the superficial ectoderm as a complex tubular branching system that invades the stroma through active growth centers, the terminal end buds (TEBs) (Russo, I.H. and Russo, J., 1978; Russo. J. and Russo, I.H., 1978; Russo, J., et al., 1979). The TEB is a primitive element of the mammary parenchyma;. at the time of pubertal growth in the rat (at about 25-35 days of age) it starts to bifurcate into alveolar buds (ABs); these, with successive estrous cycles progress to virginal lobules (Russo, J. and Russo, I.H., 1978;Russo, J. et al 1979). The administration of DMBA to virgin rats elicits a tumorigenic response whose incidence is directly proportional to the density of TEBs primed by the ovarian hormones for their differentiation to ABs (Russo, J. and Russo, I.H., 1978; Russo, J., et al., 1979). This postulate is supported by the observations that although 100% incidence of carcinomas is elicited when DMBA is administered to rats between the ages of 30 and 55 days, the highest number of tumors per animal develops when the carcinogen is given to animals when they are 40 to 46 days of age, a period when TEBs are most actively differentiating into ABs. The sharp decrease in the number of TEBs observed in animals older than 55 days is accompanied by a lower incidence of tumors, as well as a lower number of tumors per animal (Russo, J., et al., 1982; Russo, J. and Russo, I.H., 1978; 1982; 1987a).

The first lesions induced by DMBA consist in the enlargement of one or various adjacent TEBs, which appear darkly stained in whole mount preparations. These lesions, observed between 7 and 14 days post-treatment, are called intraductal proliferations (IDPs) (Russo, J. and Russo, I.H., 1978; Russo, J. et al., 1977; 1979; 1989). Lesions arising in adjacent TEBs tend to coalesce forming microtumors, which become evident after 20 days of DMBA administration (Russo, J. et al., 1977). IDPs are lined by a multilayered epithelium; when they progress to intraductal carcinomas they exhibit a marked stromal reaction with desmoplasia, and infiltration by mast cells and lymphocytes (Russo, J. et al., 1977; 1989). From these structures the fully developed or palpable tumors grow into invasive carcinomas with cribriform, comedo or papillary patterns (Russo, J., et al., 1989). Some tumors metastasize , mainly to the lungs, if the animals are allowed to live long enough (Russo, J. et al., 1989). DMBA induces an array of benign lesions, such as cysts, adenomas, alveolar hyperplasias and fibroadenomas, which are originated from more differentiated structures, such as ABs and virginal lobules. They appear much later than IDPs and intraductal carcinomas. These observations indicate that there are two different pathogenetic pathways, one for the malignant and another for the benign lesions. The fact that benign lesions appear later than the malignant ones indicate that the former are not precursors of the latter (Russo, J. et al., 1977; Russo, J. and Russo, I.H., 1987a).

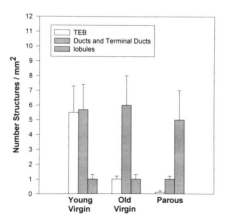

Figure 5. Structure of the nulliparous and parous rat mammary gland.

A further evidence in support of the TEB as the site of origin of mammary carcinomas has been obtained by plotting the incidence of adenocarcinomas against the percentage of TEBs, ABs and lobules present in the mammary gland at the time of carcinogen administration. A high correlation coefficient has been found between the incidence of carcinomas and the number of TEBs, but no between tumor incidence and the number of the other terminal structures (Russo, J., et al., 1977). Further evidence that it is the number of TEBs which affects the susceptibility of the mammary gland to carcinogenesis has been obtained from the study of the influence of pregnancy on mammary cancer initiation. Full term pregnancy, which completely eliminates the TEBs in the mammary gland through the induction of full differentiation, if completed prior to carcinogen administration, inhibits tumor development (Russo, J, Russo, I.H., 1980a,b; 1987a; Russo, J., et al., 1977; 1982) (Figure 5).

If pregnancy is interrupted, however, this protection is minimized or nullified (Russo, J. and Russo, I.H., 1980a,b). Hormonal treatment with estrogenic compounds (Chan and Dao, 1983; Welsch, 1985; Thompson and Ronan, 1987) or with chorionic gonadotropin (hCG) (Russo, J. et al., 1982b; Russo, J. and Russo, I.H., 1987a; Tay and Russo, 1985; Russo, I.H., et al., 1991) also reduces the number of TEBs through the induction of changes similar to those occurring with pregnancy. The degree of differentiation induced by these hormonal treatments correlates with the degree of refractoriness to undergo malignant transformation (Russo, J. and Russo, I.H., 1987a). One of the elements that influence the susceptibility of the TEB to carcinogenesis is the high proliferative activity of its epithelium (Russo, J. and Russo, I.H., 1980a,b; 1987a; Ciocca, et al., 1982) (Figure 6). Determination of the mammary gland's growth fraction has revealed that the largest compartment is in the TEBs, in which 55% of the cells are proliferating, whereas in ABs and lobules only 23% of the cells are in the proliferative pool. The growth fraction decreases with both aging and differentiation. In the mammary gland of parous animals the growth fraction is only 1% (Russo, J. and Russo, I.H., 1980a,b).

Carcinogenic initiation requires the stable alteration of DNA molecules, a process that requires that the carcinogen binds to the DNA (Russo,J. and Russo, I.H., 1980a,b; Russo, J., et al., 1982a). Maximal DNA binding occurs during DNA synthesis, thus, carcinogens damage DNA mostly during the S-phase (Berenblum, et al., 1976; Frei and Harsano, 1967; Kakunaga, 1975; Marquardt, et al., 1979). If the damage is not repaired during the G1 phase, this damage is transmitted to the daughter cells and it becomes fixed during successive S-phases of the cycle (Berenblum, et al 1976; Frei and Harsano, 1967; Kakunaga, 1975; Marquardt, et al., 1979). We have demonstrated that the uptake of ^{3}H-DMBA is selectively higher in TEBs than in other structures of the mammary gland; this uptake, expressed as the number of grains per nucleus, highly correlates with the DNA synthetic activity of the cells or DNA-LI (Russo, J., et al., 1982a). DMBA is metabolized by the mammary epithelium to both polar and phenolic metabolites. The metabolic pathway is similar in both the TEBs of virgin rats and the lobules of parous animals; however, the formation of polar metabolites is higher in the epithelial cells of TEBs, in which the binding of the carcinogen to DNA is also higher (Russo, J. and

Russo, I.H., 1987a; Tay and Russo, 1981a; 1981b). Removal of adducts from the DNA differs between TEBs and lobules; the former have a very low rate of adduct removal, whereas the latter are more efficient, indicating that the lobules repair the damage induced by the carcinogen more efficiently (Tay and Russo, 1981a; 1981b; 1985).

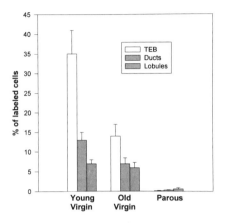

Figure 6. Proliferative activity in the nulliparous and parous rat mammary gland.

These data allowed us to conclude that the susceptibility of the mammary gland to carcinogenesis is modulated by the following parameters: 1) the presence of terminal end buds; 2) the size of the proliferative compartment; 3) the amount of binding of the carcinogen to the DNA, and 4) the ability of the cells to repair the DNA damaged by the carcinogen.

A UNIFIED CONCEPT OF MAMMARY CARCINOGENESIS

Comparative studies between humans and rodents have allowed us to determine that mammary cancer originates in undifferentiated terminal structures of the mammary gland. The terminal ducts of the Lob 1 or TDLU of the human female breast have many points in common with the TEB of the rat mammary gland. Firstly, the TEB in the rat and the Lob 1 in women are both the site of origin of ductal carcinomas. Secondly, cell replication in Lob 1 is at its peak during early adulthood, at a time during which the breast is more susceptible to carcinogenesis, decreasing considerably with aging. TEBs have also their highest proliferative activity when the animals are young, a period of greater susceptibility to undergo malignant transformation due to the greater binding of carcinogen to the DNA, and lower cell repair; aging results in decreased proliferative activity and susceptibility to carcinogens. The parallelism we have found between the TEB, that when affected by DMBA evolves to IDPs, carcinoma *in situ*, and invasive carcinoma, and the Lob 1, the site of origin of mammary carcinomas, has been further confirmed by in vitro studies, that have confirmed that like TEBs, Lob 1 have also the highest proliferative activity and greater carcinogen binding to the DNA; more importantly, when treated with carcinogens *in vitro* they express phenotypes indicative of cell transformation. These comparative studies indicate that both in rodents and in humans there is a target cell of carcinogenesis, which is found in a specific compartment whose characteristics are a determinant factor in the initiation event. These target cells will become the "stem cells" of the neoplastic event, depending upon: a) topographic location within the mammary gland tree, b) age at exposure to a known or putative genotoxic agent, and c) reproductive history of the host. Epidemiologic findings , such as the higher incidence of breast cancer in nulliparous women and in women having an early menarche support this concept, since it parallels the higher cancer incidence elicited by carcinogens when exposure occurs at a young age, and in nulliparous animals. In both cases, the mammary tissue contains predominantly undifferentiated structures. Thus, the protection afforded by early full term pregnancy in women, or full term pregnancy or hormonal treatment in rodents could be explained by the higher degree of differentiation of the mammary gland at the time in which an etiologic agent or agents act. Even though differentiation significantly reduces cell proliferation in the mammary gland, nevertheless, the mammary epithelium remains capable of responding with proliferation to given stimuli, such as a new pregnancy. Under these circumstances, however, the cells that are stimulated to proliferate are from structures that have already been primed by the first cycle of differentiation, thus creating a second type of "stem cells" that are able to metabolize the carcinogen and repair the DNA damage induced more efficiently than the cells of the virginal gland, and are, therefore, less susceptible to carcinogenesis. A carcinogenic stimulus powerful enough may overburden the system, succesfully initiating a neoplastic process. These conditions might explain the small fraction of tumors developing in the mammary gland exposed to a carcinogenic stimulus after completion of the first cycle of differentiation. The relevance of our work lies in the side to side comparison of findings in an experimental animal model and in the human breast, that validates experimental data for extrapolation to the human situation. The findings that cell proliferation is of important for cancer initiation, whereas differentiation is a powerful inhibitor provide novel tools for developing rational strategies for breast cancer prevention.

ACKNOWLEDGMENTS

This work was supported by National Cancer Institute grants CA64896 and CA67238, and NIEHS grant ESO7280.

REFERENCES

Basolo F, Elliott J, Tait L, Chen XQ, Maloney T, Russo IH, Pauley R, Momiki S, Caamano J, Klein-Szanto AJP, Koszalka M, Russo J (1991) Transformation of Human Breast Epithelial Cells by c-Ha-ras oncogene. Mol Carcinog 4:25-35.
Berenblum I (1976) A speculative review: the probable nature of promoting action, its

significance in the understanding of the mechanism of carcinogenesis. Cancer Res 14:471-476.

Boring CC, Squires TS, Tang T (1993) Cancer Statistics CA-Cancer J Clin 43:72-76.

Calaf G, Russo J (1993) Transformation of human breast epithelial cells by chemical carcinogens. Carcinogenesis 14:483-492.

Chan PC, Dao TL (1983) Effects of dietary fat on age-dependent sensitivity to mammary carcinogenesis. Cancer Letters 18:245-253.

Ciocca DR, Parente A, Russo J (1982) Endocrinological milieu and susceptibility of the rat mammary gland to carcinogenesis. Am. J. Pathol. 109:47-56.

Daling JR, Malone KE, Voigt LF, White E, Weiss NS (1994) Risk of breast cancer among young women: relationship to abortion. J Natl Cancer Inst 88:1584-1602.

De Waard F, Trichopoulos D (1988) A unifying concept of the aetiology of breast cancer. Int J Cancer 41:666-669.

Foley J, Tom T, Morompot R, Butterworth B, Goldsworthy TH (1993) Comparison of proliferating cell nuclear antigen (PCNA)/cyclin to tritiated thymidine as a marker of proliferating hepatocytes in rat. Environ Health Perspect 101: 199-206.

Frei JV, Harsano T (1967) Increased susceptibility to low doses of carcinogen of epidermal cells in stimulated DNA synthesis. Cancer Res 27:1482-1491.

Gerdes J, Becker MHG, Key G, Kattoretti G, (1992) Immunohistological detection of tumor growth fraction (ki-67 antigen) in formalin fixed and routinely processed tissues. J Pathol 168:85-86.

Henderson BE, Ross RK, Pike MC (1993) Hormonal chemoprevention of cancer in women. Science 259:633-638.

Huggins C, Grand LC, Brillantes FP (1959) Critical significance of breast structure in the induction of mammary cancer in the rat. Proc Natl Acad Sci USA 45:1294-1300.

Huggins C, Yang NC (1962) Induction and extinction of mammary cancer. Science 137:25-28.

John EM, Kelsey JL (1993) Radiation and other environmental exposures and breast cancer. Epidemiol Rev 15:157-162.

MacMahon B, Cole P, Liu M, Lowe CR, Mirra AP, Ravinihar B, Salber EJ, Valaoras VG, Yuasa S (1970) Age at first birth and breast cancer risk. Bull World Health Organ 34: 209-221.

Marquardt H, Baker S, Tierney B, Grover PL, Sims P (1979) Comparison of mutagenesis and malignant transformation by dihydrodiols of 7,12-dimethylbenz(a) anthracene. Br J Cancer 39:540-547.

Marquis ST, Rajan JV, Wynshaw-Boris A, Xu J (1995) The Developmental pattern of BRCA1 expression implies a role in differentiation of the breast and other tissues. Nature Genetics 11:17-26.

McGregor DH, Land CE, Choi K, Tokuoka S, Liu PI, Wakabayashi I, Beebe GW (1977) Breast cancer incidence among atomic bomb survivors, Hiroshima and Nagasaki 1950-1989. J Natl Cancer Inst. 59:799-811.

Newcomb PA, Storer BE, Longnecker MP,Mittendorf R, Gringberg ER, Willett WC (1996) Pregnancy termination in relation to risk of breast cancer, J Am Med Assoc 275:283-287.

Page DL, Anderson TJ (1987) "Diagnostic Histopathology of the Breast" New York:

Churchill Livingstone.

Parker SL, Tong T, Bolden S, Wingo PA (1996) Cancer statistics, 1996. CA-Cancer J Clin 65:5-27.

Rogers AE, Lee SY (1986) Chemically-induced mammary gland tumors in rats: modulation by dietary fat. In Ip C, Birt DF, Rogers AE, Mettlin C (eds) "Dietary Fat and Cancer" New York: Alan R. Liss, Inc., NY, pp 255-268.

Rosner B, Colditz GA, Willett WC (1994) Reproductive risk factors in a prospective study of breast cancer: The nurses health study. Am J Epidemiol 139:819-835.

Russo IH, Gimotty P, Dupuis M, Russo J (1989) Effect of Medroxyprogesterone Acetate on the Response of the Rat Mammary Gland to Carcinogenesis. British J. of Cancer 59:210-216.

Russo IH, Koszalka M, Russo J (1991) Comparative study of the influence of pregnancy and hormonal treatment on mammary carcinogenesis. Brit. J. Cancer 64:481-484.

Russo IH, Russo J (1978) Developmental stage of the rat mammary glan as determinant of its susceptibility to7,12-dimethylbenz(a)anthracene.J. Natl. Cancer Inst. 61:1439-1442.

Russo IH, Russo J (1988) Hormone prevention of mammary carcinogenesis: A new approach in anticancer research. Anticancer Res. 8:1247-1264.

Russo IH, Russo J (1989) Hormone prevention of mammary carcinogenesis by norethynodrel-mestranol. Breast Cancer Res Treat 14:43-56.

Russo IH, Russo J (1993) Physiological basis of breast cancer prevention. European J Cancer Prevention 2:101-111.

Russo IH, Russo J (1994) Role of hCG and inhibin in breast cancer (Review). Int. J Oncol 4: 297-306.

Russo J (1983) Basis of cellular autonomy in susceptibility to carcinogenesis. Toxicol Pathol 11:149-166.

Russo J, Calaf G, Sohi N, Tahin Q, Zhang PL, Alvarado ME, Estrada S, Russo IH. (1993a) Critical steps in breast carcinogenesis. New York Acad Sci 698:1-20.

Russo J, Calaf G, Russo IH (1993b) A critical approach to the malignant transformation of human breast epithelial cells. CRC Critical Rev Oncogen 4: 403-417.

Russo J, Gusterson BA, Rogers AE, Russo IH, Wellings SR, Van Zwieten MJ (1990) Comparative Study of Human and Rat Mammary Tumorigenesis. Lab. Invest. 62:1-32.

Russo J, Lynch H, Russo IH, (1996) Genes associated with familial breast cancer affect the pattern of breast lobular development (Submitted).

Russo J, Miller J, Russo IH (1982b) Hormonal treatment prevents DMBA induced rat mammary carcinoma. Proc. Am. Assoc. Cancer Res. 23:348a.

Russo J, Mills MJ, Moussalli MJ, Russo IH (1989a) Influence of breast development and growth properties in vitro. In Vitro Cell Develop Biol 25:643-649.

Russo J, Reina D, Frederick J, Russo IH (1988) Expression of phenotypical changes by human breast epithelial cells treated with carcinogens in vitro. Cancer Res 48:2837-2857.

Russo J, Rivera R, Russo IH (1992) Influence of age and parity on the development of the human breast. Breast Cancer Res Treat. 23:211-218.

Russo J, Romero AL, Russo IH (1994)   Architectural pattern of the normal and cancerous breast under the influence of parity. J. Cancer Epidemiol, Biomarkers & Prevention, 3:219-224.

Russo J, Russo IH, Ireland M, Saby J (1977) Increased resistance of multiparous rat mammary gland to neoplastic transformation by 7, 12-DMBA. Proc. Am. Assoc. Cancer Res. 18:140.

Russo J, Russo IH (1978) DNA-labeling index and structure of the rat mammary gland as determinant of its susceptibility to carcinogenesis. J. Natl. Cancer Inst. 61:1451-1459.

Russo J, Russo IH (1980a) Susceptibility of the mammary gland to carcinogenesis II. Pregnancy interruption as a risk factor in tumor incidence. Am. J. Pathol. 100:497-511.

Russo J, Russo IH (1980b) Influence of differentiation and cell   kinetics on the susceptibility of the rat mammary gland to carcinogenesis Cancer Res. 40:2677-2687.

Russo J, Russo IH (1982) Is Differentiation the Answer in Breast Cancer Prevention? Internat Res Com (IRCS)10:935:945.

Russo J, Russo IH (1987a) Biological and molecular bases of mammary carcinogenesis. Lab Invest 57:112-137.

Russo J, Russo IH (1987b): Development of the human mammary gland In Neville MC, Daniel C.W (eds):   The Mammary Gland Development, Regulation, and Function. New York: Plenum Pub. Corp., pp 67-93.

Russo J, Russo IH, van Zwieten MJ, Rogers AE, Gusterson B (1989) Classification of neoplastic and non-neoplastic lesions of the rat mammary gland. In Jones TC, Mohr U, Hunt RD (eds); "Integument and Mammary Glands of Laboratory Animals." Berlin: Springer Verlag, pp. 275-304.

Russo J, Russo IH (1993) Developmental pattern of the human breast and susceptibility to carcinogenesis. Europ J Cancer Prevention 2:85-100.

Russo J, Russo IH (1994) Toward a physiological approach to breast cancer prevention. Cancer Epidemiol, Biomarkers & Prevention 3:353-364.

Russo J, Russo IH (1995) Hormonally induced differentiation: A novel approach to breast cancer prevention. J. Cell Biochem 22: 58-64.

Russo J, Saby J, Isenberg W, Russo IH (1977) Pathogenesis of mammary carcinomas induced in rats by 7,12-dimethylbenz(a)anthracene. J. Natl. Cancer Inst., 59:435-445.

Russo J, Tay LK, Russo IH (1982a) Differentiation of the mammary gland and susceptibility to carcinogenesis: A Review. Breast Cancer Res. Treat., 2:5-73.

Russo J, Wilgus G, Russo IH (1979) Susceptibility of the mammary gland to carcinogenesis. I. Differentiation of the mammary gland as determinant of tumor incidence and type of lesion. Am. J. Pathol. 96:721-734.

Soule HD, Maloney TM, Wolman SR, Peterson, ND, Brenz R, McGrath CM, Russo J, Pauley RJ, Jones RF, Brooks SC (1990)   Isolation and characterization of a spontaneously immortalized human breast epithelial cell line, MCF-10. Cancer Res 50:6075-6086.

Tait LR, Soule HD, Russo J (1990) Ultrastructural and immunocytochemical characterization of an immortalized human breast epithelial cell line, MCF-10. Cancer Res 50:6087-6094.

Tay LK, Russo J (1981a) 7,12-Dimethylbenz(a)anthracene (DMBA) induced DNA binding and repair synthesis in susceptible and non-susceptible mammary epithelial cells in culture. J Natl Cancer Inst 67:155-161.

Tay LK, Russo J (1981b) Formation and removal of 7,12- dimethylbenz(a)anthracene nucleic acid adducts in rat mammary epithelial cells with different susceptibility to carcinogenesis. Carcinogenesis 2:1327-1333.

Tay LK, Russo J (1985) Effect of human chorionic gonadotropin on 7, 12-dimethylbenz (a)anthracene-induced DNA binding and repair synthesis by rat mammary epithelial cells. Chem-Biol Interact 55:13-21.

Thompson HJ, Ronan A (1987) Effect of L-a-difluoromethylornithine and endocrine manipulation on the induction of mammary carcinogenesis by 1-methyl-1-nitrosourea. Carcinogenesis 57:2003-2009.

Wellings SR (1980) Development of human breast cancer. Adv Cancer Res 31:287-299.

Wellings SR, Jensen HM, Marcum RG (1975) An atlas of subgross pathology of 16 human breasts with special reference to possible precancerous lesions. J Natl Cancer Inst 55:231-275.

Welsch CW (1985) Host factors affecting the growth of carcinogen-induced rat mammary carcinomas:a review and tribute to Charles Brenton Huggins. Cancer Res. 45:3415-3443.

Etiology of Breast and
Gynecological Cancers, pages 17–29
© 1997 Wiley-Liss, Inc.

EPIDEMIOLOGIC ANALYSIS OF BREAST AND GYNECOLOGIC CANCERS

Barbara Sorenson Hulka, M.D., M.P.H.

Epidemiology Department
The University of North Carolina at Chapel Hill
Chapel Hill, NC 27599-7400

ABSTRACT

This review focuses on etiologic factors and hormonal correlates of the three major gynecologic cancers - uterine cervix, uterine corpus and ovary - and breast cancer. The incidence rate of the three gynecologic cancers combined is only 40 percent of the breast cancer rate (43.6 vs 109.5 per 100,000), whereas the combined mortality rate is half that for breast cancer (14.3 vs 27.3 per 100,000).

Cervical cancer is distinctive in that it's hormonal correlates are few; it exhibits the epidemiologic characteristics of a sexually transmitted disease. Integration of Human Papilloma Virus DNA types 16, 18 (or other) within the cellular genome has been identified in more than 80% of high grade cervical intraepithelial neoplasias and invasive carcinomas.

Epithelial ovarian cancers occur most commonly in nulliparous, infertile women and familial carriers of BRCA1. Oral contraceptive (OC) use reduces ovarian cancer risk by at least one-half, a benefit which increases with increasing duration of use and persists for at least 15 years after discontinuation. Pregnancy and OCs suppress gonadotropin secretion, whereas fertility drugs enhance follicle-stimulating hormone production. These indicators of alterations in the hypothalmic-pituitary-ovarian axis provide some support for both the excess gonadotropin and the incessant ovulation theories of ovarian carcinogenesis.

Endometrial carcinoma is the prototype hormonally-determined disease. Increased estrogen from either endogenous or exogenous sources increases risk. Lowering the estrogen load or adding progestin reduces risk. This explains the marked protection achieved by combined estrogen/progestin OC's and the dramatic increased risk uncurred by long-term estrogen replacement therapy (ERT). Breast tissue, also a target for sex steroid hormones, displays a more complex risk profile. Current ERT use increases breast cancer risk by about 30%; adding a progestin to the estrogen does not improve the situation (40% increased risk). Furthermore, OCs do not reduce breast cancer risk, but may increase it for current OC users under age 45. The magnitude of these hormonal effects is much smaller than that exhibited with endometrial cancer.

INTRODUCTION

The most common gynecologic cancers are ovarian, endometrial and uterine cervix. Yet, in the United States (US) their combined incidence rate is only 40% of that for breast cancer and combined mortality rate is half that of breast cancer. Table 1 shows incidence and mortality rates for the three gynecologic cancers and breast cancer. For uterine corpus, the rates include both endometrial carcinomas and sarcomas. The latter account for only 1.3% of cancers of the uterine corpus, although they are relatively more common in African-Americans than Caucasians (Harlow, et al., 1986).

Table 1. Incidence and Mortality Rates per 100,000 Women (1987-91)

| | | Uterus: | |
	Breast	Cervix	Corpus	Ovary
Incidence Rates*				
White	113.2	7.8	22.2	15.6
Black	94.0	14.0	14.5	10.3
All races	109.5	8.6	21.2	14.8
Mortality Rates*				
White	27.2	2.6	3.2	8.0
Black	31.2	6.7	6.0	6.5
All races	27.3	3.0	3.5	7.8

*Age-adjusted to the 1970 U.S. standard population (Ries, et al., 1994).

CERVICAL CANCER

Cervical cancer is distinctive from the other gynecologic cancers and breast cancer in that it has the epidemiologic profile of a sexually transmitted disease. Historically, it has been associated with a number of different sexually transmitted organisms, Treponema pallidum and Herpes simplex type 2, as examples. More recently, with the availability of PCR-based laboratory techniques evidence for a causal association between specific types of Human Papilloma Virus (HPV) and invasive cervical carcinoma has become overwhelming. Types 16 and 18 are well established cancer-associated types, and additional types e.g., 31, 33, 35, 39, 35, 45, 51, etc., are continually being added to the list (Schiffman, et al., 1993). Types 16 and 18 are integrated in host cell DNA, although 16 has also been identified in episomal locations. Viral DNA enhances expression of HPV oncoproteins, E6 and E7; the former binds p53 protein and the latter binds pRB, resulting in increased cell proliferation (Werness, et al., 1993).

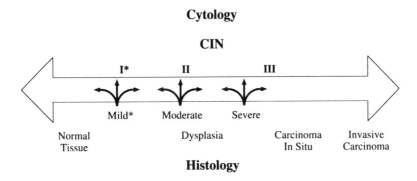

Figure 1. Pathogenesis of Invasive Cervical Cancer

The prolonged pathogenesis of cervical cancer is also distinctive. Because of this characteristic, cervical cytology, which identifies all forms of precursor lesions, has been uniquely successful in reducing the incidence of invasive, life-threatening disease. Figure 1 illustrates the pathologic and corresponding cytologic changes in the cervix during the course of cancer development. A decade or more may transpire between the initial cellular changes and the development of invasive cancer. Cancer-associated HPV types are present in a successively greater proportion of lesions as one moves from the left to the right hand side of the figure. HPV DNA has been identified in more than 80% of high grade cervical intraepithelial neoplasia (CIN) (Schiffman, et al., 1993). CIN 1 is the usual manifestation of infection with HPV types 6 or 11, which have little carcinogenic potential but are associated with anogenital warts (Daling, Sherman, 1992). Regression or persistence without progression can occur at any point in the histologic spectrum prior to the development of invasive cancer; these are the most likely outcomes in early stage lesions.

Table 2 lists the major risk factors for cervical neoplasia. However, when the effect of HPV types 16/18/etc is taken into account, the risk inferred by other factors is reduced or eliminated. Some residual effect of lifetime number of sexual partners and high parity may persist (Schiffman, et al., 1993). Cofactors such as smoking or other sexually transmitted organisms may enhance persistence of HPV and progression of neoplasia (Koutsky, et al., 1992). Both nicotine and cotinine have been identified in cervical mucus of active and passive smokers and these may serve as proxies for carcinogenic constituents of cigarette smoke (McCann, et al., 1992).

Table 2. Risk Factors for Cervical Neoplasia

Lifetime number of sex partners
Age at first intercourse (<16 or 17)
Parity (3+)
Cigarette smoking (current)
OC use
Socioeconomic status (low)
HPV types 16/18
Herpes Simplex type 2 (seropositive)
Chlamydia (seropositive)

Oral contraceptive (OC) use appears to have a different effect on risk of invasive carcinoma than on preinvasive lesions, and the direction of the association depends on whether or not the population is cytologically screened. Women receiving OCs in the US are subject to regular Pap smears, which identify all grades of CIN. Because of this screening, OCs appear to increase risk for dysplasia and carcinoma in situ (risk estimates 2 to 3-fold). Since precursor lesions are removed, invasive cancer is unlikely to develop in women using OCs, and risk estimates of <1 for invasive cancer are consistently reported. In the absence of screening, preinvasive lesions are rarely identified, since most are asymptomatic and not readily apparent on clinical examination. In unscreened populations, the invasive cancer risk estimates associated with OC use may be 2 to 3-fold. From an epidemiologic perspective, cytologic screening is inexorably confounded with OC use in populations where screening is common (Hulka, 1989).

The topic of hormone replacement therapy (HRT) and cervical neoplasia has received little research attention. Two cohort studies from England and Sweden, where cytologic screening has been much less universal than in the US, showed no increased risk for invasive cervical carcinoma with HRT use (Adami, et al., 1989; Hunt, et al., 1987).

Thus, invasive cervical cancer has become less of an epidemiologic conundrum, as a viral etiology has become established and a preventive strategy has been applied - screening for and treatment of precursor lesions. The effectiveness of this strategy has been well documented by 30 years of declining incidence and mortality rates for cervical cancer, a time period coincident with the introduction and widespread application of cytologic screening in the US.

OVARIAN CANCER

More than 85% of ovarian cancers arise from epithelial cells; serous carcinomas are the most common, followed by mucinous, endometrioid and clear cell carcinomas. The remainder are nonepithelial, originating in germ cells or stromal cells (Lee, et al., 1987). Epidemiologic analyses concentrate on the epithelial cancers, primarily because of the rarity of the other forms.

Table 3 summarizes factors that either increase or reduce risk for epithelial ovarian cancinomas. As with breast and endometrial cancer, it is a disease of older women with maximum age-specific rates in the 70 to 79 year age group. Risk varies with respect to family history of ovarian cancer. Women without such a history have a life time probability of developing the disease of about 1.6%; with one first or second degree relative the risk is 5%; and with two such relatives the life time probability is 7% (Kerlikowske, et al., 1992). Women in breast/ovarian cancer families, who carry a mutated BRCA1, experience a life time risk of 85% or more (Whittemore, 1994). The other significant risk factors are nulligravidity, which exerts a 2 to 3-fold increased risk compared to mulltigravidity, (Nason, Nelson, 1994) and infertility (Nasca, et al., 1984), the effects of which may be further enhanced by use of fertility drugs (Whittemore, et al., 1992).

Table 3. Risk Factors for Epithelial Ovarian Cancer

Risk enhancement	Risk Reduction
Older age	OC use
Caucasian vs African American and Hispanic	Gravidity
North Amercian, Northern European descent	Lactation
Family history of ovarian cancer	Tubal ligation
Breast/ovarian cancer syndrome (BRCA1)	Hysterectomy
Nulliparity	
Infertility	**No Effect on Risk**
Fertility drugs	ERT

A pooled analysis of 12 case-control studies (Whittemore, et al., 1992) showed no association between estrogen replacement therapy (ERT) and incidence of ovarian cancer. However, a recently reported cohort study showed a statistically significant increased risk of death from ovarian cancer following >10 years of ERT use (Rodriguez, et al., 1995). Methodologic arguments have been garnered to account for the differing results, but at present a relationship between ERT and ovarian cancer has not been unequivicably established.

Two factors have a major impact on risk reduction: increasing number of pregnancies, irrespective of gestation length, and long duration OC use. Prolonged laction also contributes to risk reduction, but to a lesser extent (Whittemore, 1994). As reported in the Cancer and Steroid Hormone (CASH) study, risk estimates for ovarian cancer in relation to OC use were: ever versus never use, 0.6; more than 10 years of use,

0.2 with a benefit that persisted for at least 15 years after discontinuation. All OC formulations were effective (Lee, et al., 1987). Models using modified life table methods indicate that 10 years or more of OC use could reduce the life time probability of developing ovarian cancer among women with a family history by about one half (Kerlikowske, et al., 1992).

Two theories of ovarian carcinogenesis have been proposed to account for the parity and OC effects on risk reduction. The pituitary gonadotropin theory states that increased circulating levels of gonadotropins increase risk by excessive stimulation of the ovary and follicles. Both pregnancy and OCs suppress secretion of these hormones. Fertility drugs stimulate ovulation by increasing follicular phase levels of follicle stimulating hormone. However, there are inconsistencies with this theory. Prolonged lactation reduces risk although pituitary gonadotropin levels are elevated. ERT does not protect against ovarian cancer although its use results in reduced gonadotropin production. Furthermore, a recently reported nested case control study, analysing hormone levels in prediagnotic stored sera, did not support the theory; on the contrary, a high androgen/low gonadotropin hormonal profile was associated with an increased risk of developing ovarian cancer (Helzlsouer, et al., 1995).

The second theory is that of "incessant ovulation". The theory postulates that ovulation-induced injury to ovarian epithelium is the initial step in carcinogenesis. Repetitive ovulation may produce inclusion cysts composed of mesothelial cells, which normally overlie the ovary, and as the result of unspecified subsequent events, this trapped epithelium undergoes malignant transformation. According to this theory, OCs and pregnancy protect against ovarian cancer by suppressing ovulation. The small risk reduction associated with both tubal ligation and hysterectomy could result from reduction in blood flow to the ovary and a reduced ovulatory frequency. However, the lack of a consistent association between ovarian cancer risk and ages at menarche and menopause, which together affect the number of ovulatory years, does not conform with the theory.

ENDOMETRIAL CANCER

Endometrial cancer provides a model system for hormonal effects in women. Estrogens induce endometrial proliferation and carcinomatous change, whereas progestins counteract these effects. Epidemiologic data are consistent with this model. The increased risk associated with obesity is thought to function through the increased number and size of adipose cells, which are active sites for aromatization of adrenal androstenedione to estrone, the major estrogenic compound in postmenopausal women. Obese postmenopausal women have higher serum estrone levels than comparable nonobese women and lower levels of steroid hormone-binding globulin, allowing for greater bioavailability of estrogens (Siiteri, 1987). The adverse effects of nulliparity and infertility on risk may be mediated through anovulatory menstrual cycles with elevated levels of estrogen relative to progesterone.

Use of ERT in postmenopausal women provides a classic example of a cause and effect relationship established through epidemiologic research. Estrogen alone increases risk; the magnitude of the increase being dependent on the duration and recency of use. Relative risk approximates 10-fold with 10 years of use, an effect which is moderated with increasing time since last use. Five years or more after discontinuation, the risk drops to approximately twice that of women who have never used ERT (Brinton, et al., 1993). These effects are reasonably constant irrespective of estrogen type (conjugated or nonconjugated), dose, or regimen. A daily or cyclic dose of 0.625 mg of conjugated estrogens, the most commonly used replacement estrogen in the US, is sufficient to produce the effects noted (Hulka, 1994).

An important consideration with respect to estrogen use is the type of cancer induced. Estrogen-associated cancers are disproportionately early stage and low grade (Hulka, et al., 1980; Brinton, et al., 1993). Their prognosis is better than that for carcinomas developing in the absence of estrogen therapy (Schwartzbaum, et al., 1987). However, five years or more of unopposed estrogen increases the risk for advanced stage carcinoma by at least 2-fold (Brinton, et al., 1993).

Recognition of estrogen effects on the uterus in the late 1970s and early 1980s led to changes in prescribing practices. Progestins were added to the estrogen regimen for a week or more in the monthly cycle. More recent studies have shown that 10 or more days of a progestin is required to counteract the estrogen effect on the endometrium, and even this schedule does not totally eliminate risk (Voight, et al., 1991). In the 1990s, continuous daily administration of low dose estrogen and progestin gained acceptance. However, it will be at least a decade before sufficient numbers of long-term users of the continuous combined regimen will have accrued for epidemiologic evaluation of its effect on endometrial cancer risk.

The histologic consequences of hormone use are further elucidated by the findings from the Postmenopausal Estrogen Progestin Intervention (PEPI) trial. This randomized double-blind clinical trial was undertaken to determine the effects of estrogen plus different types and regimens of progestins, estrogen alone, or placebo on lipid profiles and other cardiovascular risk factors. By means of annual endometrial aspiration, endometrial effects were identified and patient saftey was assured. By the end of the third study year, one third of the women on estrogen alone had developed precursor leisions: adenomatous hyperplasia with or without atypia. Another third had developed lesser endometrial alterations. All of these changes were infrequent in the estrogen plus progestin and placebo arms of the trial (Writing Group for PEPI Trial, 1996).

Recognizing that current hormonal contraceptives are combined estrogen and progestin (or progestin only), the effect on endometrial cancer risk might be anticipated. Ever use reduces the relative risk to about 0.5, an effect which is more pronounced among current users and persists after discontinuation for at least a decade (The Cancer and Steroid Hormone Study of the Centers for Disease Control and the National Institute of Child Health and Human Development, 1987; Hulka, et al., 1982).

Cigarette smoking is also protective (Baron, et al., 1986). Although total estrogens (primarily estrone) appear not to differ in postmenopausal smokers and nonsmokers, the competitive metabolic pathway between 16a-hydroxyestrone and 2-hydroxyestrone may be altered such that the latter compound with low estrogenic activity is favored (Cauley, et al., 1989; Michnovicz, et al., 1986). Smoking increases both the proportion of bound to unbound estradiol and the levels of steroid hormone binding globulin. These changes result in reduced levels of bioavailable estrogen (Jensen, Christiansen, 1988).

The mechanism by which full-term pregnancy protects against endometrial cancer is not immediately obvious. Pregnancy causes large increases in steroid hormones, estrogen and progesterone, and protein hormones, prolactin and chorionic gonadotropins. However, one full-term pregnancy reduces endometrial cancer risk by at least a third relative to nulliparous women (Brinton, et al., 1992).

BREAST CANCER

Breast cancer is the most common cancer in women with 182,000 new cases and 46,000 deaths projected for 1995 (Wingo, et al., 1995). The peak incidence rate is 484 per 100,000 women per year at ages 75 to 79 (Ries, et al., 1994) or almost 1 per 200 women annually. Although rates increase with advancing age, the rate of increase declines after age 50, the aproximate age of natural menopause, when ovarian function ceases and secretion of estrogen and progesterone drops.

Given the experience with hormonal effects on endometrial tissue, it was anticipated that the breast, also a target tissue for sex steroid hormones, would respond in a similar manner. However, hormonal effects on the breast, as shown in table 4, indicate that the endometrial cancer model does not translate directly to the breast. Both estrogen and progesterone appear to stimulate cell growth rather than exhibit the mutually antagonistic effects observed in the uterus. Breast cancer incidence is markedly reduced by oophorectomy at a young age. Late age at full-term pregnancy (30 years or more) increases risk compared to an early age (less than 20 years). Early age at menarche and late age at natural menopause are associated with increased risk (Hulka, Stark, 1995). Nulliparity increases risk and high parity decreases risk for postmenopausal breast cancer (Kelsey, et al., 1993; Rosner, et al., 1994). Obesity, which increases risk in postmenopausal women, is thought to operate through increased estrogen levels. Breast feeding, if continued for many months or years, appears to reduce risk in premenopausal women (Yoo, et al., 1992).

The effect of OCs and HRT on risk of breast cancer have been studied extensively. With respect to OCs, adverse effects appear to occur in women diagnosed with breast cancer at young ages, mostly less than 35. After age 45 no increased risk is evident. In fact, a small diminution in risk among prior OC users aged 45 to 54 was reported from the CASH study (Wingo, et al., 1993). These findings are consistent with a promotional action of OCs, advancing the age of onset of cancers which would otherwise present at a latter age. In a recent case control study of women under age 45, the relative risk (RR) for breast cancer associated with OC use among women younger than 35 years was 1.7 (95% CI 1.2-2.6); for those 35 to 39 years the RR was 1.4 (95% CI 1.0-1.8) and in the 40 to 44 year age group the RR was 1.1 (95% CI 0.9-1.4). In the youngest age group risk estimates were greater for recent and longterm users (Brinton, et al., 1995). These data suggest that specific subgroups of women may be adversely affected by OCs. Those with a genetic susceptibility, such as BRCA1 carriers, could be one such group. Alternatively, BRCA1 carriers in ovarian cancer families might be benefited by OC use (Kerlikowski, et al., 1992).

Table 4. Hormonally-mediated Indicators of Breast Cancer Risk

| Indicator | Risk Groups | | |
	High	Low	RR
Gender	female	male	150.0
Age	old	young	17.0
Oophorectomy before age 35	no	yes	3.0
Age at first full-term pregnancy	>30yrs	<20 yrs	2.0
Age at menarche	<12	>14	1.5
Age at menopause	>54	<45	1.5
Obesity* (Postmenopausal)	<23	>30	1.5
Parity (Postmenopausal)	nulliparous	>4	1.5
Breast Feeding (Premenopausal)	none	years	1.5
Hormonal Contraception breast cancer <45yrs	yes	no	1.5
Hormone replacement therapy	yes	no	1.5

*Body mass index (kg/m^2)
Adapted from Hulka, Cancer 1994.

Among the many studies on HRT and breast cancer, the prospectively designed Nurses Health Study is one of the largest. During 725,550 person-years of follow-up on postmenopausal women, 1935 cases of breast cancer were diagnosed. The RR for breast cancer associated with use of estrogen alone was 1.3 (95% CI 1.1 to 1.5); with use of estrogen plus progestin the RR was 1.4 (95% CI 1.2 to 1.7) (Colditz, et al., 1995), indicating that progestins are unlikely to protect the breast. Age, recency and duration of hormone use affected risk. In the oldest age group (ages 60 to 64) current use of 5 or more years duration produced a RR of 1.7. At ages 60 to 64 the baseline breast cancer incidence rate is high, 348 per 100,000 women (Ries, et al., 1994). A 70% increase in risk attributable to HRT would affect large numbers of women.

REFERENCES

Adami HO et al. (1989): Risk of cancer in woman receiving hormone replacement therapy. International Journal of Cancer 44:833-839.

Baron JA, Byers T, Greenberg ER, et al. (1986): Cigarette smoking in women with cancers of the breast and reproductive organs. J Natl Ca Inst 77:677-680.

Brinton LA, Berman ML, Mortel R, Twiggs LB, Barrett RJ, Wilbanks GD, Lannom L (1992): Reproductive, menstrual, and medical risk factors for endometrial cancer: Results from a case-control study. American Journal of Obstetrics and Gynecology 167(5):1317-1325.

Brinton LA, Barrett RJ, Berman ML, Mortel R, Twiggs LB, Wilbanks GD (1993): Cigarette smoking and the risk of endometrial cancer. American Journal of Epidemiolgy 137(3):281-291.

Brinton LA, Hoover RN, the Endometrial Cancer Collaborative Group (1993): Estrogen Replacement Therapy and Endometrial Cancer Risk: Unresolved Issues. Obstetrics and Gynecology 81(2):265-271.

Brinton LA, Daling JR, Liff JM, Schoenberg JB, Malone KE, Stanford JL, Coates RJ Gammon MD, Hanson L, Hoover RN (1995): Oral contraceptives and breast cancer risk among younger women. Journal of the Nation Cancer Insitute 87(11):827-835.

Cauley JA, Gutai JP, Kuller LH, et al. (1989): The epidemiology of serum sex hormones in postmenopausal women. American Journal of Epidemiology 129:1120-1131.

Cauley JA, Gutai JP, Kuller LH, LeDonne D, Powell JC (1989): The epidemiology of serum sex hormones in postmenopausal women. American Journal of Epidemiology 132:1120-1131.

Colditz GA, Hankinson SE, Hunter DJ, Willett WC, Manson JE, Stampfer MJ, Hennekens C, Rosner B, Speizer FE (1995): The use of estrogen and progestins and the risk of breast cancer in postmenopausal women. The New England Journal of Medicine 332(24):1589-1593.

Daling JR, Sherman KJ (1992): Relationship between human papillomavirus infection and tumours of anogenital sites other than the cervix. IARC Scientific Publications 119:223-41.

Harlow BL, Weiss NS, Lofton S (1986): The Epidemiology of Sarcomas of the Uterus. JNCI 76(3):399-402.

Helzlsouer K, Alberg A, Gordon G, Longcope C, Bush T, Hoffman SC, Comstock G (1995): Serum gonadotropic and steriod hormones and the development of ovarian cancer. JAMA 274:1926-1930.

Hulka BS, Fowler WC, Kaufman DG, Grimson RC, et al. (1980): Estrogen and Endometrial Cancer: Cases and Two Control Groups from North Carolina. American Journal of Obstetrics and Gynecology 137:92.

Hulka BS, Kaufman DG, Fowler WC Jr, Grimson RC, Greenberg BG (1980): Predominance of early endometrial cancers after long-term estrogen use. JAMA 244(21):2419-2422.

Hulka BS, Chambless LE, Kaufman DG, Fowler WC Jr, Greenberg BG (1982): Protection against endometrial carcinoma by combination-product oral contraceptives. JAMA 247(4):475-477.

Hulka BS (1989): Hormonal contraceptives and risk of cervical cancer. In: Michal F, Ed. Safety Requirements for Contrceptive Steriods. Proceedings of a Symposium on Improving Safety Requirements for Contraceptive Steriods, Cambridge University Press, Cambridge.

Hulka BS, Liu ET, Lininger RA (1994): Steriod hormones and risk of breast cancer. Cancer 74(3):1111-1124.

Hulka BS (1994): Links between hormone replacement therapy and neoplasia. Fertility and Sterility 62(6):168s-175s.

Hulka BS, Stark AT (1995): Breast cancer: cause and prevention. The Lancet 346:883-887.

Hunt K, Vessey M, McPherson K, Coleman M (1987): Long-term surveillance of mortality and cancer incidence in women receiving hormone replacement therapy. British Journal of Obstetrics and Gynecology 94:620-635.

Kelsey JL, Gammon MD, John EM (1993): Reproductive factors and breast cancer. Epidemiol Rev 15:36-47.

Kerlikowske K, Brown JS, Grady DG (1992): Should women with familial ovarian cancer undergo prophylactic oophorectomy? Obstetrics and Gynecology 80(4):700-707.

Koutsky LA, Holmes KK, Critchlow CW et al. (1992): A cohort study of the risk of cervical intraepithelial neoplasia grade 2 or 3 in relation to papillomavirus infection. N Engl J Med 327:1272-1278.

Jensen J, Christiansen C (1988): Effects of smoking on serum lipoproteins and bone mineral content during postmenopasual hormones replacement therapy. Am J Obstet Gynecol 159:820-825.

Lee NC, Wingo PA, Gwinn ML, Rubin GL, Kendrick JS, Webster LA, Ory HW (1987): The reduction in risk of ovarian cancer associated with oral-contraceptive use. The New England Journal of Medicine 316(11)650-655.

McCann MF, Irwin DE, Walton LA, Hulka BS, Morton JL, Axelrad CM (1992): Nicotine and Cotinine in the Cervical Mucus of Smokers, Passive Smokers, and Nonsmokers. Ca Epid, Biomarkers and Prevention 1:125-129.

Michnovicz JJ, Hershcopf RJ, Naganuma H, et al. (1986): Increase of 2-hydroxylation of estradiol as a possible mechanism for the anti-estrogenic effect of cigarette smoking. N Engl J Med 315:1305-1309.

Nasca PC, Greenwald P, Chorost S, Richart R Caputo T (1984): An epidemiologic case-control study of ovarian cancer and reproductive factors. American Journal of Epidemiology 119(5):705-713.

Nason FG, Nelson BE (1994): Estrogen and progestrone in breast and gynecologic cancers. Primary Care of the Mature Woman 21(2):245-270.

Ries LAG, Miller BA, Hankey BF, Kosary CL, Harras A, Edwards BK (1994): SEER Cancer Statistics Review, 1973-1991: Tables and Graphs, National Cancer Institute. Bethesda, Maryland: NIH Pub. No. 94-2789.

Rodriguez C, Calle EE, Coates RJ, Miracle-McMahill HL, Thun MJ, Heath CW Jr. (1995): American Journal of Epidemiology 141(9):828-835.

Rosner B, Colditz G, Willet W (1994): Reproductive risk factors in a prospective study of breast cancer: the nurses' health study. Am J Epidemiol 139:819-835.

Schiffman MH, Bauer HM, Hoover RN, Glass AG, Cadell DM, Rush BB, Scott DR, Sherman ME, Kurman RJ, Wacholder S, Stanton CK, Manos MM (1993): Epidemiologic Evidence Showing That Human Papillomaus Infection Causes Most Cervical Intrapithelial Neoplasia. JNCI 85(12):958-964.

Siiteri PK (1987): Adipose as a source of hormones. American Journal of Clinical Nutrition 45:277-282.

Simpson ER, Mendelson CR (1990): The role of adipose tissue in estrogen biosynthesis in the human. In: Frisch RE, ed. Adipsoe tissue and reproduction. New York: Krager Publishing Co.

Schwartzbaum JA, Hulka BS, Fowler WC, Kaufman DG, Hoberman D (1987): The influence of exogenous estrogen use on survival after diagnosis of endometrial cancer. American Journal of Epidemiology 126(5):851-860.

The Cancer and Steriod Hormone Study of the Centers for Disease Control and the National Institute of Child Health and Human Development (1987): Combination oral contraceptive use and the risk of endometrial cancer. JAMA 257(6):796-800.

The Writing Group for the PEPI Trial (1996): Effects of hormone replacement therapy on endometrial histology in post-menopausal women: the post-menopausal estrogen/progestin intervention (PEPI) trial. JAMA: In press.

Voight LF, Weiss NS Chu J, Daling JR, McKnight B, Van Belle G (1991): Progestagen supplementation of exogenous oestrogens and risk of endometrial cancer. Lancet 338:274-277.

Werness BA, Levine AJ, Howley PM (1990): Association of Human Pappilomavirus Types 16 and 18 E6 Proteins with p53. Science 248:76-79.

Whittemore AS, Harris R, Itnyre J, the Collaborative Ovarian Cancer Group (1992): Characteristics relating to ovarian cancer risk: collaborative analysis of 12 US case-controls studies. II. Invasive epithelial ovarian cancers in white women. American Journal of Epidemiology 136(10):1184-1203.

Whittemore AS (1994): Characteristics relating to ovarian cancer risk: implications for prevention and detection. Gynecology and Oncology 55:s15-s19.

Wingo PA, Lee NC, Ory HW, Beral V, Peterson HB, Rhodes P (1993): Age-specific differences on the relationship between oral contraceptive use and breast cancer. Cancer supplement 71(4):1506-1517.

Wingo, PA, Tong T, Bolden S (1995): Cancer Statistics, 1995. CA-A Cancer Journal for Clinicians 45(1):8-30.

Yoo KY, Tajima K, Kuroishi T et al. (1992): Independent protective effects of lactation against breast cancer: a case-control study in Japan. Am J Epidemiol 135:726-733.

Etiology of Breast and
Gynecological Cancers, pages 31–51
© 1997 Wiley-Liss, Inc.

RECENT ADVANCES IN THE MOLECULAR GENETICS OF HEREDITARY BREAST AND OVARIAN CANCER

Johnathan M. Lancaster and Roger W. Wiseman

Laboratory of Molecular Carcinogenesis,
National Institute of Environmental Health Sciences,
National Institutes of Health, Research Triangle Park,
North Carolina 27709, USA

INTRODUCTION

Approximately 1 in 3 Americans will develop cancer at some point in their lifetime, and 1 in 6 will die of the disease. Over the past 60 years the total cancer incidence in the United States has increased steadily, with notable increases in breast cancer in females, prostate cancer in males, and lung cancer in both sexes (Ries, 1995). Despite the multitude of factors including environment, hormones, behaviour and inheritance that have been linked to the disease, a unifying theory of carcinogenesis remains elusive (Varmus and Weinberg, 1993). What is clear, however, is that cancer is fundamentally a disease of DNA, and with technological advances in molecular biology, the number of cancers in which distinct genetic defects are identifiable continues to increase rapidly. In this review we will first give an overview of the classes of genes involved in cancer predisposition and illustrate how defects in such genes can lead to a wide range tumors. We will then focus on two specific genes, BRCA1 and BRCA2, involved in hereditary breast and ovarian cancer.

Proto-Oncogenes and Tumor Suppressor Genes

Central to the biology of cancer is loss of cellular growth control. Such loss of control could be due to the removal of growth inhibiting/differentiation-inducing signals, or increase in growth stimulating signal. Such an edict, leads to the concept at a molecular genetic level, of genes which are stimulatory - proto-oncogenes, or inhibitory - tumor suppressor genes (Bishop, 1991). Proto-oncogenes are normal cellular genes, which code for proteins that stimulate growth during the normal cell cycle. Activation of these genes - to oncogenes - by mutation or amplification, results in unrestrained cell growth and tumorigenesis. As only one copy of an oncogene needs to be "activated" for loss of growth control, oncogenes are said to act dominantly at a cellular level. With the exception of the RET proto-oncogene, which functions as a receptor tyrosine kinase and gives rise to the Multiple Endocrine Neoplasia (MEN2) syndrome (Smith et al., 1994), oncogenes are not thought to play a role in inherited predispositions to cancer. A mutated oncogene carried in the germline would presumably be incompatible with conception or normal fetal development. Tumor suppressor genes encode proteins which are inhibitory to cell proliferation, functioning in the control of cell growth and differentiation and maintenance of genomic integrity. Both copies of the gene are required to be inactivated, either by gene deletion, mutations, rearrangements or loss of expression. As such, they are said to act recessively at a cellular level. It is the germline inheritance of defects in tumor suppressor gene that is responsible for many of the cancer predisposition syndromes. In addition, somatic mutations in these hereditary cancer predisposition genes are responsible for a significant number of sporadic cancers that arise in the absence of a family history (Greenblatt et al., 1994). The products of tumor suppressor genes are involved at many levels in growth control, including signal transduction, cytoskeletal integrity, transcription and cell cycle control, and mismatch repair. Several of these genes are described in further detail below.

Cancer Predisposition Genes

An early paradigm of cancer predisposition genetics was that of retinoblastoma (RB) (Knudson, 1978). Autosomal inheritance of defects in this gene leads to ocular tumors in early childhood, with 90% penetrance, as well as increased incidence of osteosarcoma and soft-tissue sarcoma in later life (Abramson et al., 1984). Retinoblastoma studies led to the development of the Knudson "two-hit" hypothesis that both gene copies must be mutated during neoplastic development, now a fundamental principle in the understanding of tumor suppressor genes (Knudson, 1985). RB produces a 110 kD nuclear phosphoprotein, the phosphorylation-status of which, varies throughout the cell cycle and appears to control the G1/S phase transition and thus cell growth (Charollais et al., 1994).

Inactivation of the p53 tumor suppressor gene on chromosome 17p13.1 is the most frequently defined genetic alteration in human cancer and a wide variety of tumor types are affected (Greenblatt et al., 1994). Most p53 mutations in sporadic cancers are somatic events, in individuals with wild-type germline p53. In the rare Li Fraumeni Syndrome (LFS) however, germline mutations in p53 produce a dominantly inherited cancer predisposition characterized by mesenchymal and epithelial tumors including soft tissue sarcomas, breast carcinomas, brain tumors, leukemias, osteosarcoma, and adrenocortical carcinomas (Li et al., 1969; Malkin et al., 1990). Most p53 alterations are missense mutations located in four evolutionarily conserved domains of the protein. Analysis of the p53 mutation spectra of tumor types has implicated specific carcinogenic agents (Greenblatt et al., 1994). The p53 gene product appears to regulate cell growth by binding to DNA and other gene products such as mdm2 (Momand et al., 1992). p53 is also known to transcriptionally activate the p21 gene, which encodes an inhibitor of Cdk2 - a cyclin dependent kinase - resulting in a block of DNA synthesis and cell division (El-Deiry et al., 1993). Inactivation of p53 in thymocytes results in failure to undergo apoptosis, and suggests that p53 may also play a role in apoptosis induction (Lowe et al., 1993). p53 increases in response to irradiation-induced G1 arrest, a checkpoint absent in cancer-prone patients with ataxia telangiectasia, implying that p53 protects cells from entering S phase with damaged DNA (Kastan et al., 1992).

Another protein known to bind to Cdk4 and contribute to the cell cycle regulatory pathway with RB, is p16 (Serrano et al., 1993). The gene which codes for this protein is postulated to be a tumor suppressor gene located on 9p, named Multiple Tumor Suppressor 1 (MTS1), and shows high frequency of loss of heterozygosity in tumors of bladder, brain, lung, breast, bone, skin, kidney, ovary, and lymphocyte (Kamb et al., 1994). Linkage studies on families with multiple cases of cutaneous malignant melanoma indicated that an area on 9p13-22 was likely the locus of a familial melanoma susceptibility gene, MLM (Cannon-Albright et al., 1992). Germline MTS1 mutations in 9p21-linked melanoma families supports that this is the responsible susceptibility gene in this syndrome (Hussussian et al., 1994). However, the rate of MTS1 point mutations in tumors with allele loss at 9p21 is low, suggesting that other mechanisms may be responsible for inactivation of the remaining allele (Cairns et al., 1994, 1995). Indeed, methylation of 5' CpG islands in p16 has been described in up to 20% of primary tumors relative to normal surrounding tissue. This hypermethylation, and homozygous deletion may be other ways in which this tumor suppressor gene is inactivated in the absence of point mutations (Merlo et al., 1995).

Several cancer susceptibility genes have been implicated in the genesis of urological malignancies. Cytogenetic studies of families with an inherited predisposition to Wilm's tumor (WT), led to the cloning of WT1 on 11p13, that encodes a zinc finger transcription factor (Gessler et al., 1993; Ton et al., 1991.). Mutations in the DNA binding region abrogate its regulatory role and result in tumors of the kidney and urogenital abnormalities in heterozygotes, though carriers do not appear to be at any increased risk for other tumor types (Coppes et al., 1993). The Von Hippel-Lindau (VHL) gene was cloned recently, and inactivating mutations predispose to central nervous system hemangioblastomas, renal cell carcinomas, pancreatic cysts and pheochromocytomas (Latif et al., 1993). Based on its ability to specifically bind and inhibit the cellular transcription factor Elongin SIII, and thus inhibit transcription elongation, the VHL protein appears to be an important factor in the transcriptional regulatory network. (Duan et al., 1995).

Germline mutations in neurofibromatosis I and II (NFI and NFII) genes, on 17q11 and 22q12 respectively, give rise to multiple tumors of neuronal and several other tissue types (Trofatter et al., 1993). NFI gene product, neurofibromin, has GTPase-activating properties, and may act as a regulator of RAS^{GTP} (O'Connell et al., 1992; Bourne et al., 1990). The NF II protein is localized to the membrane-cytoskeletal interface, and thought to play a role in maintenance of cellular structure (Trofatter et al., 1993).

Numerous genes are known to be responsible for colorectal cancer predisposition. Germline mutations in the familial adenomatous polyposis coli (APC) gene, located at 5q21 are responsible for a syndrome of multiple early onset adenomatous polyps in the colon, and thus profound predisposition to cancer (Groden et al., 1991; Kinzler, 1991.). Somatic mutations in the gene are also responsible for sporadic colon cancers (Nakamura et al., 1992; Kinzler, 1991.). The gene product is a 312 kD cytoplasmic protein of unknown function, though it is speculated that it plays a role in cell adhesion or cytoskeletal integrity. Like mutant p53, truncated APC protein acts in a dominant negative fashion to bind wild-type protein (Su et al., 1993).

Clearly then, alterations at a genetic level are integral to the development of cancer in the colon. The potential harm to a multicellular organism of critical genetic changes is such that extensive repair mechanisms have evolved to protect the genome. These systems are responsible for replacing mismatched base pairs and the excision of insertions that can occur during replication and recombination. Study of these systems in E. Coli led to the discovery of four critical proteins - MutH, MutS, MutL, and MutU, that form active complexes, bind to DNA and repair defects in response to specific methylation patterns (Cox, 1976). The realization that defects in the DNA repair system in the human, could play a role in carcinogenesis, has stimulated further interest in this field. Human cancer cell lines and tumors characteristic for their hypermutability were shown to be defective in their ability to repair mismatches (Parsons et al., 1993; Umar et al., 1994). Further, human lymphoblastoid cell lines deficient in mismatch repair were resistant to the effects of alkylating agents that would normally result in such DNA damage as to kill the cell (Kat et al., 1993). This suggested that the mechanism was also involved in the cell death that results when mutation levels rise above a critical point (Goldmacher et al., 1986).

Study of the genes integral to mismatch repair in humans - MSH2, MLH1, PMS1, and PMS2 - led to the identification of mutations responsible for another familial syndrome of colorectal cancer; the hereditary nonpolyposis colorectal cancer syndrome (HNPCC)/ Lynch II syndrome, in which tumors also develop in small intestine, endometrium, ovary, stomach, kidney, and ureter (Fishel et al., 1993; Leach et al., 1993; Nicolaides et al., 1994). Recent preliminary evidence suggests that breast cancer may also be implicated in this syndrome (Risinger et al, 1996). These genes are also mutated in a small subset of sporadic colorectal cancers (Aaltonen et al., 1994; Borresen et al., 1995). Certain regions of the genome contain blocks of DNA which are repeated a variable number of times in different individuals. These simple sequence repeats, or microsatellites, challenge the fidelity of DNA polymerase proof-reading/repair and are frequently altered in individuals with impaired DNA repair machinery. HNPCC tumors are characteristic for the hypermutability of their microsatellite repeat sequences (Aaltonen et al., 1993). The repair gene defect is carried in the germlines of these patients and passed on as an autosomal dominant trait. In a small number of carriers, normal tissue, with one normally functioning allele, has an increased level of mutability, but less so than the tumor tissue, in which both alleles are inactivated and therefore unable to fulfill DNA repair functions (Parsons et al, 1995). Doubtless the list of mismatch repair genes will grow - GTBP is the newest member of the family to be identified - and their role in other forms of cancer will become clear (Papadopoulos et al., 1995). It is easy to see how somatic loss of ability to repair DNA, with consequent increased mutability of genes involved in cell growth control, could lead to cancer development, and why individuals carrying germline defects in these genes are predisposed to a wide variety of cancers (Modrich, 1994).

Hereditary Breast and Ovarian Cancer

Perhaps the most heralded developments in the molecular genetics of human cancer in recent years were the isolation of the familial breast/ovarian cancer susceptibility genes, BRCA1 and BRCA2 (Miki et al., 1994; Wooster et al., 1995). As with the cancer predisposition genes described above, these genes are also believed to be tumor suppressors. In the remainder of this chapter, we will focus on BRCA1 and BRCA2 studies that illustrate some of the challenges of molecular genetics, several features of familial cancer predisposition, and multiple non-scientific/social consequences of genetic testing.

Approximately 184,000 new cases of breast cancer, and 21,000 new cases of ovarian cancer are diagnosed in the USA each year. Breast cancer is the most common malignancy in women, and ovarian cancer remains the leading cause of death due to gynecologic malignancy. Many factors influence a woman's risk of developing breast and/or ovarian cancer, and family history is the most important predictor of risk for both malignancies. However, familial breast and ovarian cancer account for only 5 - 10% of total cases of the disease (Lynch et al., 1987; Claus et al., 1991). That is to say, 90% of cases of breast and ovarian cancer are sporadic, and have no familial etiology. Despite this, many families are known to exist in which multiple generations have been afflicted with early onset breast and/or ovarian cancer. Study of many such families reveals a pattern of disease compatible with the transmission of an autosomal dominant gene. Hereditary breast cancer families can be divided into site-specific breast only, breast/ovarian - in which increased rates of early onset breast and ovarian cancer are observed, and Li-Fraumeni syndrome families, as above (Li et al., 1969; Malkin et al., 1990). Breast cancer families have also been reported to be associated with the estrogen receptor gene, though no mutations have been identified (Zuppan et al, 1991). Familial forms of ovarian cancer appear to be divided into site specific ovarian cancer families (SSOC), in which other malignancies do not appear to occur in the family at any greater rate than in the general population, breast/ovarian cancer families (as above), and hereditary non-polyposis colorectal cancer (HNPCC)/Lynch II syndrome, described above (Lynch et al., 1991; Bewtra et al., 1992). More rarely, non-epithelial ovarian cancers are seen in association with Peutz-Jeghers and basal cell nevus familial syndromes (Spigelman et al., 1989; Kraemer et al., 1984).

BRCA1

In 1990, using genetic linkage analysis to study a series of breast cancer families, the long arm of chromosome 17 was identified as the location of the BRCA1 gene, which causes a dominantly inherited predisposition to early onset breast cancer (Hall et al., 1990). Soon after this, it was shown that several ovarian cancer families were also linked to the 17q locus (Narod et al., 1991), and that this gene was likely to be a tumor suppressor gene, since the wild-type allele is always lost in breast and ovarian tumors of women who carry a germline mutation (Smith et al., 1992). Loss of heterozygosity studies in sporadic brest and ovarian tumors suggested that this gene, as well as being responsible for a large proportion of cases of familial breast/ovarian cancer, was also involved in the more common non-heredirary forms of the disease (Jacobs et al., 1993; Smith et al., 1992; Futreal et al., 1992). After an intensive search by research groups around the world, the identification of the BRCA1 gene was announced in September 1994 (Miki et al., 1994).

BRCA1 is a large gene consisting of 22 coding exons, distributed over approximately 80,000 base pairs of genomic DNA. It encodes a protein of up to 1863 amino acids, which can be alternatively spliced in several ways. Within its amino-terminal region - exons 2 to 5 - there is a C3HCH RING finger motif predicted to bind zinc atoms. A family of more than 50 genes from a wide variety of species contain homologous RING domains. Since many RING finger genes act as transcription factors, it has been proposed that BRCA1 may play a role in the control of gene expression, consistent with this concept (Miki et al., 1994).

More recently it has been reported that the BRCA1 protein exhibits sequence homology and biochemical analogy to a family of acidic secretory proteins, known as granins, found in the golgi apparatus and secretory granules (Jensen et al., 1996). Using two antibodies against the C-terminal, and one against the N-terminal the group demonstrate that BRCA1 is located predominantly in the membrane fraction, with little in the nucleus and none in the cytoplasm. Further, using immunogold electron microscopy they were able to demonstrate that BRCA1 localizes to membrane bound vesicles in apical cytoplasm at the tips of microvilli. These findings suggests that BRCA1 functions as a novel secreted growth inhibitor, and raises exciting pharmacological possibilities. These findings are preliminary and await confirmation by other groups.

The mutations identified to date, number over 100, and appear to be distributed throughout the gene. There are several mutation "hot-spots" - in exons 2, 5, 11 and 20, which account for about one quarter of all alterations (Futreal et al., 1994; Merajver et al., 1995; Hosking et al., 1995; Takahashi et al., 1995; Castilla et al., 1994; Simard et al., 1994; Friedman et al., 1994; Shattuck-Eidens et al., 1995; Hogervorst et al., 1995; Struewing et al., 1995; Couch et al., 1995; Lancaster et al., 1996). Mutations producing premature stop codons (nonsense and frameshift mutations due to insertion or deletion of any number of basepairs not divisible by three), produce a truncated protein product, and are responsible for approximately ~90% of mutations identified (Couch et al., 1996). Little correlation has been observed between genotype and phenotype, though preliminary evidence suggests that mutations within the 3' end of the gene may be associated with a lower incidence of ovarian cancer (Shattuck-Eidens et al.,; Gayther et al., 1995; Holt et al., 1996). Conversely, Friedman et al report a family with 7 cases of early onset breast cancer, carrying a germline mutation in exon 24, that produces a protein product truncated by only the final 10 amino acids (Friedman et al., 1994). This contrasts with lessor affected families carrying one of the more common BRCA1 mutations - 185DelAG - which produces a protein product only 35 amino acids long, due to this deletion in exon 2. Further, considerable variation in penetrance exists *between* different families carrying the 185DelAG mutation.

Carriers of germline BRCA1 mutations have a considerably elevated risk of developing breast and ovarian cancer, estimated at 54% and 30% respectively by age 60 (Ford et al., 1994; Easton et al., 1995). Preliminary data also indicate that BRCA1 mutation carriers have a 4.1 relative risk of developing colon cancer, and males have a 3.3 relative risk of developing prostate cancer (Easton et al., 1993). No excesses in cancer risk has been seen in other anatomical sites. It is important to note that, these estimates have been obtained from families selected on the basis of their high incidence of breast and ovarian cancers. It is quite possible therefore, that families exist, carring germline BRCA1 mutations with low penetrance. The risk of developing a malignancy due to such BRCA1 mutations could be significantly lower than in those families studied to date, and it may be difficult to recognize these individuals based on the pattern of inheritance. It will be some time before the complete BRCA1 mutation spectrum will be known, such that accurate estimates of penetrance and consequent risk of malignancy can be established. Likewise, studies of lifestyle factors and genes that may modify penetrance are ongoing. To date the only gene demonstrated to modify risk in BRCA1 carriers is HRAS1 (Phelan et al., 1996). A variable number of tandem repeats (VNTR) polymorphism 1 kb downstream of HRAS1 exists in a common and rare form. Individuals who have the rare allele are known to have an increased risk of certain types of cancer, including breast cancer. Phelan et al. (1996) studied 307 female BRCA1 mutation carriers at this locus, and demonstrated an increased risk for ovarian cancer of 2.11 for BRCA1 carriers with the rare HRAS allele. The group claim that this is the first study to show the effect of a modifying gene on the penetrance of an inherited cancer syndrome.

In 1995 the first human known to be homozygous for a BRCA1 mutation was reported (Boyd et al., 1995). The patient, a woman who developed breast cancer at age 32, carried the same 2800delAA mutation in both copies of BRCA1. Haplotype analysis revealed that she was also homozygous for 5 BRCA1 flanking markers. The statistical probability of an individual inheriting two mutated BRCA1 genes, from the chance meeting of two *unrelated* parents, range from 1:40,000 to 1:360,000 depending on the estimated population frequency of germline BRCA1 mutations. Recently, Gowen et al. (1996) reported the development of the first BRCA1 deficient mice, which carry one inactivated BRCA1 allele. Mice carrying one inactivated BRCA1 allele remained phenotypically normal at 5 months. Mice homozygous for the introduced mutation die at approximately 10 - 13 days in-utero with severe disruption to development of neural tube structures seen in 40% of cases. The apparent lethality in-utero for mouse but not human BRCA1 mutation homozygosity remains to be explained.

The majority of the mutations identified to date have been carried in patients germline; the remaining good copy of BRCA1 is inactivated by deletion of all, or part of the chromosome arm. It was predicted that BRCA1, like other familial cancer predisposition genes, would also prove to be mutated in sporadic, ie non-familial, forms of the disease (Nakamura et al. 1992). To date however, of approximately 300 sporadic ovarian cancers screened for BRCA1 alterations, only 5 somatic and 18 germline mutations have been identified. In addition, 9 germline but no somatic mutations have been identified in 184 sporadic breast cancers screened (Futreal et al., 1994; Merajver et al., 1995; Hosking et al., 1995; Takahashi et al., 1995; Lancaster et al., 1996a). Interestingly, preliminary data suggests that germline mutations in BRCA1 may be responsible for a sizeable proportion (10-20%) of early onset ovarian cancers, and that the average age of patients with somatic mutations causing ovarian cancer is up to 20 years greater than those with cancer caused by germline mutations (Lancaster et al., 1996a). This is consistent with the fact that in a germline mutation carrier, only a single somatic event is necessary to inactivate BRCA1. In a normal individual, born with two functional gene copies, 2 somatic events in a specific clone of cells are required to inactivate the gene, thus taking many more years to occur. If this is the case, then it is possible that part of the reason that few somatic BRCA1 mutations have been identified to date, is that researchers have so far concentrated screening efforts on individuals who have developed cancer at a young age, in the hope of increasing the probability of detecting mutations. Though in familial forms of the disease, this may well be true, screening an older population with sporadic breast or ovarian cancer may be more fruitful in the search for somatic mutations.

Thompson et al. (1995) have reported that in sporadic breast cancer tissue, BRCA1 mRNA expression levels may be diminished by 5 to 20 fold, compared to normal breast tissue. Decreased BRCA1 expression mediated by antisense oligonucleotides is associated with an increased proliferative rate *in vitro* for normal mammary epithelial cells and MCF7 breast cancer cells. Further, Holt et al. (1996) demonstrated that retroviral transfer of wild-type BRCA1 gene inhibited growth *in vitro*, of breast and ovarian cancer cell lines, while mutant BRCA1 genes have no effect on breast cancer cell lines. Interestingly, a mutation in the 3', but not the 5' end of the gene inhibit ovarian cancer cell line growth. Preliminary evidence suggests that families with mutations in the 3' end of BRCA1 have a lower incidence of ovarian cancer (Gayther et al., 1996). Holt et al. (1996) went on to demonstrate inhibition of MCF-7 tumors in nude mice transfected with wild-type BRCA1, and increased survival in mice with established tumors following peritoneal treatment with retro-viral vector expressing wild-type BRCA1.

Clearly, although these reports are preliminary and require further investigation in larger studies, it is becoming evident that BRCA1 may well play a significant role in the biology of sporadic breast cancer despite the lack of somatic inactivating mutations identified.

BRCA2

BRCA1 is responsible for most families with multiple cases of both early-onset breast and ovarian cancer and approximately 45% of families with breast cancer only, but very few families with both female and male breast cancer. Many of the families not linked to BRCA1 were found to be linked to a second breast cancer susceptibility gene BRCA2, localized to a region of 6 million base pairs on 13q12-13, between D13S289 and D13S267 in September 1994 (Wooster et al, 1994). This region was rapidly narrowed to approximately 600 kb with a set of Icelandic families, and more finely localized when Schutte et al. (1995) identified a 300kb homozygous somatic deletion in a pancreatic carcinoma, the centromeric boundary of which was 300 kb centromeric to D13S171, and the telomeric boundary closely centromeric to D13S171 (Figure 1). Concentrating efforts on this region led to the isolation of BRCA2 in December 1995 (Wooster et al., 1995). They described inactivating germline mutations in probands from six families exhibiting strong linkage to microsatellite markers in the region. Each mutation caused serious disruption to the open reading frame, providing strong evidence that the gene identified was indeed BRCA2. Other studies have since confirmed this finding (Phelan et al., 1996; Tavigian et al., 1996; Thorlacius et al., 1996; Couch et al., 1996). Subsequent to the identification of BRCA2, we studied its role in sporadic disease, and identified only one germline and one somatic alteration in 70 sporadic breast cancers, and none in 55 sporadic ovarian cancers, indicating thus far that mutational inactivation of BRCA2 does not play a significant role in sporadic disease (Lancaster et al., 1996c).

BRCA2 is a large gene spanning approximately 200 kb basepairs of genomic DNA with an estimated transcript size of 10-12 kb, that encodes a protein of 3,418 amino acids. Carriers of germline BRCA2 mutations are highly predisposed to early onset female breast cancer, and moderately predisposed to ovarian cancer. Carriers are also at increased risk of male breast, pancreatic, prostate, colon cancers and ocular melanoma (Phelan et al., 1996).

Similarity Between BRCA1 and BRCA2

Comparison of BRCA1 and BRCA2 is of interest. Both are sizeable genes containing a large exon 11 of 3,426 and 4,932 bp respectively. The translational start

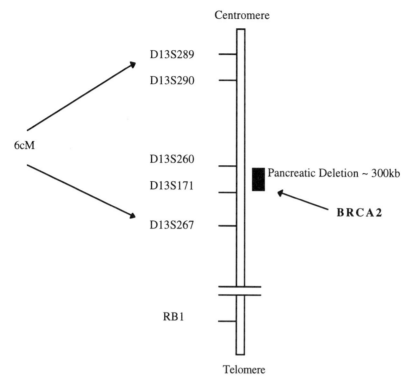

Figure 1: Relative positions of microsatellite markers, the RB1 gene and the pancreatic homozygous somatic deletion in the BRCA2 region of chromosome 13q.

sites are both in exon two, producing large, negatively charged proteins that are most highly expressed in testis. Mutations in BRCA1 are distributed throughout the gene, and initial screening suggests that this is also true for BRCA2. In both genes the vast majority of mutations identified to date appear to produce premature truncation of protein synthesis. BRCA2 appears to have an excess of deletions relative to BRCA1, which has an approximately equal number of deletions to point mutations and insertions (Wooster et al., 1995; Tavtigian et al., 1996; Couch et al., 1996). BRCA2, like BRCA1 exhibits some sequence homology to the granin family, and may imply a similar biological function related to regulated secretion (Jensen et al., 1996).

Genetic Screening

Until the cloning of BRCA1 and BRCA2, geneticists relied on genetic linkage analysis to assess members of high risk families for the probability of developing breast and ovarian cancer (Easton et al., 1993). Multiple affected family members were required for analysis, and result were not definitive. With the identification of BRCA1 and BRC2, it has become possible to directly screen affected individuals for mutations in these genes. If a specific mutation is identified, it is technically straightforward to determine which other family members also carry the alteration, and are therefore strongly predisposed to cancer development. Non-carriers can be reassured that they are at no greater risk of developing cancer than the general population.

At present screening for BRCA1 and BRCA2 mutations is confined to research protocols, and remains technically challenging. The incidence of false positive and negative results make the currently available screening tools inadequate for widespread clinical use. However, as the spectrum of mutations in these genes becomes saturated, and the extent of other external control defects is established, it may be possible to consider large scale screening of high risk individuals within the population. A completely reliable screening test remains elusive. The ultimate goal is to develop a highly reliable assay to assess the functional integrity of the BRCA1 and BRCA2 gene products.

As the number of cancer predisposition genes identified continues to grow, the need for efficient and sensitive techniques to identify inactivating mutations also increases. In many ways, direct DNA sequencing is viewed as the "gold-standard" for identifying or characterizing all possible sequence alterations. Other techniques can be applied to rapidly screen large numbers of samples, but limited DNA sequencing is still required to characterize the specific DNA alteration. Though highly sensitive, DNA sequencing is expensive, limited in terms of sample numbers, and time consuming to perform and analyze.

When a specific predisposing mutation has been identified in a particular family, or if the spectrum of mutations in a specific ethnic group is limited, allele specific oligonucleotide hybridization can be used to screen other family or populations members. This method is not applicable to screen large genes such as BRCA1 and BRCA2 for unknown mutations, as the mutation spectrum is great, and distributed throughout the gene.

One of the most widely used techniques in mutation detection currently, is single strand conformation polymorphism analysis (SSCP) (Orita et al., 1989) This technique relies on the differences in the spacial conformation that a PCR product acquires when denatured and allowed to form intra-strand hydrogen bonds. Remarkably, molecules with single base substitutions tend to form unique conformations that migrate at different rates through electrophoretic gels, allowing subtle sequence alterations to be localized. SSCA can detect most missense, nonsense and frameshift mutations under optimal conditions, it allows large numbers of samples to be examined simultaneously in an economical and technically straightforward manner. The sensitivity of the technique is diminished with PCR products greater than 250 basepairs, and radiolabeling is required to obtain maximum sensitivity (Qiang and Sommer, 1994).

More than 90% of the mutations identified in BRCA1 lead to premature termination of protein synthesis, and initial results with BRCA2 suggest a similar pattern. Detection of such nonsense and frameshift mutations is possible using the protein truncation test (PTT), which detect differences in protein sizes caused by the presence of premature stop codons. PTT is a sensitive screening technique that allows high sample throughput.

However, it relies on use of RNA to screen the entire coding region of BRCA1 and BRCA2, which is not always readily available. Certain mutations decrease the stability of mRNA and may consequently decrease the sensitivity of this the technique. Missense mutations, which represent a small but significant subset of the BRCA1 mutation spectrum cannot be detected by PTT. The ability of PTT to detect all truncated proteins may also be limited by gel resolution of near full-length products and loss of small peptide fragments from the gel. This technique has been used extensively to analyze the APC gene, and is being applied increasingly to BRCA1 and BRCA2 (Van Der Luijt et al., 1994; Hogervorst et al., 1995, Lancaster et al, 1996a & c).

Multiplex Heteroduplex Analysis (MHA) has been described as an initial analytical step to screen for frequently occurring BRCA1 mutations (Gayther et al., 1996). Using this technique, one quarter of the coding region can be screened, encompassing 50% of BRCA1 mutations reported to date. This technique is particularly applicable, as 97% of the mutations within this region are either insertions or deletions. Gayther et al. report that in 60 families screened using MHA, sensitivity was equivalent to direct sequence analysis.

Dideoxy fingerprinting (DDF), is a more novel mutation detection technique, which represents a hybrid of SSCA and dideoxy sequencing reactions (Sarkar et al., 1992). Native gel electrophoresis of radiolabelled fragments resulting from a sequencing reaction with a single dideoxy nucleotide increases the sensitivity of the SSCA element by inducing multiple band shifts in the presence of an alteration. DDF can be exceedingly sensitive BRCA1 screening technique, but is labor intensive (Lancaster et al., submitted).

The choice of mutation detection technique has to be made considering the type of mutations being sought, the size of the gene and distribution of mutations, the resources and time available, and the required detection sensitivity.

Clinical Management Options

Identification of BRCA1 and BRCA2 mutation carriers, allows close monitoring for early signs of malignancy. Unfortunately however, no established or proven monitoring protocol exists. For breast disease the monitoring offered may include instruction in breast self-examination, regular clinical examinations in combination with annual or semi-annual mammograms beginning as early as 25 - 30 years of age (Hoskins et al., 1995). The effect of the additional radiation exposure on such individuals is unknown, and carries a theoretical risk of increasing the rate at which the remaining wild-type BRCA1 allele is inactivated. Preventative measures at present include prophylactic mastectomy or chemoprevention, within controlled research protocols. The effect of prophylactic surgery on mortality and morbidity is yet to be established. As it is impossible to remove every single cell of breast tissue, the risk of developing breast cancer - although reduced - remains, after mastectomy.

Screening options for ovarian cancer may include annual pelvic examinations, vaginal ultrasound and CA125 monitoring from the mid 20's or 5 years prior to the earliest age of ovarian cancer in the family (NIH Consensus Development Panel on Ovarian Cancer, 1995). Some women may elect to undergo prophylactic oophorectomy after completing childbearing. Again, such monitoring and prophylactic surgery has not been *proven* to decrease mortality or morbidity from the disease. The effect of screening for ovarian cancer in the general population with ultrasound and CA125 independently, has been shown in studies to lead to a very high false positive rate, and subsequent unnecessary laparotomies (Jacobs et al., 1996.) Reports exist of intra-abdominal carcinomatosis following prophylactic oophorectomy, likely due to "tiny" remnants of ovarian tissue left at oophorectomy, and thus, this procedure does not exclude the possibility of ovarian cancer developing (Struewing et al., 1995). In addition, debate continues over the use of hormone replacement in these women. The consequences of a premature menopause, in terms of osteoporosis and cardiovascular disease must be balanced against the possible increased risk of hormones on breast cancer development (Berchuck et al. 1996). Likewise, in a female who declines prophylactic surgery, the recognized protective benefit of oral contraceptives on ovarian cancer may be outweighed by detriment to breast cancer risk. (Hunt et al., 1994; McKeon et al., 1994; Khoo et al., 1992)

Disease patterns within BRCA1 families show that additional factors influence the age at which cancer develops in a carrier (Phelan et al, 1996). Identification of the these genetic or environmental factors will enable appropriate advice to be given in terms of risk and avoidance behaviour. At this point however, counseling such women on clinical management is difficult, as sufficient data does not exist to support or refute many of the options available.

DILEMMAS OF GENETIC TESTING

The ability to screen for mutations highlights some of the dilemmas common to genetic testing; dilemmas amplified in testing for late onset disease (Schneider et al., 1995). Even when testing families using linkage analysis, problems of confidentiality arose within the families. By definition for this type of analysis, multiple family members need to be involved. Such confidentiality worries are common in testing for genetic disease. The threat to a person's self image and plans for the future are considerble. Feelings of guilt emerge in siblings found not to be mutation carriers, and in combination with the anger, dispare and depression experienced by carriers, can destroy family dynamics. In studies of individuals diagnosed as carriers of defects in the Huntington's Disease gene, up to 15% were at risk of suicide (Adams et al., 1993). Such risks would likely also apply to BRCA1 and BRCA2 carriers.

As the number of presymptomatic individuals identified as BRCA1 and BRCA2 mutation carriers rises, obstetricians will certainly receive requests for BRCA1 and BRCA2 prenatal testing. Knowledge of the precise family mutation means that prenatal testing using fetal cells is relatively straightforward and a result could be obtained in a few days allowing for pregnancy termination if desired. Whether a fetus with a BRCA1 or BRCA2 mutation should be aborted is a matter that the parents should decide after receiving adequate education and counseling. The justification for aborting a fetus with a mutant BRCA1 or BRCA2 gene might seem marginal as that individual is likely to be unaffected by cancer until late in life. Conversely, termination of a pregnancy that carries mutant BRCA1 or BRCA2 might be viewed as justified by women who have lost multiple family members at young ages to breast and/or ovarian cancer; all in the context of a society in which thousands of undesired pregnancies are aborted electively every year. Assisted reproductive technology has advanced to the point where selective implantation of embryos with normal BRCA1 and BRCA2 genes is feasible, for those who object to termination of an affected pregnancy. A more detailed discussion of the issues surrounding prenatal testing for BRCA1 can be found in our recent clinical commentary devoted to the subject (Lancaster et al., 1996b).

Outside the family environment, issues of confidentiality become even more pertinent. The potential for loss of - or inability to obtain - health, life and disability insurance is great, as is the risk of discrimination in work, education and social intercourse. Such issues must be discussed fully during pre- and post- screen counseling. Thus, genetic testing for BRCA1 mutations should only be undertaken if appropriate support services can be offered to an individual. The emergence of "high-risk" breast and ovarian cancer clinics provides the ideal setting for this, such that individuals have access to experts in breast/ovarian cancer screening and treatment, genetics, birth control as well as the ethical, legal and social issues associated with testing (Schneider et al., 1995).

FUTURE DIRECTIONS

The availability of reliable mutation screening tests for BRCA1, BRCA2 and other cancer predisposition genes will facilitate the identification of high risk individuals. This in turn will lead to greater knowledge of penetrance and disease behaviour, and hence will allow more informed counseling for high risk families. At present, it is apparent that even within a single family, individuals carrying the identical mutation in BRCA1, develop different malignancies at significantly different ages. It is feasible that environmental, hormonal, reproductive and behavioural factors influence this. Examining such factors in large numbers of BRCA1 and BRCA2 kindreds, for carriers and non-carriers, affected and non-affected individuals, will reveal what, if any, measures are possible to diminish a BRCA1 or BRCA2 carrier's chances of developing a malignancy. It is hoped that the development of BRCA1 and BRCA2-deficient mice with gene targeting techniques will allow investigation of different mutation phenotypes, the effect of external factors and behaviour on disease development, and the role of chemopreventative and chemotherapeutic agents in the management of these patients.

Currently, non-surgical treatment of cancer is based on principles of "cell killing". This may take the form of chemical agents which interfere with cellular metabolism or division, or radiation damage to cellular genetic material to toxic levels. In both cases, the therapeutic benefit to the patient is based on the balance of tumor cell death to normal cell death. Unfortunately, many agents which damage tumor cells are also toxic to normal cells, and it is this toxicity that limits therapy. Side effects are severe; bone marrow supression and neutropenia leading to susceptibility to infection, excessive nausea and vomiting caused by gastro-intestinal cell death and central stimulation of vomiting centres, as well as toxicity to other systems including renal, hepatic and neurological. The more selective the anticancer agent is to malignant cells, the less effect it has on normal cells, and the less severe the side effect profile. It could be said, however, that these approaches are not aimed at the underlying molecular cause for the loss of growth control, and therefore doomed to limited success. As the biology of BRCA1 and BRCA2 is further elucidated, their interactions with other genes established, and the functions of the protein products identified, it will become possible to determine precisely how defects in the genes result in loss of growth control. With this knowledge we will hopefully begin to move towards controlling these cancers. This may involve restoring levels of functional protein by genetically manipulating mutation carriers to correct the defect, by replacing the defective gene in patients with viral vectors, or by administration of exogeneous protein or synthetic substitutes. Quite how rapidly therapeutics will develop in this area is difficult to predict. Clearly though, it is only with full understanding of the underlying biology that more effective prevention and treatment of breast and ovarian cancer can be developed.

REFERENCES

Aaltonen LA, Peltomaki P, Leach FS, Sistonen P, Pylkkanen L, Mecklin JP, Jarvinen H, ,kPowell SM, Jen J, Hamilton SR (1993): Clues to the pathogenesis of familial colorectal cancer. Science 260:812-816.

Aaltonen LA, Peltomaki P, Mecklin JP, Jarvinen H, Jass Jr, Green JS, Lynch Ht, Watson P, Tallqvist G, Juhola M (1994): Replication errors in benign and malignant tumors from hereditary nonpolyposis colorectal cancer patients. Cancer Res 54:1645-1648.

Abramson DH, Ellsworth RM, Kitchin FD, Tung G (1984): Second nonocular tumors in retinoblastoma survivors. Are they radiation induced? Ophthalmology 91:1351-1355.

Adams S, Wiggins S, Whyte P, Bloch M, Shokeir MH, Soltan H, Meschino W, Summers A, Suchowersky O, WL Welch JP (1993): Five year study of prenatal testing for Huntington's disease: demand, attitudes, and psychological assessment. J Med Genet 30:549-356.

Bewtra C, Watson P, Conway T,Read-Hippee C, Lynch HT (1992): Hereditary ovarian cancer: a clinicopathological study. Int J Gynaecol Pathol 11:180-187.

Bishop MJ (1991): Molecular themes in carcinogenesis. Cell 64:235-248.

Borresen AL, Lothe RA, Meling GI, Lystad S, Morrison P, Lipford J, Kane MF, Rognum TO, Kolodner RD (1995): Somatic mutations in the hMSH2 gene in microsatellite unstable colorectal carcinomas. Hum Mol Genet 4:2065-2072.

Bourne H, Sanders D, McCormick F (1990). The GTPase superfamily: A conserved switch for diverse cell functions. Nature 348:125-132.

Boyd M, Harris, McFarlane R, Davidson RH, Black DM (1995): A human BRCA1 gene knockout. Nature 375:541-542.

Cairns P, Mao L, Merlo A, Lee DJ, Schwab D, Eby Y, Tokino K, van-der-Riet P, Blaugrund JE, Sidransky D (1994): Rates of p16 (MTS1) mutations in primary tumors with 9p loss. Science 265:415-416.

Cairns P, Polascik TJ, Eby Y, Tokino K, Califano J, Merlo a, Mao L, Herath J, Jenkins R, Westra W (1995): Frequency of homozygous deletion at p16/CDKN2 in primary human tumors. Nat Genet 11:210-212.

Cannon-Albright LA, Goldgar DE, Meyer LJ, Lewis CM, Andersn DE, Fountain JW, Hegi ME, Wiseman RW, Petty EM, Bale AE (1992): Assignment of a locus for familial melanoma MLM, to chromosome 9p13-22. Science 258:1148-1152.

Cannon-Albright L, Larsson C, Goldgar DE, Narod SA (1996): Ovarian cancer risk in BRCA1 carriers is modified by the HRAS1 variable number of tandem repeat (VNTR) locus. Nat Genet 12:309-311.

Castilla LH, Couch FJ, Erdos MR, Hoskins KF, Calzone K, Garber JE, Boyd J, Lubin MB, Deshano ML, Brody LC (1994): Mutations in the BRCA1 gene in families with early-onset breast and ovarian cancer. Nat Genet 8:387-391.

Charollais RH, Tiwari S, and Thomas NS (1994). Into and out of G1: the control of cell proliferation. Biochimie 76:887-894.

Claus EB, Thompson N, Risch N (1991): Genetic analysis of breast cancer and steroid hormone study. Am J Hum Genet 48:232-242.

Collins N, McManus R, Wooster R, Mangion J, Seal S, Lakhani SR, Ormiston W, Daly PA, Ford D, Easton DF (1995): Consistent loss of the wild type allele in breast cancers from a family linked to the BRCA2 gene on chromosome 13q12-13. Oncogene 10:1673-1675.

Coppes MJ, Campbell CE, Williams BRG (1993): The role of WT1 in Wilms tumorigenesis. FASEB J 7:886-895.

Couch FJ, Weber BL, and the Breast Cancer Information Core (1996): Mutations and Polymorphisms in the familial early onset breast cancer (BRCA1) gene. Human Mutation (In press).

Couch FJ, Farid LM, DeShano ML, Tavtigian SV, Calzone K, Campeau L, Peng Y, Bogden B, Chen Q, Neuhausen S, Shattuck-Eidens D, Godwin AK, Daly M, Radford DM, Sedlacek S, Rommens J, Simard J, Garber J, Merajver S, Weber BL (1996). BRCA2 germline mutations in male breast cancer cases and breast cancer families. Nat Genet 13:123-125.

Cox EC (1976): Bacterial mutator genes and the control of spontaneous mutation. Annu Rev Genet 10:135-156.

Duan DR, Pause A, Burgess WH, Aso T, Chen DY, Garrett KP, Conaway RC, Conaway JW, Linehan WM, Klausner RD (1995): Inhibition of transcription elongation by the VHL tumor suppressor protein. Science 269:1402-1406.

Easton DF, Bishop DT, Ford D, Crockford GP, Breast Cancer Linkage Consortium (1993): Genetic linkage analysis in familial breast and ovarian cancer: results from 214 families. Am J Hum Genet 52:678-701.

Easton DF, Ford D, Bishop DT, and the Breast cancer Linkage Consortium (1995): Breast and ovarian cancer incidence in BRCA1-mutation carriers. Am J Hum Genet 56:265-271.

El-Deiry WS, Tokino T, Velculescu VE, Levy DB, Parsons R, Trent JM, Lin D, Mercer WE, Kinzler KW, Vogelstein B (1993): WAF1, a potential mediator of p53 tumor suppression. Cell 75:817-825.

Fishel R, Lescoe MK, Rao MR, Copeland NG, Jenkins NA, Garber J, Kane M, Kolodner R (1994): The human mutator gene homolog MSH2 and its association with hereditary nonpolyposis colon cancer. Cell 75:1027-1038.

Ford D, Easton DF, Bishop DT, Narod SA, Goldgar DE (1994): Risks of cancer in BRCA1-mutation carriers. Breast Cancer Linkage Consortium. Lancet 343:692-695.

Friedman LS, Ostermeyer EA, Szabo CI, Dowd P, Lynch ED, Rowell SE, King MC (1994): Confirmation of BRCA1 by analysis of germline mutations linked to breast and ovarian cancer in ten families. Nat Genet 8:399-404.

Futreal PA, Soderkvist P, Marks JR, Iglehart JD, Cochran C, Barrett JC, Wiseman RW (1992): Detection of frequent allelic loss on proximal chromosome 17q in sporadic breast carcinoma using microsatellite length polymorphisms. Cancer Res 52:2624-2627.

Futreal PA, Liu Q, Shattuck-Eidens D, Cochran C, Harshman K, Tavtigian S, Bennett LM, Haugen-Strano A, Swensen J, Miki Y (1994): BRCA1 mutations in primary breast and ovarian carcinomas. Science 266:120-122.

Gayther SA, Warren W, Mazoyer S, Russell PA, Harrington PA, Chiano M, Sel S, Hamoudi R, van-Rensberg EJ, Dunning AM (1995): Germline mutations of the BRCA1 gene in breast and ovarian cancer families provide evidence for a genotype-phenotype correlation. Nat Genet 11:428-433.

Gayther SA, Harrington P, Russell P, Kharkevich G (1996): Rapid detection of regionally clustered germ-line BRCA1 mutations by multiplex heteroduplex analysis. Am J Hum Genet 58:451-456.

Gessler M, Konig A, Moore J, Qualman S, Arden K, Cavenee W, Bruns G (1993): homozygous inactivation of WT1 in Wilms tumor associated with the WAGR syndrome. Genes Chromosomes Cancer 7:131-136.

Goldmacher VS, Cuzick RA Jr, Thilly WG (1986): Isolation and partial characterization of human cedll mutants differing in sensitivity to killing and mutation by methylnitrosourea and N-methyl-N'-nitro-N-nitrosoguanidine. Biol Chem. 261:12462-12471.

Gowen LC, Johnson BL, Latour AM, Sulik KK, Koller BH (1996): BRCA1 deficiency results in early embryonic lethality characterized by neuroepithelial abnormalities. Nat Genet 12:191-194.

Greenblatt MS, Bennett WP, Hollstein M, and Harris CC. Mutations in the p53 tumor suppressor gene (1994):Clues to cancer etiology and molecular pathogenesis. Cancer Res 54:4855-4878.

Groden J, Thliveris A, Samowitz W, Carlson M, Gelbert L, Albertsen H, Joslyn G, Stevens J, Spirio L, Robertson M (1991): Identification and characterization of the familial adenomatous polyposis coli gene. Cell 66:589-600.

Hall JM, Lee MK, Newman B, Morrow JE, Anderson LA, Bing H, King MC (1990): Linkage of early-onset familial breast cancer to chromosome 17q21. Science 250:1684-1689.

Han HJ, Yanagisawa A, Kato Y, Park JG, Nakamura Y (1993): Genetic instability in pancreatic cancer and poorly differentiated type of gastric cancer. Cancer Res 53:5087.

Holt JT, Thompson ME, Szabo C, Robinson-Benion C, Arteaga CL, King MC, Jensen RA (1996): Growth retardation and tumor inhibition by BRCA1. Nat Genet 12:298-302.

Hogervorst FBL, Cornelis RS, Bout M, van Vliet M, Oosterwijk JC, Olmer R, Bakker B, Klijn JG, Vasen HF, Meijers Hf, Meijers-Heijboer H (1995):et al(1995). Rapid detection of BRCA1 mutations by the protein truncation test. Nat Genet 10:208-212.

Hosking L, Trowsdale J, Nicolai H, Solomon E, Foulkes W, Stamp G, Signer E, Jeffreys A (1995): A somatic BRCA1 mutation in an ovarian tumor. Nat Genet 9:343-344.

Hoskins KF, Stopfer MS, Calzone KA, Merajver SD, Rebbeck TR, Garber JE, Weber BL (1995): Assessment and counseling for women with a family history of Breast Cancer. JAMA 273:577-585.

Hunt K (1994): Breast cancer risk and hormone replacement therapy: a review of the epidemiology. Int J Fertil Menopausal Stud 39 Suppl 2:67-74.

Hussussian CJ, Struewing JP, Goldstein AM, Higgins PA, Ally DS, Sheahan MD, Clark WH Jr, Tucker MA, Dracopoli NC (1994): Germline p16 mutations in familial melanoma. Nat Genet 8:15-21.

Jacobs IJ, Smith SA, Wiseman RW, Futreal PA, Harrington T, Osborne RJ, Leech V, Molyneux A, Berchuck A, Ponder BA (1993): A deletion unit on chromosome 17q in epithelial ovarian tumors distal to the familial breast/ovarian cancer locus. Cancer Res 53:1218-1221.

Jacobs IJ and Lancaster JM (1996):The molecular genetics of sporadic and famiiial epithelial ovarian cancer. International Journal of Gynecological Cancer 6 (In Press)

Jensen RA, Thompson ME, Jetton TL, Szabo CL, van der Meer R, Helou B, Tronick SR, Page DL, King MC, Holt JT (1996): BRCA1 is secreted and exhibits properties of a granin. Nat Genet 12:303-308.

Kamb A, Gruis NA, Weaver-Feldhaus J, Liu Q, Harshman K, Tavtigian SV, Stockert E, Day RS 3rd, Johnson BE, Skolnick MH (1994): A cell cycle regulator potentially involved in genesis of many tumor types. Science 264:436-440.

Kastan MB, Zhan Q, el-Deiry WS, Carrier F, Jacks T, Walsh WV, Plunkett BS, Vogelstein B, Fornace AJ Jr (1992): A mammalian cell cycle checkpoint pathway utilizing p53 and GADD45 is defective in ataxia-telangiectasia. Cell 71:587-597.

Kat A, Thilly WG, Fang WH, Longley MJ, Li GM, Modrich P (1993): An alkylation-tolerant, mutator human cell line is deficient in strand-specific mismatch repair. Proc Natl Acad Sci USA 90:6424-6428.

Khoo SK, Chick P (1992): Sex steroid hormones and breast cancer: is there a link with oral contraceptives and hormone replacement therapy? Med J Aust 156:124-132.

Kinzler KW (1991): Identification of a gene located at chromosome 5q21 that is mutated in colorectal carcinomas. Science 251:1366-1370.

Knudson AG (1971): Mutation and cancer: A statistical study of retinoblastoma. Proc Natl Acad Sci USA. 68:820-823.

Knudson AG (1978): Retinoblastoma:a prototypic hereditary neoplasm. Semin Oncol 5:57-60.

Knudson AG (1985): Hereditary cancer, oncogenes, and antioncogenes. Cancer Res 45:1437-1443.

Kolodner RD (1995): Mismatch repair: mechanisms and relationship to cancer susceptibility. Trends Biochem Sci 20:397-401.

Kraemer BB, Silva EG, Sneige N (1984): Fibrosarcoma of ovary. A new compnent in the nevoid basal-cell carcinoma syndrome. Am J Surg Pathol 8:231-236.

Lancaster JM, Cochran C, Brownlee HA, Evans C (1996): Detection of BRCA1 mutations in women with early onset ovarian cancer using the protein truncation test. JNCI 8:552-554.

Lancaster JM, Wiseman RW and Berchuck A (1996): An inevitable dilemma: Prenatal Testing for Mutations in the BRCA1 Breast/Ovarian Cancer Susceptibility Gene. Obstet Gynecol 87:306-309.

Lancaster JM, Wooster R, Mangion J, Phelan CM (1996): BRCA2 Mutations in Primary Breast and Ovarian Cancer. Nat Genet (In Press).

Lancaster JM, C Cochran, A Futreal, A Berchuck and RW Wiseman. BRCA1 Mutation Detection: Sensitivity of Dideoxy Fingerprinting and Single Strand Conformation Analysis. Molecular Carcinogenesis (Submitted).

Latif F, Tory k, Gnarra J, Yao M, Duh FM, Orcutt ML, Stackhouse T, Kuzmin I, Modi W, Geil L (1993): Identification of the von Hippel-Lindau disease tumor suppressor gene. Science 260:1317-1320.

Leach FS, Nicolaides NC, Papadopolous N, Liu B, Jen J, Parsons R, Peltomaki P, Sistonen P, Aaltonen LA, Nystrom-Lahti M (1993): Mutational analysis of mutS homolog in hereditary nonpolyposis colorectal cancer. Cell 75:1215-1225.

Li FP, Fraumeni JF Jr (1969): Soft tissue sarcomas, breast cancer, and other neoplasms, a familial syndrome? Ann Int Med 71:747-751.

Loeb LA (1994): Microsatellite instability: marker of a mutator phenotype in cancer. Cancer Res 54:5059-5063.

Lowe SW, Schmitt EM, Smith SW, Osborne BA, Jacks T (1993): P53 is required for radiation induced apoptosis in mouse thymocytes. Nature 362:847-849.

Lynch HT, Bewtra C, Wells IC, Schuelke GS (1987): Hereditary ovarian cancer: clinical and biomarker studies. In Cancer Genetics in Women. Edited by Lynch HT, Kullander S. Boca Raton: CRC Press, Inc. 49-97.

Lynch HT, Lanspa S, Smyrk T, Boman B, Watson P, Lynch J (1991): Hereditary nonpolyposis colorectal cancer (Lynch Syndromes I & II): genetics, pathology, natural history and cancer control, part I. Cancer Genet Cytogenet 53:143-160.

Malkin D, Li FP, Strong LC, Fraumeni JF, Nelson CE, Kim DH, Kassel J, Gryca MA, Bischoff FZ, Tainsky MA, Friend SH (1990): Germline p53 mutations in a familial syndrome of breast cancer, sarcomas, and other neoplasms. Science 250:1233-1238.

McKeon VA (1994): Hormone replacement therapy: evaluating the risks and benefits. J Obstet Gynecol Neonatal Nurs 23:647-657.

Merajver SD, Pham TM, Caduff RF, Chen M, Poy EL, Cooney KA, Weber BL, Collins FS, Johnston C, Frank TS (1995): Somatic mutations in the BRCA1 gene in sporadic ovarian tumors. Nat Genet 9:439-443.

Merlo A, Herman JG, Mao L, Lee DJ, Gabrielson E, Burger PC, Baylin SB, Sidranksky D (1995): 5'CpG island methylation is associated with transcriptional silencing of the tumor suppressor p16/CDKN2/MTS1 in human cancers. Nature Medicine 1:686-692.

Meselson M (1988): In Recombination of Genetic Material, KB Low (ed). San Diego: Academic Press inc., pp 91-113.

Miki Y, Swensen J, Shattuck-Eidens D, Futreal PA, Harshman K, Tavtigian S, Liu Q, Cochran C, Bennett LM, Ding W, Bell R, Rosenthal J, Hussey C, Tran T, McClure M, Frye C, Hattier T, Phelps R, Haugen-Strano A, Katcher H, Yakumo K, Gholami Z, Shaffer D, Stone S, Bayer S, Wray C, Bogden R, Dayanath P, Ward J, Tonin P, Narod S, Bristow P, Norris F, Helvering L, Morrison P, Rosteck P, Lai M, Barrett JC, Lewis C, Neuhausen S, Cannon-Albright L, Goldgar D, Wiseman R, Kamb A, Skolnick MH (1994): A strong candidate for the breast and ovarian cancer susceptibility gene BRCA1. Science 266:66-71.

Modrich P (1994): Mismatch Repair, genetic stability and cancer. Science 226:1959-1960

Momand J, Zambetti GP, Olson DC, George D, Levine AJ (1992): The mdm2 oncogene product forms a complex with the p53 protein and inhibits p53-mediated transactivation. Cell 69:1237-1245.

Nakamura Y, Nishisho I, Kinzler, Vogelstein, Miyoshi Y, Miki Y, Ando H, Horii A (1992): Mutations of the APC (adenomatous polyposis coli) gene in FAP (familial polyposis coli) patients and in sporadic colorectal tumors. Tohoku J Exp Med 168:141-147.

Narod SA, Feunteun J, Lynch HT, Watson P, Conway T, Lynch J, Lenoir GM (1991): Familial breast-ovarian cancer locus on chromosome 17q12-q23. Lancet 338:82-83.

Nicolaides NC, Papadopoulos N, Liu B, Wei YF, Carter Kc, Ruben SM, Rosen CA, Haseltine WA, Fleischmann RD, Fraser CM (1994): Mutations of two PMS homologues in hereditary nonpolyposis colon cancer. Nature 371:75-80.

NIH Consensus Development Panel on Ovarian Cancer: Ovarian Cancer Screening, Treatment, and Follow-up (1995). JAMA 273:491-497.

O'Connell P, Cawthon R, Xu GF, Li Y, Viskochil D, White R (1992): The neurofibromatosis type 1 (NF1) gene: identification and partial characterization of a putative tumor suppressor gene. J Dermatol 19:881-884.

Orita M, Iwahana H, Kanazawa H, Hayashi K, Sekiya T (1989): Detection of polymorphisms of human DNA by gel electrophoresis as single-strand conformation polymorphisms. Proc Nat Acad Sci USA 86:2766-2770.

Papadopoulos N, Nicolaides NC, Liu B, Parsons R, Lengauer C, Palombo F, D'Arrigo A, Markowitz S, Willson JK, Kinzler KW (1995): Mutations of GTBP in genetically unstable cells.Science 268:1915-1917.

Parsons R, Li GM, Longley MJ, Fang WH, Papadopolous N, Jen J, de la Chapelle A, Kinzler KW, Vogelstein B, Modrich P (1993): Hypermutability and mismatch repair deficiency in RER+ tumor cells. Cell 75:1227-36.

Parsons R, Li GM, Longley M, Modrich P, Liu B, Berk T, Hamilton SR, Kinzler KW, Vogelstein B (1995): Mismatch repair deficiency in phenotypically normal human cells. Science 268:738-740.

Phelan CM, Lancaster JM, Tonin P, Gumbs C, Cochran C, Carter R, Ghadirian P, Perret C, Moslehi R, Dion F, Faucher MC, Dole K, Karimi S, Lounis H, Warner E, Goss P, Anderson D, Larsson C, Narod SA, Futreal PA (1996): Mutation analysis of the BRCA2 gene in 49 site-specific breast cancer families. Nat Genet 13:120-122.

Phelan CM, Rebbeck TR, Weber BL, Devilee P, Ruttledge MH, Lynch HT, Lenoir GM, Stratton MR, Easton DF, Ponder BA, Cannon-Albright L, Larsson C, Goldgar DE, Narod SA (1996): Ovarian cancer risk in BRCA1 carriers is modified by the HRAS1 variable number of tandem reeat (VNTR) locus. Nat Genet 12:309-311.

Qiang L and Somer SS (1994): Parameters affecting the sensitivity of dideoxy fingerprinting and SSCP. PCR Methods and Applications 4:97-108.

Ries LAG (1995): NCI Surveillance Epidemiology and End Results (SEER) Program.Ranking for top 5 cancers based on rates in 1992. In: JNCI 87:867.

Risinger, J. I., Barrett, J. C., Watson, P., Lynch, H. T. and Boyd, J. Molecular genetic evidence for the occurance of breast cancer as an integral tumor in the hereditary nonpolyposis colorectal cancer syndrome. (In Press, Cancer, 1996).

Sarkar G, Yoon HS, Sommer S (1992): Dideoxy Fingerprinting (ddF): A rapid and efficient screen for the presence of mutations. Genomics 13:441-443.

Schneider KA, Patenaude AF and Garber JE (1995): Testing for cancer genes: Decisions, decisions. Nature Medicine 1:302-303.

Serrano M, Hannon GJ, and Beach D (1993): A new regulatory motif in cell-cycle control causing specific inhibition of cyclin D/CDK4. Nature 366:704-707.

Shattuck-Eidens D, McClure M, Simard J, Labrie F, Narod S, Couch F, Hoskins K, Weber B, Castilla L, Erdos M (1995): A collaborative survey of 80 mutations in the BRCA1 breast and ovarian cancer susceptibility gene. JAMA 273:535-541. Simard J, Tonin P, Durocher F, Morgan K, Rommens J, Gingras S, Samson C, Leblanc JF, Belanger C, Dion F (1994): Common origins of BRCA1 mutations in Canadian breast and ovarian cancer families. Nat Genet 8:392-398.

Smith SA, Easton DF, Evans DGR, Ponder BA (1992): Allele losses in the region 17q12-21 in familial breast and ovarian cancer involve the wild-type chromosome. Nat Genet 2:128-131.

Smith DP, Eng C, Ponder BA (1994): Mutations of the RET proto-oncogene in the multiple endocrine neoplasia type 2 syndromes and Hirchsprung disease. J Cell Sci Suppl 18:43-49.

Spigelman AD, Murday V, Phillips RK (1989): Cancer and the Peutz-Jeghers syndrome. Gut 30:1588-1590.

Struewing JP, Brody LC, Erdos MR, Kase RG, Giambarresi TR, Smith SA, Collins FS, Tucker MA (1995): Detection of eight BRCA1 mutations in ten breast/ovarian cancer families, including one family with male breast cancer. Am J Hum Genet 57:1-7.

Su LK, Johnson KA, Smith KJ, Hill DE, Vogelstein B, Kinzler KW (1993): Association between wild type and mutant APC gene products. Cancer Res 53:2728-2731.

Takahashi H, Behbakht K, McGovern PE, Chui HC, Couch FJ, Weber BL, Friedman LS, King MC, Furusato M, LiVolsi VA (1995): Mutation Analysis of the BRCA1 Gene in Ovarian Cancers. Cancer Res 55:2998-3002.

Tavtigian SV, Simard J, Rommens J, Couch F, Shattuck-Eidens D, Neuhausen S, Merajver S, Thorlacius S, Offit K, Stoppa-Lyonnet D, Belanger C, Bell R, Berry S, Bogden R, Chen Q, Davis T, Dumont M, Frye C, Hattier T, Jammulapati S, Janecki T, Jiang P, Kehrer R, Leblanc JF, Goldgar DE. (1996): The complete BRCA2 gene and mutations inchromosome 13q-linked kindreds. Nat Genet 12: 333-337.

Thompson ME, Jensen RA, Obermiller PS, Page DL, Holt JT(1995): Decreased expression of BRCA1 accelerates growth and is often present during sporadic breast cancer progression. Nat Genet 9:444-450.

Thorlacius S, Olafsdottir G, Tryggvadottir L, Neuhausen S, Jonasson JG, Tavtigian SV, Tulinius H, Ogmundsdottir and Eyfjord JE. (1996): A single BRCA2 mutation in male and female breast cancer families from Iceland with varied cancer phenotypes. Nat Genet 13:117-119.

Ton CC, Huff V, Call KM, Cohn S, Strong LC, Housman DE, Saunders GF (1991): Smallest region of overlap in Wilms tumor deletions uniquely implicates an 11p13 zinc finger gene as the disease locus. Genomics 10:293-297.

Trofatter J, MacCollin MM, Rutter JL, Murrell JR, Duyao MP, Parry DM, Eldridge R, Kley N, Menon AG, Pulaski K (1993): A novel moesin-, ezrin-, radixin-like gene is a candidate for the nearofibromatosis 2 tumor suppressor. Cell 72:791-800.

Van Der Luijt R, Khan PM, Vasen H, van-Leeuwen C, Tops C, Roest P, den-Dunnen J, Fodde R (1994): Rapid detection of translation-terminating mutations at the adenomatous polyposis coli (APC) gene by direct protein truncation test. Genomics 20:1-4.

Umar A, Boyer JC, Thomas DC, Nguyen DC, Risinger JI, Boyd J, Ionov Y, Perucho M, Kunkel TA (1994): Defective mismatch repair in extracts of colorectal and endometrial cancer cell lines exhibiting microsatellite instabillity. J Biol Chem 269:14367-14370.

Varmus H and Weinberg RA (1993): Genes and the Biology of Cancer. New York: Scientific American Library.

Wooster R, Neuhausen SL, Mangion J, Quirk Y, Ford D, Colins N, Nguyen K, Seal S, Tran T, Averill D (1994): Localization of a breast cancer susceptibility gene, BRCA2, to chromosome 13q12-13. Science 265:2088-2090.

Wooster R, Bignell G, Lancaster J, Swift S, Seal S, Mangion J, Collins N, Gregory S, Gumbs C, Micklem G, Barfoot R, Hamoudi R, Patel S, Rice C, Biggs P, Hashim Y, Smith A, Connor F, Arason A, Gudmundson J, Ficenec D, Kelsell D, Ford D, Tonin P, Bishop DT, Spurr NK, Ponder BAJ, Eeles R, Peto J, Devilee P, Cornelisse, C, Lynch H, Narod S, Lenoir G, Egilsson V, Barkadottir RB, Easton DF, Bentley DR, Futreal PA, Ashworth A, Stratton MR (1995): Identification of the breast cancer susceptibility gene BRCA2. Nature 378:789-92.

Zuppan P, Hall JM, Lee MK, Ponglikitmongkol M, King MC (1991): Possible linkage of the estrogen receptor gene to breast cancer in a family with late-onset disease. Am J Hum Gen 48:1065-1068.

Etiology of Breast and
Gynecological Cancers, pages 53–61
© 1997 Wiley-Liss, Inc.

DEFINING ETIOLOGIC HETEROGENEITY IN BREAST CANCER USING GENETIC BIOMARKERS

Timothy R. Rebbeck, Amy H. Walker, Catherine M. Phelan, Andrew
K. Godwin, Kenneth H. Buetow, Judy E. Garber, Steven A. Narod,
Barbara L. Weber

Departments of Biostatistics and Epidemiology (TRR, AHW), Medi-
cine and Genetics (BLW), University of Pennsylvania School of
Medicine, Philadelphia, PA 19104; Department of Medical Genet-
ics, Montreal General Hospital, Montreal, Quebec H3G 1A4 (CMP);
Fox Chase Cancer Center, Philadelphia, PA 19111 (AKG, KHB);
Dana-Farber Cancer Institute, Boston, MA 02115 (JEG); Women's
College Hospital, Toronto, Ontario M5G 1N9 (SAN).

INTRODUCTION

Most breast cancer cannot be explained by a single gene or a single environmental
exposure. Instead, breast cancer may result from the interactions of multiple genetic
and environmental factors over time. This complex, multifactorial etiology implies
that there will be etiologic heterogeneity among breast cancer cases in the general
population. The ability to identify etiologically heterogeneous breast cancer cases
may aid the search for genetic and environmental factors involved in breast cancer
etiology. This may in turn have implications for optimizing breast cancer prevention,
detection, and treatment strategies.

We consider two classes of biomarkers that may be involved in breast cancer
etiology and may define heterogeneous groups of breast cancer cases in the general
population: biomarkers of genetic susceptibility and biomarkers of genetic effect
(National Research Council, 1987, Schulte and Perera, 1993). Biomarkers of genetic
susceptibility are defined here as those that regulate an individual's ability to
metabolize environmental carcinogens or steroid hormones. Biomarkers of genetic
effect are defined here as somatic genetic damage that may be the result of exposure
to environmental agents. Examples of this latter class of biomarker are sister
chromatid exchange, DNA adducts, and loss of constitutional heterozygosity (LOH).
We present a biological motivation for pursuing these biomarkers in studies to identify
etiologic heterogeneity in breast cancer, and provide two examples that illustrate
these concepts.

Genetic Biomarkers of Breast Carcinogenesis

Allelic variability in genes that regulate the metabolism of environmental
carcinogens (i.e., biomarkers of genetic susceptibility) may determine the rate at
which somatic mutations occur in tumor suppressor genes in response to environmental exposures. Likely candidates for this class of genes include those that regulate the

phase I monooxygenation and phase II conjugation of potentially carcinogenic compounds. Figure 1 illustrates how these genes may act to predispose an individual to develop breast cancer in response to carcinogenic environmental exposures.

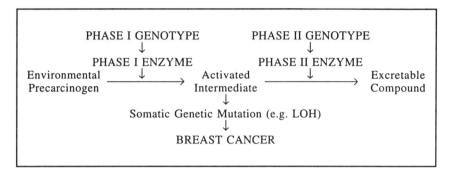

Figure 1: Phase I and II Metabolism

In phase I metabolism of environmental carcinogens, substrates are processed into biologically active forms by the phase I monooxygenation enzymes. These enzymes, primarily members of the cytochrome P450 family, convert numerous environmental substrates to a reactive (monooxygenated) form. The substrates for phase I enzymes include carcinogenic compounds found in the diet or workplace (Nebert and Gonzalez, 1987). The phase I enzymes also metabolize steroid hormones (Metzler and McLachlan, 1978). The hypothesis implied by this model is that a genotype associated with increased phase I enzyme activity increases breast cancer risk or may modify age of breast cancer onset.

In phase II metabolism, activated carcinogenic intermediates are detoxified to more hydrophilic forms by the phase II conjugation enzymes. The substrates for the phase II enzymes include carcinogenic compounds that have been activated by the phase I enzymes. The hypothesis implied by this model is that a genotype associated with decreased phase II enzyme activity increases breast cancer risk or may modify age of breast cancer onset.

As indicated in Figure 1, genetic control of interindividual variability in the phase I and II enzymes may result in an increased accumulation of somatic mutation at these tumor suppressor or oncogene loci with accumulating environmental exposures over time. Substantial interindividual heterogeneity in LOH has been reported that could be explained in part by exposure to environmental carcinogens and their metabolism (Sato et al. 1990, Rebbeck, et al., 1994a). This observation is consistent with the multistage model of carcinogenesis (Knudson, 1971): the phase I and II enzymes could affect the rate at which individuals who inherited a "first hit" at a tumor suppressor gene would somatically acquire the "second hit" required for tumorigenesis. Breast cancer etiology may therefore be explained by inherited predisposition to develop a tumor, inherited predisposition to accumulate somatic mutation, and exogenous exposures. This model also implies that not all breast cancer will be caused by the same set of etiologic agents. Therefore, etiologic heterogeneity may exist in the general population: different combinations of etiologic agents may produce breast cancer in different population subgroups.

Significance of Genetic Biomarkers in the General Population

The genes involved in breast cancer etiology may be classified according to their allele frequencies and the size of effects of these alleles on cancer risk. This information can then be used to estimate the proportion of breast cancer in the general population that may be attributable to specific candidate genotypes. First, there may be a few genes with allelic variants that have large effects on an individual's breast cancer risk. In general, these allelic variants are expected to be relatively rare in the general population. However, the risk of developing breast cancer is high for those individuals who carry these alleles. These genes will be denoted here as "major" genes based on the size of their effect on an individual's cancer risk. An example of this class of genes is the hereditary breast and ovarian cancer susceptibility gene *BRCA1*. Second, there may be a large number of genes with relatively common allele frequencies, each of which confers a small to moderate cancer risk. These genes will be denoted here as "polygenes" based on their allele frequencies and smaller size of effects on an individual's cancer risk. Both major genes and polygenes may play an important role in breast cancer etiology. From a population perspective, "polygenes" may explain a larger proportion of breast cancer in the general population than "major" genes. Using published rare allele frequencies and relative risk estimates, a hypothetical calculation of population cancer risk attributable to a "major" gene (the breast cancer susceptibility gene *BRCA1*) and a "polygene" (glutathione-S-transferase-, denoted here as *GSTM1*) is presented in Table 1.

Table 1: Attributable Risk

GENE	RARE ALLELE FREQUENCY	POPULATION SIZE OF EFFECTS	ATTRIBUTABLE RISK
BRCA1	.005	RR=8.5	3.6%
GSTM1	.50	RR=1.5	20.0%

Table 1 indicates that the size of effects (here, relative risk) on individual breast cancer risk is large for *BRCA1*, but mutations at this locus are rare. Thus the proportion of breast cancer explained by a gene such as *BRCA1* may be small in the general population. In contrast, the size of effects of a carcinogen metabolizing gene such as *GSTM1* is relatively small, but these mutations are common. A relatively large proportion of breast cancer in the general population may be attributed to genes such as *GSTM1* compared with *BRCA1*. Therefore, studies of the genetic etiology of breast cancer may need to consider both "major" genes as well as "polygenes" to explain the etiology of breast cancer in the general population.

EXAMPLES

The following two examples illustrate the ability to define etiologic heterogeneity in a sample of breast cancer cases by using genetic biomarkers. A case series design (Begg and Zhang, 1994) was employed in each example. The first study (Rebbeck, et al., 1995) describes etiologic heterogeneity defined by family history, age at diagnosis, and candidate susceptibility genotypes. The second study (Rebbeck, et al., 1996) describes etiologic heterogeneity defined by somatic genetic mutation and candidate susceptibility genotypes. In both studies, there was evidence for etiologic heterogeneity when phenotypes (age at diagnosis, LOH) were stratified by candidate genotypes.

Example 1: Heterogeneity in Age at First Breast Cancer Diagnosis

Hereditary breast cancer is hallmarked by multiple early onset, multifocal breast tumors. However, the penetrance of breast cancer is not uniform across all high-risk women in these families. We examined whether glutathione-S-transferase µ (*GSTM1*) or θ (*GSTT1*) genotypes influence the penetrance of breast cancer. Deletion polymorphisms exist in *GSTM1* and *GSTT1* that may hinder the metabolic detoxification of some environmental carcinogens (Fryer, et al., 1993, Pemble, et al. 1994). We hypothesize that women who carry deletions (*del*) in *GSTM1* or *GSTT1* may be more susceptible to the effects of environmental carcinogens than women who carry wild-type (*wt*) alleles, and may therefore manifest breast cancer at an earlier age.

To address this hypothesis, we studied 151 breast cancer cases with a positive family history of breast cancer ascertained through hereditary breast cancer clinics (Rebbeck, et al., 1995). Age at first breast cancer diagnosis was obtained on all study subjects. Approximately 40% of subjects were diagnosed before age 40, with a mean age at diagnosis of 46.8 years. PCR-based assays were used to identify deletion carriers at *GSTM1* and *GSTT1* using published protocols (Fryer, et al. 1993, Pemble, et al., 1994). Approximately half (50.3%) of study subjects carried homozygous deletions at *GSTM1*, and 19.2% carried homozygous deletion mutations at *GSTT1*.

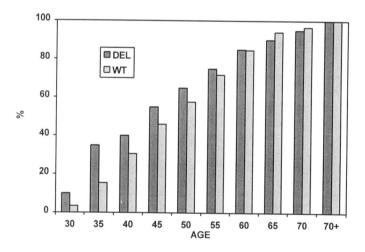

Figure 2: Cumulative Age of First Breast Cancer Diagnosis, Stratified by *GSTT1* Genotype

Kaplan-Meier survival models were fitted using this distribution to compare age at breast cancer diagnosis across *GSTT1* and *GSTM1* genotypes. The mean age at diagnosis was significantly earlier in *GSTT1-del* carriers (42.6 yrs) than in *GSTT1-wt* carriers (47.2 yrs; χ^2 = 4.41, df=1, p=0.035). When stratified by age at first breast cancer diagnosis, the effect of *GSTT1* was not significant in women diagnosed after age 40 (χ^2 = 0.37, df=1, p=0.848). In women diagnosed before age 40, the mean age at diagnosis was significantly earlier in *GSTT1-del* carriers (31.3 yrs) than in *GSTT1-wt* carriers (34.6 yrs; χ^2= 8.58, df=1, p=0.003). This represented a 22% difference across the observed age range (25-40 yrs) by *GSTT1* genotype. The cumulative distribution of age at first breast cancer diagnosis is presented in Figure 2. No associations with age at diagnosis were observed with *GSTM1* genotypes alone, nor were significant interactions of *GSTM1* and *GSTT1* observed. These findings may define heterogeneity in the age at first breast cancer diagnosis based on *GSTT1* genotype in women from hereditary breast cancer families.

Example 2: Biomarkers of Genetic Susceptibility and Effect

The model presented in Figure 1 suggests that rates of somatic genetic mutation may be influenced by the ability to metabolize environmental carcinogens by way of the phase I and II metabolism pathways. To address this hypothesis, twenty eight patients diagnosed as having primary ductal carcinomas of the breast were ascertained at the Fox Chase Cancer Center (FCCC) in 1993 (Rebbeck, et al., 1994b). These women were ascertained without respect to family history, tumor stage or grade, or age at diagnosis. Women who were surgically treated for breast cancer were ascertained through FCCC medical records. Women were asked to participate in this study at the time of their follow-up clinic visit. If they agreed, normal and tumor tissue samples were obtained and genomic DNA prepared. Tumor histopathological classifications were determined according to the typing scheme of the World Health Organization.

All genotype data were generated by polymerase chain reaction (PCR) techniques. Highly polymorphic tetranucleotide repeat markers generated by the Cooperative Human Linkage Center (CHLC) were used to measure LOH on 33 chromosome arms. Markers were selected in two ways. First, markers were selected that were located in regions in which elevated proportions of LOH have been previously reported in breast tumors. In those regions in which no elevated LOH has been reported, the most telomeric CHLC marker available on that chromosomal arm was chosen. The candidate susceptibility genotypes studied here were generated by PCR-based assays at *CYP1A1* (Rebbeck, et al., 1994b), *CYP2D6* (Gough, et al., 1990), *EH* (Rosvold, et al., 1995), *NQO1* (Traveler, et al., 1992), and *GSTM1* (Comstock, et al., 1990).

Proportion of LOH was defined as the observed number of tumors that had lost heterozygosity at a particular locus divided by the number of matched (normal) tissue samples with heterozygous constitutional genotypes at that locus. Individuals with homozygous or unknown constitutional genotypes at a particular locus were not counted in this denominator. Analyses of variance were used to evaluate the relationship between the proportion of LOH in an individual and discrete variables such as hormone receptor status.

Figure 3 summarizes the variability in LOH among individuals. The proportion of LOH ranged from 0-67%. Twenty-two tumors were observed to have LOH at less than 20% of all loci studied. Six tumors were observed to have LOH at greater than

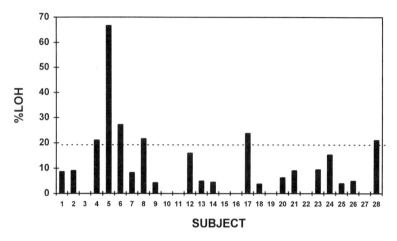

Figure 3: Inter-Individual Variability in LOH

20% of all loci studied. The number of positive lymph nodes on biopsy was not positively correlated with proportion of LOH (rank correlation = -.495, Cochran-Mantel-Haenszel statistic = 2.813, df=1, p = .144). The proportion of LOH in estrogen receptor (ER) positive tumors was half that in ER negative tumors (7.6% LOH in ER positive tumors, n=17 vs. 14.5% in ER negative tumors, n=10). However, this was not a statistically significant difference ($F_{1,27}$ = 1.55, p = .225). There was no observed difference in progesterone receptor (PR) positive vs. PR negative tumors (10.0% LOH in PR positive tumors (n=13) vs. 11.1% in PR negative tumors (n=13), $F_{1,26}$ = .03, df=1, p = .856).

The relationship between the proportion of LOH and genotypes at *CYP1A1*, *CYP2D6, EH, GSTM1*, and *NQO1* is presented in Figure 4. There was a twofold difference in the proportion of LOH for genotypes at *CYP2D6* (16.8% for 1/- genotypes vs. 7.6% for 2/2 genotypes), *GSTM1* (14.5% for "null" genotypes vs. 6.8% for wild type genotypes), and *NQO1* (13.4% for 2/- genotypes vs. 5.8% for 1/1 genotypes). These comparisons achieved p-values suggestive of genotypic effects on LOH in the range of 0.11 to 0.16. No elevated proportion of LOH was observed for genotypes at *CYP1A1* (11.9% for 1/2 genotypes vs. 10.2% for 1/1 genotypes) or *EH* (10.5% for 1/1 genotypes vs. 10.2% for 1/2 genotypes). These results provide preliminary evidence for etiological heterogeneity in somatic mutation across candidate susceptibility genotypes.

SUMMARY

Most breast cancer has a complex, multifactorial etiology. One consequence of this multifactorial phenomenon is that etiological heterogeneity may exist. This heterogeneity implies simply that two or more groups of breast cancer cases in the general population may have been caused by different sets of events. The ability to define etiologically heterogeneous subgroups in the population may facilitate a number of research and clinical issues. Studying etiologically homogeneous sub-

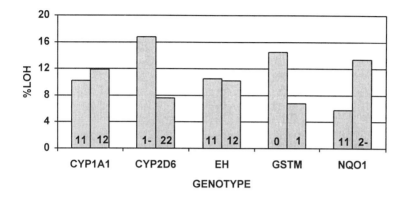

Figure 4: Inter-Individual Variability in LOH across Candidate Genotypes

groups in the general population may improve the ability to identify etiologic agents. Identification of a homogeneous group of breast cancer cases may also aid breast cancer diagnosis or treatment, and may allow a more effectively application of cancer prevention and control strategies.

Defining etiologic heterogeneity in the general population is one initial step in the process of understanding cancer etiology. Using knowledge such as that provided in the two examples presented here, formal case-control or cohort studies can be undertaken to examine whether the factors that define etiologic heterogeneity are involved in etiology. Furthermore, the results of studies of etiologic heterogeneity can point toward potential gene-gene or gene-environment interactions. The type of studies presented here can therefore serve a useful role in leading to more formal molecular epidemiological analyses.

ACKNOWLEDGMENTS

This research was supported by grants from the Public Health Service (CA60798 and ES08031 to TRR, CA67403 to FJC, CA57601 and CA61231 to BLW, and CA60643 to AKG) and a grant from the University of Pennsylvania Cancer Center.

REFERENCES

Begg CB, Zhang Z-F (1994): Statistical analysis of molecular epidemiology studies employing case-series. Cancer Epid. Biom. Prev. 3:173-175.

Board PG, Coggan M, Johnson P, Ross V, Suzuki T, Webb G (1990): Genetic heterogeneity of the human glutathione transferases: a complex of gene families. Pharmac Ther, 48:357-69.

Comstock KE, Sanderson BJ, Claglin G and Henner WD GST1 gene deletion determined by polymerase chain reaction (1990): Nucleic Acids Res 18:3670.

Daniel WW (1990): "Applied Nonparametric Statistics", 2nd Edition. Boston: PWS-KENT Publishing Co.

Fryer AA, Zhao L, Alldersea J, Pearson WR, Strange RC (1993): Use of site-directed mutagenesis of allele-specific PCR primers to identify the GSTM1 A, GSTM1 A,B and GSTM1 null polymorphisms at the glutathione-S-transferase, GSTM1 locus. Biochem. J. 295: 313-315.

Gough AC, Miles JS, Spurr NK, Moss JI, Gaedigk A, Eichelbaum M, Wolf CR (1990): Identification of the primary gene defect at the cytochrome P450 CYP2D locus. Nature. 347: 773-6.

Knudson AG (1971): Mutation and Cancer: Statistical study of retinoblastoma. Proc Nat Acad Sci USA 69(4):820-3.

Metzler M, McLachlan JA (1978): Oxidative metabolism of diethylstilbestrol and steroidal estrogens as a potential factor in their fetotoxicity. In: "Role of Pharmacokinetics in Prenatal and Perinatal Pharmacology". Neubert D, Merker HJ, Nau H, J Langman, eds, Stuttgart Georg Thieme, pp. 157-63.

Miki Y, Swensen J, Shattuck-Eidens S, Futreal A, et al. (1994): A strong candidate gene for the breast and ovarian cancer susceptibility gene BRCA1. Science 266:66-71.

National Research Council (1987): Biological markers in environmental health research. Envir Health Perspect 74:1-191.

Nebert DW, Gonzalez FJ (1987): P450 genes: structure evolution and regulation. Ann Rev Biochem, 56:945-93.

Omenn GS (1991): Future research in cancer ecogenetics. Mut Res, 247:291-3.

Pemble S, Schroeder KR, Spencer SR, Meyer DJ, Hallier E, Bolt HM, Ketterer B, Taylor JB (1994): Biochem J 300:271-276.

Rebbeck TR, Godwin A, Rosvold EA, McGlynn KA, Lustbader ED, Buetow KH (1994a) Inter- and intra-individual variability in somatic allele loss in ductal carcinoma of the breast, Am J Hum Genet, 55(3):A68.

Rebbeck TR, Rosvold EA, Duggan DJ, Zhang J, Buetow KH (1994b): Genetics of CYP1A1: Coamplification of Specific Alleles by Polymerase Chain Reaction and Association with Breast Cancer. Cancer Epid Biom Prev 3: 511-514.

Rebbeck TR, Walker AH, Hoskins K, Phelan C, Narod SA, Garber JE, Weber BL (1995) Modification of Familial Breast Cancer Penetrance by Glutathione-S-Transferase Genotypes. *American Journal of Human Genetics,* 57(4):A4.

Rosvold EA, McGlynn KA, Lustbader ED, Buetow KH (1995): Identification of an NAD(P)H: Quinone oxidoreductase polymorphism and its association with lung cancer and smoking. Pharmacogenet 5(4):199-206..

Schulte, PA, Perera FP (1993): "Molecular Epidemiology: Principles and Practices". San Diego: Academic Press.

Sato T, Tanigami A, Yamakawa K, Akiyama F, Kasumi F, Sakamoto G, Nakamura Y (1990): Allelotype of breast cancer: Cumulative allele losses promote tumor progression in primary breast cancer. Cancer Res 50:7184-7189.

Traveler RD, Tetsuro H, Danenberg KD, Stadlbauer THW, Danenberg PV, Ross D, and Gibson NW (1992): NAD(P)H:quinone oxidoreductase gene expression in human colon carcinoma cells: characterization of a mutation which modulates DT-Diaphorase activity and mitomycin sensitivity. Cancer Res 52:797-802.

Etiology of Breast and
Gynecological Cancers, pages 63–82
© 1997 Wiley-Liss, Inc.

THE GENETICS OF SPORADIC BREAST CANCER

Andrew J. Brenner and C. Marcelo Aldaz

Department of Carcinogenesis, University of Texas M.D. Anderson Cancer
Center, Science Park-Research Division, Smithville, Texas 78957

INTRODUCTION

Breast cancer which affects as many as one in eight women, is the most common
malignancy of women in the industrialized countries of the Western hemisphere (Feuer,
1993; Boring, 1994). To expedite the development of new treatment strategies, increased
emphasis has been placed on understanding the cellular and molecular events that lead to
malignancies of the breast. Over the past few years, numerous advances have been made in
the elucidation and characterization of genes whose mutation predisposes individuals to
risk of developing familial breast cancer. These genes include the recently cloned *BRCA1*
and *BRCA2* (Miki et al., 1994; Wooster et al., 1995). However, while these genes have been
shown to be frequently affected in inheritable forms of breast cancer, there is yet no conclusive
evidence to suggest that these genes are also responsible for sporadic breast cancer which
accounts for approximately 90% of breast cancer cases. To provide insight into the aberrations
responsible for the genesis of sporadic breast cancer, ongoing work is attempting to identify
genomic regions frequently affected. In this chapter, we will focus on the known somatic
genetic aberrations of sporadic breast cancer.

CYTOGENETICS OF BREAST CANCER

Numerous attempts have been made toward characterization of aberrations at the
chromosomal level in breast cancer. However, as is the case with other solid tumors of
epithelial origin, it has been difficult to discern any characteristic primary cytogenetic changes
among the large number of apparently random alterations. This is due to the inherent
difficulties in obtaining high-quality metaphases from solid tumors as well as their
characteristic clonal heterogeneity. In addition, of the tumors that have been karyotyped,
the vast majority are of the more advanced invasive stages, since the less advanced "in situ"
carcinomas tend to be much smaller, thereby making it even more difficult to obtain high-
quality metaphase cells. Nevertheless, several genetic changes with a relatively higher
prevalence have been identified. Overall, the most frequent tend to be numerical alterations

of whole chromosome copy number including trisomies of 7 and 18 and monosomies of 6, 8, 11, 13, 16, 17, 22, and X (reviewed by Devilee and Cornelisse, 1994). The most common aberrations in near-diploid tumors without metastases are loss of chromosomes 17 and 19, trisomy of chromosome 7, and overrepresentation of 1q, 3q, and 6p (Thompson et al., 1993). Structural alterations include terminal deletions and unbalanced nonreciprocal translocations, most frequently involving chromosomes 1, 6, and 16q. Breakpoints of structural abnormalities cluster to several segments, including 1p22-q11, 3p11, 6p11-13, 7p11-q11, 8p11-q11, 16q, and 19q13 (Thompson et al., 1993). Tumors from patients with metastatic breast carcinoma display a different pattern of abnormalities with structural alterations and numerous numerical alterations affecting various chromosomes (Trent et al., 1993).

A recently developed technique, comparative genomic hybridization (CGH), allows analyses of chromosome copy number abnormalities involving segments of at least 10 Mb (Kallioniemi et al., 1992A). Since CGH involves hybridizing differentially labeled genomic DNA from a tumor and a normal cell population to the same normal metaphase, it circumvents some of the difficulties encountered in conventional karyotyping. Through such analyses, nearly every tumor analyzed revealed increased or decreased DNA sequence copy number (Kallioniemi et al., 1994). The most common regions of increased copy number in breast cancer as determined by CGH include 1q, 8q, 17q22-24, and 20q13. Increased copy number at 17q was previously determined through gene fluorescence *in situ* hybridization (FISH) analysis to be 50 to 100-fold amplification of *ERBB2* (Kallioniemi et al., 1992B), a gene known to be overexpressed and amplified in a considerable percentage of breast cancers. Amplifications at region 8q would analogously be *MYC*, another gene known to be overexpressed in some breast cancers (Shiu, Watson, and Dubik, 1993). No candidate gene has yet been identified for region 20q13 amplification. Regions of decreased DNA copy number were also observed and include 3p, 6q, 8p, 11p, 12q, 13q, and 17p (Gray et al., 1994). For some of these regional losses, candidate genes exist that may be the target of deletion in the progression to a malignant phenotype (Table 1). More specifically, both *RB1* (13q) and *TP53* (17p) have been shown extensively to undergo deletion in a significant fraction of breast cancers (Cox, Chen, and Lee, 1994). Interestingly, when both loss and gain of DNA copy number as determined by CGH were compared with survival data in a series of node negative breast tumors, only copy number losses were significant for recurrence and for overall survival (Isola et al., 1995). However, as is the case with conventional cytogenetics, CGH has yet to reveal any characteristic abnormalities that occur in the majority of breast tumors and which abnormalities if any, could be considered "primary".

ONCOGENES

The proto-oncogenes encode proteins involved in a cascade of events leading to growth in response to mitogenic factors. Alteration in the normal function of proto-oncogenes, through mutation or increased expression can result in a constant growth stimulus and a constitutive mitogenic response. Aberration of a single allele of an ocogene can be sufficient to lead to altered signal and as such is dominant. In human solid tumors, the most common aberration affecting oncogenes appears to be gene amplification.

Genetic Region	Cytogenetic[1] Finding	CGH[2] Finding	Invasive[3] LOH (%)	DCIS[3] LOH (%)	Possible Targets
1p	-1p		32	8	
1q	+1q	+1q	30	16	
3p		-3p	22	0	
3q			25	0	
4p	-4p		2[1]	0[†]	
5p			18[1]	0[†]	
5q			13[1]	0[†]	
6p	-6	+6p	30	0	
6q	-6, -6q	-6q, +6q	26	8	
7p	+7	+7p	32	32	
7q	+7		25	24	
8p	-8, -8p	-8p	18	10	
8q	-8, +8q	+8q	20	22	*MYC*
9p	-9p		58	30	$p16^{INK4a}$
9q			24[1]	0[†]	
10p			11[1]	0[†]	
10q			15[1]	0[†]	
11p	-11, -11p	-11p	28	0	
11q	-11, -11q	+11q	30	12	*CCND1*
12p			8[1]	0[†]	
12q		+12q	4[1]	0[†]	
13q	-13	-13q	30	18	*RB1, BRCA2, Brush*
16p	-16		40	0	
16q	-16, -16q		48	27	*CDH1?*
17p	-17, -17p	-17p	57	33	*TP53*
17q	-17	+17q	36	31	*BRCA1,NME1 ERBB2*
18p			25	0	
18q			48	12	
19p			18[1]	0[†]	
19q		+19q	14[1]	0[†]	
20q		+20q13	17[1]	6[†]	
21q			17[1]	5[†]	
22q	-22		36	0	
Xp	-X		22[1]		
Xq	-X		8[1]		

Table 1. Summary of genetic abberrations affecting sporadic breast cancer ([1] Devilee and Cornelisse [1994], Thompson et. al. [1993]; [2] Gray et. al. [1994]; [3] Aldaz et. al. [1995]; [†] Radford et. al. [1995]).

Current data suggests of the numerous oncogenes described to date, that only a few may have a role in breast tumorigenesis. Of these, *ERBB2* remains the oncogene most studied in breast cancer. Also known as *HER2* or neu, *ERBB2* encodes a tyrosine kinase growth factor receptor with high homology to epidermal growth factor receptor (43% in the extracellular domain and 82% in the tyrosine kinase domain; Coussens et al., 1985; Jardines et al., 1993). However, while these two receptors share homology, their ligand specificity is distinct since neither epidermal growth factor nor transforming growth factor-α bind *ERBB2*. Activation or overexpression of *ERBB2* in transgenic mice results in the genesis of mammary tumors (Brouchard et al., 1989; Muller et al., 1988). As mentioned previously, FISH analysis has shown that *ERBB2* is amplified. Prior analysis by other means had shown amplification of *ERBB2* in 25-30% of breast cancers with concomitant overexpression, implicating its involvement in breast tumorigenesis (Berger et al., 1988; Zhou et al., 1987). Early studies reported a prognostic value of *ERBB2* overexpression in node-negative breast cancer. However, more recent studies using larger data sets do not support these early observations and question the prognostic role for *ERBB2* expression in node-positive breast cancer. Expression of *ERBB2* may have value in predicting response to specific therapies, but additional studies are needed to confirm these preliminary findings (reviewed by Ravdin and Chamness, 1995).

Similar to *ERBB2*, the *MYC* gene has been shown to be amplified in approximately 25% of breast carcinomas. Although the functions of *Myc* are not yet clearly understood, c-*Myc* has been shown to heterodimerize with Max (c-Myc-associated protein X), positively and negatively regulating the expression of various genes in apoptosis and cell cycle progression (Ryan and Birnie, 1996). Overexpression of *c-Myc* in transgenic mice results in mammary tumors (Muller et al., 1988), and amplification of *c-Myc* has been associated with high grade tumors in humans (Varley et al., 1987). However, when lymph node metastases from patients whose primary tumor showed amplification are examined, the metastatic cells do not show amplification, suggesting that amplification occurs before invasion and is not a prerequisite for a metastatic phenotype (Shiu et al., 1993). Of additional interest, *c-Myc* expression is modulated by the presence of estrogen in estrogen-responsive cell lines, and constitutively high *c-Myc* expression is observed in hormone-dependent lines, probably because of increased stability of the transcript (Shiu et al., 1993).

Chromosome region 11q13 has also been reported to be amplified in 15-20% of breast cancers (Lammie and Peters, 1991). The cyclin D1 (*CCND1*) gene, located in the region, is thought to be the target of such amplification. Cyclin D1 is a direct regulator of the cell cycle and is overexpressed in 45% of breast carcinomas, most of which are both estrogen and progesterone receptor positive (Gillet et al., 1994; Bartkova et al., 1994). Studies show that transgenic mice homozygously null for *CCND1* fail to undergo proliferative changes of the mammary epithelium associated with pregnancy, thereby indicating a role for *CCND1* in steroid-induced proliferation of the mammary epithelium (Sicinski et al., 1995). Transgenic mice overexpressing *CCND1* have been shown to develop mammary carcinomas (Wang et al., 1994). Analysis of *CCND1* expression by mRNA *in situ* hybridization has shown a dramatic increase of *CCND1* expression in 76% of low grade carcinoma *in situ*, further suggesting a role for *CCND1* in the tumorigenesis of the breast (Weinstat-Saslow et al., 1995).

TUMOR SUPPRESSORS AND LOSS OF HETEROZYGOSITY

Although the first tumor suppressor gene, *RB1*, was not identified until 1987, the existence of a genetic element with growth suppressive properties had been shown nearly two decades earlier. When Harris et al. fused normal mouse fibroblasts with highly malignant tumor cells, the resultant hybrids lost all tumorigenic capacity (Harris et al, 1969). Further, passage *in vitro* resulted in segregants that reverted to malignant phenotype upon loss of chromosomes (Harris et al., 1969; Klein et al., 1971). Two years later, Knudson, on the basis of statistical analysis of clinical observations, was the first to suggest retinoblastoma was a cancer caused by two mutational events (Knudson, 1971). In the hereditary form, one mutation was germinal; thus only a single additional somatic mutation was required. This results in early onset and a tendency toward bilateral tumorigenesis. In the sporadic form, both mutations are somatic, resulting in a tendency toward unilaterally and late onset. Comings later suggested that these two mutational events could occur within separate alleles of a regulatory gene (Comings, 1973). Indeed, cytogenetic analysis of retinoblastoma revealed characteristic deletions of the long arm of chromosome 13. Subsequent analysis of this region led to the identification of *RB1* and elucidation of aberrant transcripts encoded from the remaining allele (reviewed by Goodrich and Lee, 1993). Hence, a precedent emerged where inactivation of one allele of a tumor suppressor is accomplished by mutation, leading to the eventual deletion of the remaining normal allele through chromosomal aberrations and loss of heterozygosity (LOH) is thereby observed in the suppressor locus. This precedent is now considered the convention for suppressor inactivation and similar observations have been made for several other suppressive genes (e.g., *APC, DCC, VHL, TP53*; reviewed by Cox, Chen, and Lee, 1994). Further, LOH is considered indirect evidence for the existence of a suppressor gene within the affected region.

Allelotype of Breast Cancer

Because the mechanisms by which loss of heterozygosity occurs tend to involve large segments of DNA, it is possible to utilize the neighboring genes or known noncoding sequences as indicators to identify deleted regions harboring putative suppressor genes whose loss may be important in the genesis of the tumor. One such genetic marker is naturally occurring simple sequence length polymorphisms (SSLPs). SSLPs consist mainly of dinucleotide repeats, primarily $(CA)_n$, which are repeated in tandem at variable number (n) interspersed throughout the genome. To date, more than 5,000 such SSLPs with length polymorphisms of approximately 10-60 repeats, termed polymorphic microsatellites, have been identified (Dib et al., 1996; Litt and Luty, 1989). These polymorphic microsatellites have a mean heterozygosity of 70% at an average interval size of 1.6 cM. Through known linkage maps and comparison to physical maps, it is possible to select highly polymorphic microsatellites at any position within the genome. Further, through PCR amplification of these microsatellites and comparison with normal DNA from the same patient, it is possible to generate a comprehensive map of allelic imbalances (allelotype) occurring in a neoplasm (Weber and May, 1989).

Allelotyping of breast cancer has been reported in numerous studies, and numerous regions of allelic imbalance have been described using microsatellites as well as the older restriction fragment length polymorphism analysis. As reviewed by Deville and Cornelisse, compilation of data from more than 30 studies reveals a consensus of imbalances affecting more than 11 chromosome arms at a frequency of more than 25% (Table 1). Chromosome arms 1p, 1q, 3p, 6q, 8p, 11p, 13q, 17q, 18q, and 22q were affected at a frequency of 25-40%, whereas chromosome arms 16q and 17p were affected in more than 50% of tumors (Devilee and Cornelisse, 1994). In addition, chromosome arm 9p, which was not evaluated in these studies most likely because of lack of previous cytogenetic data implicating it, has recently been shown by our laboratory to be affected in 58% of breast carcinomas (Brenner and Aldaz, 1995). The loss of generic material in many of these regions has been corroborated by either CGH or classic cytogenetic data (Devilee and Cornelisse, 1994; Trent et al 1993). Further, some of these regions are known to harbor tumor suppressive genes whose loss has been demonstrated through a variety of techniques, including Southern blot analysis and FISH using gene-specific single-copy probes (Cox, Chen, and Lee, 1994).

While there is overwhelming evidence that these genetic losses occur, inherent difficulties exist in determining the relevance of such losses to breast tumorigenesis. In most cases, the tumors analyzed were of the invasive type and/or advanced stages of progression, leading to the question whether these losses are causative factors of tumorigenesis or consequences of the general genomic instability inherent to tumors. Further, it is possible that certain losses may be selected for in the progression or clonal evolution of a tumor to a more advanced type but not necessary for the genesis of the tumor. Some of these questions could be addressed in part through comparative allelotyping of both noninvasive and invasive tumors.

To address the relative timing and frequency of allelic losses of commonly affected regions in breast cancer, microsatellite length polymorphism analysis was performed in a series of preinvasive ductal carcinomas (DCIS) and invasive ductal and lobular carcinomas (Aldaz et al, 1995). Twenty different loci were examined in each group. As expected, frequencies of regional losses in invasive ductal carcinomas were similar to those in the aforementioned compilation by Devilee and Cornelisse of analyses from more than 30 studies. However, allelotyping of DCIS samples revealed that chromosomal regions 3p, 3q, 6p, 11p, 16p, 18p, 18q, and 22q were not affected by a high frequency of loss, while analyses of these same regions of invasive tumors showed them to be affected in 10-40% of cases (Aldaz et al., 1995). Our findings are in agreement with those of Radford et. al. who examined 61 DCIS samples (Radford et al, 1995). Because allelic losses affecting these regions were not frequently observed at the noninvasive (DCIS) stage it can be concluded that alterations of these regions are late events in breast cancer progression. More importantly, allelic imbalances observed on chromosome arms 7p, 7q, 16q, 17p, and 17q (Aldaz et al., 1995), as well as 9p as reported by others (Fujii et al., 1996), appear to be early abnormalities because they occur in approximately one third of DCIS samples.

Lobular carcinomas constitute approximately 10-15% of all breast cancers (Tavassoli, 1992). Histologically, lobular carcinomas have a very distinctive infiltrative growth pattern and metastatic pattern (Tavassoli, 1992). In addition, patients with invasive lobular carcinoma have been reported to have a higher risk of developing multifocal and contralateral breast cancer than those patients with invasive ductal carcinoma (Silverstein et al., 1994). To determine whether ductal and lobular carcinomas are subject to the same pattern of allelic loss, comparative allelotyping of the two subtypes was also conducted in our laboratory. Losses of chromosome arms 1p, 3q, 11q, and 18q were more prevalent for invasive ductal carcinoma than for invasive lobular carcinoma (Aldaz et al., 1995). However, 8p losses or imbalances were observed in 36% of invasive lobular tumors but only 14% of invasive ductal carcinomas. Interestingly, microsatellite instability was observed in almost 40% of lobular carcinomas, but only 13% of ductal carcinomas (Aldaz et al., 1995). This phenomenon of microsatellite instability, also known as RER+ phenotype, is identified by allele size differences between tumor and matching normal controls. First described as a characteristic of tumors from patients carrying an autosomal dominant predisposition to tumors of the colon and endometrium, microsatellite instability has been linked to defects in a group of human mismatch repair genes: h*MSH2*, h*MLH1*, h*PMS1*, and h*PMS2* (Aaltonen et al., 1993; Fischel et al., 1993; Bronner et al., 1994). Resultant errors in DNA repair are believed to be the cause of the observed genomic instability phenomenon. These data suggest that invasive lobular carcinomas may arise by a mechanism of carcinogenesis different from that of ductal breast carcinomas and appear to constitute a distinct pathologic entity.

Targets of Allelic Loss

Chromosome arm 17p, as previously discussed, is subject to allelic loss in more than 50% of invasive ductal carcinomas, and approximately 30% of noninvasive ductal carcinomas (Radford et al., 1993; Aldaz et al., 1995; Radford et al., 1995). This high frequency of allelic loss suggests that a tumor suppressor of relevance to breast tumorigenesis resides in this region. Indeed, tumor suppressor *p53* is located in this chromosome arm and is known to harbor somatic mutation in 25 to 45% of primary breast carcinomas (Osborne et al., 1991). In addition, germline *p53* mutations have been detected and shown to be causative in families with Li-Fraumeni cancer predisposition syndrome (Malkin et al., 1990; Srivastava et al., 1990). Breast cancer is one of the neoplasms affecting patients with this syndrome. In tumors from patients with Li-Fraumeni syndrome, loss of the wild-type allele is observed with retention of the mutant *p53* allele. Functional studies of cells with mutant *p53* indicate a change of phenotypes, including cellular immortalization, loss of growth suppression, and fourfold increase in protein half-life which leads to *p53* accumulation. Accumulation of *p53* protein, observed by immunohistochemical analysis in roughly 30-50% of sporadic breast carcinomas, was proposed to be an indicator of higher risk of recurrence in patients with tumors positive for *p53* expression (reviewed by Ozbun and Butel, 1995). It is possible that early in breast tumor development, *p53* inactivation through mutation and LOH may be intrinsically linked to the development of subsequent further genomic instability as suggested by findings in experimental model of carcinogenesis (Donehower et al., 1995).

Although *p53* is the most likely candidate for allelic loss on 17p, other reports indicate that there may exist another distinct locus that may be a target of allelic loss. In an analysis of 141 breast tumors, Cornelis et al. observed a strong association between *p53* mutation and allelic loss of the *p53* locus (Cornelis et al., 1994). However, in cases where *p53* mutation was not observed, allelic loss of distal region 17p13.3 was always observed, sometimes without p53 allele loss. Similar findings of distal deletion of 17p were also observed in DCIS (Radford et al., 1995). While these findings support the existence of a second gene as target of allelic loss, further studies are needed to address this issue.

The long arm of chromosome 17, also frequently affected by allelic imbalance in both familial and sporadic breast cancers, has recently been subjected to extensive analysis because 17q has been linked to familial breast cancer (Hall et al., 1990). As a result, the *BRCA1* gene was isolated by positional cloning and mutations found to cosegragate with the predisposing haplotype in affected kindreds (Miki et al., 1994). However, when sporadic breast tumors with allelic loss of 17q were examined for *BRCA1* coding sequence alterations, only about 10% of those with LOH revealed any change of sequence, and those mutations were found to be germinal (Futreal et al., 1994). Cellular mislocalization of the *BRCA1* protein has since been reported in sporadic breast tumors, although other groups have not been able to confirm these results (Chen et al., 1995). It remains to be determined what role, if any, *BRCA1* plays in sporadic breast cancer. Another known suppressive gene localized in this region, nm23 or *NME1*, has been shown to undergo allelic loss in as much as 60% of breast carcinomas (Leone et al., 1991). However, analysis of *NME1* has not revealed evidence of mutations (Cropp et al., 1994). An additional possible explanation for allele loss is the existence of a yet-unidentified gene within this region as the target of allelic loss.

Loss of the *RB1* region 13q14 has been reported for numerous neoplasms including small cell lung carcinoma, bladder carcinoma, osteosarcoma, and breast carcinoma (reviewed by Cox, Chen and Lee, 1994). These losses appear to be relatively early losses in some tumors since 15-20% of tumors at the DCIS stage reveal allelic loss of 13q (Aldaz et al., 1995; Radford et al., 1995). However, when allelic loss and expression are examined in the same breast tumors, no correlation between the two is observed, suggesting that Rb inactivation is not acquired by allelic loss and that another gene may be the target of such inactivation (Borg et al., 1992). More recently, linkage analysis of high-risk breast cancer families localized a second breast cancer susceptibility locus, *BRCA2*, to chromosome 13q12-13 (Wooster et al., 1994). This suggested that the *BRCA2* gene may be involved in sporadic breast cancer as well. However, similar to the findings with *BRCA1* on 17q, when sporadic breast tumors were analyzed for mutation of BRCA2, mutations were infrequent, indicating that *BRCA2* is not the gene being targeted by loss (Miki et al., 1996; Teng et al., 1996; Lancaster et al., 1996). Brush-1 is another gene that has been mapped to 13q12-13, proximal to *RB1*. Analysis of Brush-1 expression indicated it to be low to absent in 6 of 13 breast cancer lines and decreased in four of four tumors showing LOH of 13q12-13 (Schott et al., 1994). However, no sequence analysis has yet been reported, and the question of whether decreased expression of Brush-1 results from allelic loss involving large regions of another gene has yet to be addressed.

Chromosomal region 9p21, as previously discussed, has been shown to be affected by allelic loss in 58% of invasive ductal carcinomas and 30% of DCIS, suggesting it may be involved in breast tumorigenesis (Brenner and Aldaz, 1995; Fujii et al., 1996). Previously, the p16^{INK4a}/MTS1/CDKN2 tumor suppressor gene has been identified within this region by positional cloning and shown to be affected in 60% of breast carcinoma lines (Kamb et al., 1994). However, when primary breast tumors were analyzed in our laboratory for mutation of the *CDKN2* coding region, few mutations were found (Brenner and Aldaz, 1995). More recent analysis, including FISH determination of gene copy number, methylation of the 5' region, and analysis of expression, indicate that *p16* is indeed affected in 40 - 60% of breast tumors (Brenner et al., 1996). This observation of inactivation substantiates a role for *p16* inactivation in the tumorigenesis of the breast and as a target of 9p allelic loss.

Chromosome 16q has been suggested as a site for the occurrence of primary cytogenetic structural abnormalities in the development of breast cancer (Dutrillaux, Gerbault-Seureau, and Zafrani, 1990; Pandis et al., 1992). In particular the long arm of chromosome 16 was shown to systematically participate in nonrandom translocations with chromosome 1 and 16q deletions were also frequently observed. Breast cancer allelotypic studies have also systematically shown the common occurrence of allelic losses affecting the long arm of chromosome 16 (Sato et al., 1990; Tsuda et al., 1994; Cleton-Jansen et al., 1994). In addition to our observations (Aldaz et al., 1995), other investigators have also reported the occurrence of frequent allelic losses affecting chromosome 16q in DCIS (Tsuda et al., 1994; Radford et al., 1995).

It has been suggested that probably more than one putative tumor suppressor locus of interest in breast cancer resides in 16q. At least two regions of chromosome 16q have consistently been previously reported to show LOH: 16q21 and 16q24.2-qter (Tsuda et al., 1994; Cleton-Jansen et al., 1994; Sato et al., 1990). Very recently, by performing a high-resolution allelotype of chromosome 16 in DCIS lesions, we have identified three distinct regions with a very high incidence (about 70% or more) of allelic losses among informative DCIS samples (Chen et al., 1996). Two of the regions agree with previously described areas: 16q21 at locus D16S400 and 16q24.2 at locus D16S402. However, the region with the highest incidence of LOH observed in our study lies between markers D16S515 and D16S516 (Figure 1). Within this region the D16S518 locus was the most frequently affected: 20 of 26 DCIS tumors (77%) showed LOH at this locus. These observations strongly suggest that a putative tumor suppressor gene(s) may possible be harbored at or in the vicinity of this locus. On the basis of a YAC contig spanning the region of interest ,we can estimate that the minimum region with the highest frequency of LOH is no larger than 2-3 Mb. (Chen et al., 1996). Furthermore, on the basis of the cytogenetic location of markers D16S504 and D16S516 and the distance to D16S518, this area should be contained within bands 16q23.3-q24.1. This region appears different from another area of frequent LOH more distally located at locus D16S402 in band 16q24.2. Both areas are 17 cM apart according to the Genethon Linkage Map (March 1996) and several megabases away according to a comprehensive chromosome 16 physical and genetic map. Further studies are necessary to identify the target gene(s).

It will be particularly important to analyze for the occurrence of allelic losses at the mentioned chromosome 16 regions in other less advanced hyperplastic breast lesions. This analysis will be useful in our understanding of breast carcinogenesis and may help in the identification of markers with diagnostic or prognostic significance.

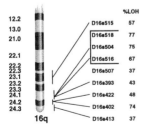

Figure 1. Chromosome arm 16q allelic loss in preinvasive breast carciomas.

CELL CYCLE IN BREAST CANCER

Normal cell division in eukaryotes proceeds through an orderly cascade of events manifested as a cell cycle. The machinery responsible for such progress includes a hierarchy of proteins and complexes each exerting an effect on the next. At the top of this hierarchy are the cyclin subunits, whose expression and stability oscillate in a phase-dependent manner. Further, the expression of certain cyclin genes can be upregulated by different mitogenic stimuli, for example, the upregulation of cyclin D1 by estrogen (Altucci et al., 1996). Each of these cyclins can associate in a non-promiscuous manner with specific cyclin-dependent kinases (CDKs). When bound, the cyclins result in activation of CDK activity. However, these cyclins are in competition with CDK inhibitors, which have the ability to displace the cyclin and form an inactive complex with the CDKs. When CDKs are active, they phosphorylate, and hence inactivate, other proteins with transcription-repressing activity (Reviewed by Sherr et al., 1994).

Of the restriction points, G1 to S is best characterized in breast cancer. The players involved in this restriction point include cyclins D1-D3; CDKs 4 and 6, the inhibitors of those CDKs *p15*, *p16*, and *p18*; and the substrate of the CDKs, the *Rb* protein (Figure 2). Collectively, these proteins are known elements responsible for regulation of progression through G1, and loss of function or disregulation of expression of an individual protein can lead to loss of cell cycle regulation and proliferation. Of these proteins, the Rb protein, cyclin D1, and *p16* have all been observed to be affected in breast tumorigenesis. As previously mentioned, cyclin D1 has been shown to be both amplified in 10-20% of breast tumors and overexpressed in the majority of breast tumors (Gillet et al., 1994; Bartkova et al., 1994; Weinstat-Saslow et al., 1995). When cyclin D1 is over-abundant, it competes with *p16* for heterodimerization with the CDKs; when cyclin D1 is bound to a CDK, it positively regulates the activity of the CDK which is able to phosphorylate and inactivate *Rb*. Inactivation of *Rb* itself has been described in breast cancer, and when multiple modes of inactivation are accounted for, *Rb* is inactivated in approximately 20% of breast cancers (Borg et al., 1992; Varley et al., 1989). In addition, analyses of *Rb* and *p16* have shown an inverse relationship in expression of the two genes in the vast majority of tumor lines studied (Okamoto et al., 1994; Parry et al., 1995). This is true in breast tumor cell lines as well: in those lines retaining *Rb* expression, *p16* is deleted, mutated, or otherwise affected, and its expression is often undetectable. In contrast, those cell lines retaining *p16* expression often lack expression of *Rb*. Further, when primary breast tumors are analyzed for *p16* expression, approximately 50% show loss of expression due to homozygous deletion, methylation of the 5' region, and rarely by mutation (Brenner et al., 1996). While *CDK4* has not been extensively studied in breast cancer, other neoplasms show overexpression or mutation of the *p16* binding site (He et al., 1994; Zuo et al., 1996). Thus, it appears that mutation or disruption of either *Rb* or *p16* expression or overexpression of cyclin D1 or possibly *CDK4* is sufficient to eliminate this pathway's control of cell cycle progression. The high cumulative rate of alterations affecting these proteins in breast cancer suggests that abrogation of the G1 restriction point may be necessary for breast tumorigenesis.

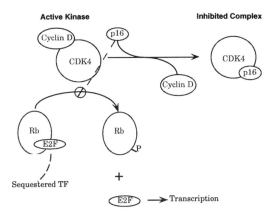

Figure 2. Schematic representation of G1/S restriction point interactions.

The CDK inhibitor $p21$WAF1/CIP1 is known to be another negative regulator of the cell cycle. Unlike $p16$, it is known to be a universal inhibitor of CDKs thereby inducing arrest at both the G1/S and G2/M restriction points (Xiong et al., 1993). Further, $p21$ also complexes with proliferating cell nuclear antigen *in vitro,* resulting in inhibition of DNA replication (Waga et al., 1994). Because $p21$ gene transcription is regulated by $p53$, it has been suggested that $p53$-dependent cell cycle arrest is mediated by $p21$. Indeed, $p21$ nullizygous mice fibroblasts fail to undergo G1 arrest following DNA damage although apoptosis is unaffected in these same cells (Brugarolas et al., 1995). As previously mentioned, positive $p53$ gene detection has been shown in as much as half of breast carcinomas, and $p53$ has been shown to be associated with $p53$ mutation and a higher risk of recurrence (reviewed by Ozbun and Butel, 1995). This would suggest that an additional possible consequence of $p53$ inactivation in the tumorigenesis of the breast is the abrogation of cell cycle arrest through loss of transcriptional activation of $p21$.

SUMMARY

Breast cancer is a complex disease in which numerous genetic aberrations occur. It is unclear which, if any, of these abnormalities are causative of breast tumorigenesis. However, on the basis of the currently accepted view of breast cancer as a multistep process, it is possible that specific abnormalities may be required in the progression from a normal breast epithelial cell to an invasive tumor cell. Figure 3 shows a schematic putative model of breast cancer progression based primarily on epidemiological and histopathological studies (Page and DuPont, 1992). Advances in methodology have allowed us to more precisely determine the approximate chronology of some of these aberrations and the possible roles each plays in the formation of malignancy. Simplistically, one could speculate that it is the early loss of cell cycle control in the presence of a mitogenic stimulus that allows a cell to divide unchecked. Such uncontrolled proliferation in the absence of wild type p53 would yield a high level of genomic instability. As proliferation continues, numerous additional chromosomal abnormalities occur, and increased tumor heterogeneity would be observed as distinct subpopulations emerge in the evolution toward a progressively more aggressive phenotype. However, much still remains to be learned to gain a full understanding of the key players behind the genetic evolution of breast cancer. Only by analyzing preinvasive and putative early stages of breast cancer will we be able to characterize the most probable sequence of genomic abnormalities.

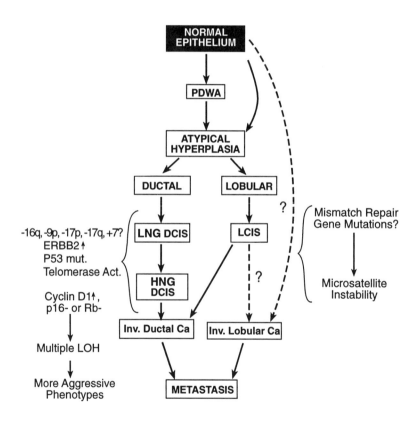

Figure 3. Schematic putative model of breast cancer progression.

ACKNOWLEDGEMENTS

The authors wish to thank contributing colleagues Taiping Chen, Andzrej Bednarek, Abhaya Paladugu, Hui Wang, and Qiao Ying Liao, and Michelle Gardiner for her secretarial assistance. This work was supported by Grants DAMD 17-94-J-4078 and DAMD 17-96-1-6252 from the U.S. Army Breast Cancer Program and NIH Grant R01 CA59967.

REFERENCES

Aaltonen LA, Peltomaki P, Leach FS, Sistonen P, Pylkkanen L, Mecklin JP, Jarvinen H, Powell SM, Jen J, Hamilton SR, et al (1993): Clues to the pathologenesis of familial colorectal cancer. Science 260:812-816.

Aldaz CM, Chen T, Sahin A, Cunningham J, Bondy M (1995): Comparative allelotype of *in situ* and invasive human breast cancer: High frequency of microsatellite instability in lobular breast carcinomas. Cancer Res 55:3976-3981.

Altucci L, Addeo R, Cicatiello L, et al (1996): 17β-estradiol induces cyclin D1 gene transcription, p36D1-p34cdk4 complex activation and p105Rb phosphorylation during mitogenic stimulation of G(1)-arrested human breast cancer cells. Oncogene 12:2315-2324.

Bartkova J, Lukas J, Muller H, Lutzhft D, Strauss M, Bartek J (1994): Cyclin D1 protein expression and function in human breast cancer. Intl J Cancer 57:353-361.

Berger MS, Locher GW, Saurer S, Gullick WJ, Waterfield MD, Groner B, Hynes NE (1988): Correlation of C-ERBB-2 gene amplification and protein expression in human breast carcinoma with nodal status and nuclear grading. Cancer Res 48:1238-1243.

Borg A, Zhang Q-X, Alm P, Olsson H, Sellberg G (1992): The retinoblastoma gene in breast cancer: allele loss is not correlated with loss of gene protein expression. Cancer Res 52:2991-2994.

Boring CC (1994): Cancer statistics. CA Cancer J Clin 44:7-26.

Bouchard L, Lamarre L, Tremblay PJ, Jolicoeur P (1989): Stochastic appearance of mammary tumors in transgenic mice carrying the MMTV/C-NEU oncogene. Cell 57:931-936.

Brenner AJ, Aldaz CM (1995): Chromosome 9p allelic loss and *p16/CDKN2* in breast cancer and evidence of *p16* inactivation in immortal breast epithelial cells. Cancer Res 55:2892-2895.

Brenner AJ, Paladugu A, Wang H, Olopade OI, Dreyling MH, Aldaz CM (1996): Loss of p16 is preferential over alternative p19 in breast cancer. Clinical Cancer Res (in press).

Bronner CE, Baker SM, Morrison PT, Warren G, Smith LG, Lescoe MK, Kane M, Earabino C, Lipford J, Lindblom A, Tannergard P, Bollag RJ, Godwin AR, Ward DC, Nordenskjold M, Fishel R, Kolodner R, Liskay RM (1994): Mutation in the DNA mismatch repair gene homologue *hMLH1* is associated with hereditary non-polyposis colon cancer. Nature 368:258-261.

Brugarolas J, Chandrasekaran C, Gordon JI, Beach D, Jacks T, Hannon GJ (1995): Radiation-induced cell cycle arrest compromised by p21 deficiency. Nature. 377(6549):552-7.

Chen T, Sahin A, and Aldaz CM (1996): Deletion Map of Chromosome 16q in Ductal Carcinoma *In Situ* of the Breast: Refining a Putative Tumor Suppressor Gene Region. (Submitted for publication).

Chen Y, Chen CF, Riley DJ, Allred DC, Chen PL, Von Hoff D, Osborne CK, Lee WH (1995): Aberrant subcellular localization of BRCA1 in breast cancer. Science 270:789-791.

Cleton-Jansen AM, Moerland EW, Kuipers-Dijkshoorn NJ, Callen DF, Sutherland GR, Hansen B, Devilee P, Cornelisse CJ (1994): At least two different regions are involved in allelic imbalance on chromosome arm 16q in breast cancer. Genes, Chromos. & Cancer, 9:101-107.

Comings DE (1973): A general theory of carcinogenesis. Proc Natl Acad Sci USA 70:3324-3328.

Cornelis RS, van Vliet M, Vos CBJ, Cleton-Jansen A-M, van de Vijver MJ, Peterse JL, Khan PM, Borresen A-L, Cornelisse CJ, Devilee P (1994): Evidence for a gene on 17p13.3, distal to TP53, as a target for allele loss in breast tumors without *p53* mutations. Cancer Res 54:4200-4206.

Coussens L, Yang-Feng TL, Liao YC, Chen E, Gray A, McGrath J, Seeburg PH, Libermann TA, Schlessinger J, Francke U, et al (1985): Tryosine kinase receptor with extensive homology to EGF receptor shares chromosomal location with Neu oncogene. Science 230:1132-1139.

Cropp CS, Lidereau R, Leone A, Liscia D, Cappa APM, Campbell G, Barker E, Le Doussal V, Steeg PS, Callahan R (1994): NME1 protein expression and loss of heterozygosity mutations in primary human breast tumors. J. Natl. Cancer Inst. 86:1167-1169.

Cox LA, Chen G, Lee E Y-H P (1994): Tumor suppressor genes and their roles in breast cancer. Breast Cancer Res Treat 32:19-38.

Devilee P, Cornelisse CJ (1994): Somatic genetic changes in human breast cancer. Biochimica et Biophysica Acta 1198:113-130.

Dib C, Fauré S, Fizames C, Samson D, Drouot N, Vignal A, Millasseau P, Marc S, Hazan J, Seboun E, Lathrop M, Gyapay G, Morissette J, Weissenbach J (1996): A comprehensive genetic map of the human genome based on 5,264 microsatellites. Nature 380:152-154.

Dickson C, Fantl V, Gillett C, Brookes S, Bartek J, Smith R, Fisher C, Barnes D, Peters G (1995): Amplification of chromosome band 11q13 and a role for cyclin D1 in human breast cancer. Cancer Let 90:43-50.

Donehower LA, Godley LA, Aldaz CM, Pyle R, Shi YP, Pinkel D, Gray J, Bradley A, Medina D, Varmus HE (1995): Deficiency of p53 accelerates mammary tumorigenesis in Wnt-1 transgenic mice and promotes chromosomal instability. Genes & Development. 9(7):882-95.

Dutrillaux B, Gerbault-Seureau M, Zafrani B (1990): Characterization of chromosomal anomalies in human breast cancer. A comparison of 30 paradiploid cases with few chromosome changes. Cancer Genet Cytogenet 49:203-217.

Easton DF, Bishop DT, Ford D, Crockford GP (1993): Genetic linkage analysis in familial breast and ovarian cancer: results from 214 families. The Breast Cancer Linkage Consortium. Am J Hum Gene 52:678-701.

Feuer EJ (1993): The lifetime risk of developing breast cancer. J Natl Cancer Inst 85:892-897.

Fishel R, Lescoe MK, Rao MRS, Copeland NG, Jenkins NA, Garber J, Kane M, Kolodner R (1993): The human mutator gene homolog *MSH2* and its association with hereditary nonpolyposis colon cancer. Cell 75:1027-1038.

Fujii H, Marsh C, Cairns P, Sidransky D, Gabrielson E (1996): Genetic divergence in the clonal evolution of breast cancer. Cancer Res 56:1493-1497.

Futreal PA, Liu Q, Shattuck-Eidens D, Cochran C, Harshman K, Tavtigian S, Bennett LM, Haugen-Strano A, Swensen J, Miki Y, Eddington K, McClure M, Frye C, et al (1994): *BRCA1* mutations in primary breast and ovarian carcinomas. Science 266:120-122.

Gillett C, Fantl V, Smith R, Fisher C, Bartek J, Dickson C, Barnes D, Peters G (1994): Amplification and overexpression of cyclin D1 in breast cancer detected by immunohistochemical staining. Cancer Res 54:1812-1817.

Goodrich DW, Lee W-H (1993): Molecular characterization of the retinoblastoma susceptibility gene. Biochimica et Biophysica Acta 1155:43-61.

Gray JW, Collins C, Henderson IC, Isola J, Kallioniemi A, Kallioniemi O-P, Nakamura H,

Pinkel D, Stokke T, Tanner M, Waldman F (1994): Molecular Cytogenetics of Human Breast Cancer. 645-652.

Hall JM, Lee MK, Newman B, Morrow JE, Anderson LA, Huey B, King MC. (1990): Linkage of early-onset familial breast cancer to chromosome 17q21. Science 250:1684-1689.

Harris H, Miller OJ, Klein G, Worst P, Tachibana T (1969): Suppression of malignancy by cell fusion. Nature 223:363-368.

He J, Allen JR, Collins VP, Allalunis-Turner MJ, Godbout R, Day III RS, James CD (1994): CDK4 amplification is an alternative mechanism to p16 gene homozygous deletion in glioma cell lines. Cancer Res 54:5804-5807.

Isola JJ, Kallioniemi OP, Chu LW, Fuqua SA, Hilsenbeck SG, Osborne CK, Waldman FM (1995): Genetic aberrations detected by comparative genomic hybridization predict outcome in node-negative breast cancer. Am J Path 147:905-911.

Jardines L, Weiss M, Fowble B, Greene M (1993): neu(c-erbB-2/HER2) and the epidermal growth factor receptor (EGFR) in breast cancer. Pathobiology 61:268-282.

Kallioniemi A, Kallioniemi O-P, Piper J, Tanner M, Stokke T, Chen L, Smith HS, Pinkel D, Gray JW, Waldman FM (1994): Detection and mapping of amplified DNA sequences in breast cancer by comparative genomic hybridization. Proc Natl Acad Sci USA 91:2156-2160.

Kallioniemi A, Kallioniemi O-P, Sudar D, Rutovitz D, Gray JW, Waldman F, Pinkel D (1992a): Comparative genomic hybridization for molecular cytogenetic analysis of solid tumors. Science 258:818-820.

Kallioniemi OP, Kallioniemi A, Kurisu W, Thor A, Chen LC, Smith HS, Waldman FM, Pinkel D, Gray JW (1992b): ERBB2 amplification in breast cancer analyzed by fluorescence in situ hybridization. Proc Natl Acad Sci USA 89:5321-5325.

Kamb A, Gruis N, Weaver-Feldhaus J, Qingyun L, Harshman K, Tavtigian S, Stockert E, Day R, Johnson B, Skolnick M (1994): A cell cycle regulator potentially involved in genesis of many tumor types. Science 264:436-440.

Klein G, Bregula U, Wiener F (1971): The analysis of malignancy by cell fusion. J Cell Sci 8:659-672.

Knudson AG (1971): Mutation and Cancer: Statistical study of retinoblastoma. Proc Natl Acad Sci USA 68:820-823.

Lammie GA, Peters G (1991): Chromosome 11q13 abnormalities in human cancer. Cancer

Cells 3:413-420.

Lancaster JM, Wooster R, Mangion J, et al (1996): BRCA2 mutations in primary breast and ovarian cancers. Nature Genetics 13:238-240.

Leone A, McBride OW, Weston A, Wang MG Anglard P, Cropp CS, Goepel JR, Lidereau R, Callahan R, Linehan WM, Rees RC, Harris CC, Liotta LA, and Steeg PS (1991): Somatic allelic deletion of nm23 in human cancer. Cancer Res 51:2490-2493.

Litt M, Luty JA (1989): A hypervariable microsatellite revealed by in vitro amplification of a dinucleotide repeat within the cardiac muscle actin gene. Am J Hum Genet 44:397-401.

Malkin D, Li FP, Strong LC, Fraumeni JF Jr, Nelson CE, Kim DH, Kassel J, Gryka MA Bischoff FZ, Tainsky MA, et al (1990): Germ line p53 mutations in a familial syndrome of breast cancer, sarcomas, and other neoplasms. Science 250:1233-1238.

Miki Y, Katagiri T, Kasumi F, Yoshimoto T, Nakamura Y (1996): Mutation analysis in the BRCA2 gene in primary breast cancers. Nature Genetics 13:245-247.

Miki Y, Swensen J, Shattuck-Eidens D, Futreal PA, Harshman K, Tavtigian S, Liu Q, Cochran C, Bennett LM, et al (1994): A strong candidate for the breast and ovarian cancer susceptibility gene BRCA1. Science 266:66-71.

Muller WJ, Sinn E, Pattengale PK, Wallace R, Leder P (1988): Single-step induction of mammary adenocarcinoma in transgenic mice bearing the activated c-neu oncogene. Cell 54:105-115.

Okamoto A, Demetrick DJ, Spillare EA, Hagiwara K, Hussain SP, Bennett WP, Forrester K, Gerwin B, Serrano M, Beach DH, Harris CC (1994): Mutations and altered expression of p16INK4 in human cancer. Proc Natl Acad 91:11045-11049.

Osborne RJ, Merlo GR, Mitsudomi T, Venesio T, Liscia DS, Cappa APM, Chiba I, Takahashi T, Nau MM, Callahan R, Minna JD (1991): Mutations in the p53 gene in primary human breast cancers. Cancer Res 51:6194-6198.

Ozbun MA, Butel JS (1995): Tumor suppressor p53 mutations and breast cancer: a critical analysis. Adv Cancer Res 66:71-141.

Page DL, Dupont WD (1992): Benign breast disease: indicators of increased breast cancer risk. Cancer Detection & Prevention 16:93-97.

Pandis N, Heim S, Bardi G, et al (1992): Whole-arm t(1;16) and i(1q) as sole anomalies identify gain of 1q as a primary chromosomal abnormality in breast cancer. Genes Chromosomes & Cancer, 5:235-238.

Parry D, Bates S, Mann DJ, Peters G (1995): Lack of cyclin D-Cdk complexes in Rb-negative cells correlates with high levels of p16$^{INK4/MTS1}$ tumour suppressor product. EMBO J 14:503-511.

Radford DM, Fair KL, Phillips NJ, Ritter JH, Steinbrueck T, Holt MS, Donis-Keller H (1995): Allelotyping of ductal carcinoma *in situ* of the breast: deletion of loci on 8p, 13q, 16q, 17p and 17q. Cancer Res 55:3399-3405.

Radford DM, Fair K, Thompson AM, Ritter JH, Holt M, Steinbrueck T, Wallace M, Wells SA Jr, Donis-Keller HR (1993): Allelic loss on a chromosome 17 in ductal carcinoma in situ of the breast. Cancer Res 53:2947-2949.

Ravdin PM, Chamness GC (1995): The c-*erbB-2* proto-oncogene as a prognostic and predictive marker in breast cancer: a paradigm for the development of other macromolecular markers - a review. Gene 159:19-27.

Ryan KM, Birnie GD (1996): Myc oncogenes: the enigmatic family. Biochem J 314:713-721.

Sato T, Tanigami A, Yamakawa D, et al (1990): Allelotype of breast cancer: cumulative allele losses promote tumor progression in primary breast cancer. Cancer Res., 50:7184-7189.

Schott DR, Chang JN, Deng G, Kurisu W, Kuo WL, Gray J, Smith HS (1994): A candidate tumor suppressor gene in human breast cancers. Cancer Res 54:1393-1396.

Sherr CJ (1994): G1 phase progression: cycling on cue. Cell 79:551-555.

Shiu RPC, Watson PH, Dubik D (1993): c-*myc* oncogene expression in estrogen-dependent and -independent breast cancer. Clin Chem 39:353-355.

Sicinski P, Donaher JL, Parker SB, Li T, Fazeli A, Gardner H, Haslam SZ, Bronson RT, Elledge SJ, Weinberg RA (1995): Cyclin D1 provides a link between development and oncogenes in the retina and breast. Cell 82:621-630.

Silverstein MJ, Lewinsky BS, Waisman JR, Gierson ED, Colburn WJ, Senofsky GM, Gamagami P (1994): Infiltrating lobular carcinoma. Is it different from infiltrating duct carcinoma? Cancer 73:1673-1677.

Silverstein MJ, Lewinsky BS, Waisman JR, Gierson ED, Colburn WJ, Senofsky GM, Gamagami P (1994): Infiltrating lobular carcinoma. It is different from infiltrating duct carcinoma? Cancer 73:1673-1677.

Srivastava S, Zou ZQ, Pirollo K, Blattner W, Chang EH (1990): Germ-line transmission of a mutated p53 gene in a cancer-prone family with Li-fraumeni syndrome. Nature 348:747-749.

Tavassoli FA (1992): Pathology of the Breast, Norwalk, CT: Appleton & Lange.

Tavtigian SV, Simard J, Rommens J, et al (1996): The complete BRCA2 gene and mutations in chromosome 13q-linked kindreds. Nature Genetics 12:333-337.

Teng DH, Bogden R, Mitchell J, et al (1996): Low incidence of BRCA2 mutations in breast carcinoma and other cancers. Nature Genetics 13:241-244.

Thompson F, Emerson J, Dalton W, Yang J-M, McGee D, Villar H, Knox S, Massey K, Weinstein R, Bhattacharyya A, Trent J (1993): Clonal chromosome abnormalities in human breast carcinomas I. Twenty-eight cases with primary disease. Genes, Chromo Cancer 7:185-193.

Trent J, Yang J-M, Emerson J, Dalton W, McGee D, Massey K, Thompson F, Villar H (1993): Clonal chromosome abnormalities in human breast carcinomas II. Thirty-four cases with metastatic disease. Genes, Chromo Cancer 7:194-203.

Tsuda H., Callen DF, Fukutomi T., Nakamura Y, Hirohashi S (1994): Allele loss on chromosome 16q24..2-qter occurs frequently in breast cancer irrespectively of differences in phenotype and extent of spread. Cancer Tes., 54:513-517.

Varley JM, Armour J, Swallow JE, Jeffreys AJ, Ponder BA, T'Ang A, Fung YK, Brammar WJ, Walker RA (1989): The retinoblastoma gene is frequently altered leading to loss of expression in primary breast tumours. Oncogene 4:725-729.

Varley JM, Swallow JE, Brammar WJ, Whittaker JL, Walker RA (1987): Alterations to either C-ERBB-2 (NEU) or C-MYC proto-oncogenes in breast carcinomas correlate with poor short-term prognosis. Oncogene 1:423-430.

Waga S, Hannon GJ, Beach D, Stillman B (1994): The p21 inhibitor of cyclin-dependent kinases controls DNA replication by interaction with PCNA Nature. 369:574-578.

Wang TC, Cardiff RD, Zukerberg L, Lees E, Arnold A, Schmidt EV (1994): Mammary hyperplasia and carcinoma in MMTV-cyclin D1 transgenic mice. Nature 369:669-671.

Weber JL, May PE (1989): Abundant class of human DNA polymorphisms which can be typed using the polymerase chain reaction. Am J Hum Genet 44:388-396.

Weinstat-Saslow D, Merino MJ, Manrow RE, Lawrence JA, Bluth RF, Wittenbel KD, Simpson JF, Page DL, Steeg PS (1995): Overexpression of cyclin D mRNA distinguishes invasive and in situ breast carcinomas from non-malignant lesions. Nature Med 1:1257-

1260.

Wooster R, Neuhausen SL, Mangion J, Quirk Y, Ford D, Collins N, Nguyen K, Seal S, Tran T, Averill D, Fields P, Marshall G, Narod S, et al (1994): Localization of a breast cancer susceptibility gene, *BRCA2*, to chromosome 13q12-13. Science 265:2088-2090.

Wooster R, Bignell G, Lancaster J, Swift S, Seal S, Mangion J, Collins N, et al (1995): Identification of the breast cancer susceptibility gene BRCA2. Nature 378:789-792.

Xiong Y, Hannon GJ, Zhang H, Casso D, Kobayashi R, Beach D (1993): p21 is a universal inhibitor of cyclin kinases. Nature 366(6456):701-704.

Yeager T, Stadler W, Belair C, Puthenveettil J, Olopade O, Reznikoff C (1995): Increased p16 levels correlate with pRb alterations in human urothelial cells. Cancer Res 55:493-497.

Zhou D, Battifora H, Yokota J, Yamamoto T, Cline MJ (1987): Association of multiple copies of the c-erbb-2 oncogene with spread of breast cancer. Cancer Res 47:6123-6125.

Zuo L, Weger J, Yang Q, Goldstein AM, Tucker MA, Walker GJ, Hayward N, Dracopoli NC (1996): Germline mutations in the *p16INK4a* binding domain of CDK4 in familial melanoma. Nature Genetics 12:97-99.

Etiology of Breast and
Gynecological Cancers, pages 83–99
© 1997 Wiley-Liss, Inc.

MOLECULAR EPIDEMIOLOGY OF BREAST CANCER

Christine B. Ambrosone and Peter G. Shields

Division of Molecular Epidemiology (CBA)
National Center for Toxicological Research
3900 NCTR Road
Jefferson, AR 72079

Laboratory of Human Carcinogenesis
National Cancer Institute
Building 37, Room 2C16
Bethesda, MD 20892

INTRODUCTION

Breast cancer is the most commonly occurring cancer among women in the United States, except for non-melanotic skin cancer, and is second only to lung cancer as a cause of cancer death in women (Boring et al., 1992). Breast cancer incidence has increased dramatically over the last ten years, and it is currently estimated that as many as one of every eight women in the United States will develop breast cancer during her lifetime (Feuer et al., 1993).

In addition to the dramatic increase in breast cancer incidence in the last decade, there is a disparity in rates between geographic regions within this country. Risk appears to be highest among women in the northeast, particularly for those in urban areas (Marshall, 1993). Differences also exist between countries, some with a five to tenfold magnitude (Willett, 1989). Migrant studies have also shown that breast cancer incidence rates change as women move from low-risk countries to those with higher rates (Buell, 1973). Underdeveloped countries with traditionally low incidence rates are also experiencing a rise in breast cancer incidence (Boyle, 1988).

For the most part, the etiology of breast cancer remains unknown. Some risk factors for breast cancer have been elucidated, mostly related to hormonal status or family history, yet these explain only a portion of the variability in disease incidence (Madigan et al., 1996). Although variations in dietary, socioeconomic, and reproductive factors may partially explain geographic differences in breast cancer incidence rates, they do not appear to fully account for geographic and temporal disparities. It is plausible that environmental contaminants and dietary carcinogens that are associated with a more westernized lifestyle, that include exposures to aryl and heterocyclic aromatic amines, nitro- and polycyclic aromatic hydrocarbons, and N-nitroso compounds, may be related to breast cancer risk.

While epidemiological studies generally have not implicated specific environmental or chemical etiologies, it is our hypothesis that these exposures can contribute to human breast cancer risk. It is well known that there is a wide interindividual variation (Harris, 1989) in cancer risk related to carcinogen metabolism. Given this, and data showing that carcinogenesis is a multistage complex process, we believe that there are susceptible subgroups of women to particular carcinogens based on specific heritable susceptibilities. When these subgroups are grouped together, however, as in population-based studies, the effects of a particular exposure may not be observable above the background of other exposures and susceptibilities. In this case, the effects may be diluted and thus, not statistically significant. Molecular epidemiological approaches that stratify women on the basis of carcinogen metabolizing capacity, for example, is one method that can categorize susceptible groups of women. The basis of our hypothesis, which focuses on tobacco use, and the use of molecular epidemiological methods, is detailed below.

CHEMICAL CARCINOGENS AND HUMAN BREAST CANCER

Several lines of evidence indicate that chemical carcinogens can reach the breast in laboratory animals and humans. Many are lipophilic substances, and may be stored in the adipose tissue of the breast (Obana et al., 1981; Morris, Seifter, 1992). Also, work by Petrakis and colleagues showed that levels of cotinine, a metabolite of nicotine, were higher in nipple fluid aspirate than in serum of women who smoked (Petrakis et al., 1978). Additionally, nipple fluid aspirate had mutagenic activity in the Ames' *Salmonella typhimurium* assay that was sensitive to aromatic amines (Petrakis et al., 1980). Heterocyclic amines administered to nursing rat dams were found at high levels in the breast tissue, and were excreted in the milk (Ghoshal, Snyderwine, 1993). Other lines of evidence indicate that breast tissues can metabolically activate chemical carcinogens, and increase the biologically effective dose. Two recent studies have identified DNA adducts in normal breast tissue from women with and without breast cancer (Perera et al., 1995; Li et al., 1996), some of which were putatively related to tobacco smoking. The mutational spectrum of the p53 gene also supports a role for chemical carcinogens in breast cancer risk, because the pattern of mutation in breast cancer is quite similar to that for lung cancer, in which chemical carcinogens are known to be etiologically related (Biggs et al., 1993). Therefore, it is reasonable to suspect that these carcinogens may be involved in human breast cancer.

N-Nitroso compounds, PAHs and aryl aromatic and heterocyclic amines also are present in cigarette smoke. If these compounds are human mammary carcinogens, one would expect to see an association between smoking and breast cancer risk. As reviewed by Palmer and Rosenberg, however, in the majority of epidemiologic studies, an association between smoking and breast cancer risk has not been found (Palmer, Rosenberg, 1993). Some studies have found smoking to be associated with slightly elevated breast cancer risk, while others report a decreased risk. Interestingly, a recent study by Morabia and colleagues used an innovative methodologic approach to study cigarette smoking and breast cancer risk

(Morabia et al., 1996) . Because exposure to passive smoke has been found to be associated with breast cancer risk to a greater degree than active smoking, Morabia hypothesized that inclusion of passive smokers in the reference category of non-smokers would dilute estimates of risk associated with active smoking. In a large case-control study of breast cancer, with a reference category only of women exposed to neither active nor passive cigarette smoke, a clear dose-response association was observed between lifetime smoking and breast cancer risk, with an odds ratio of 4.6 (95% confidence interval 2.2-9.7) in the highest quartile of use. It is possible that previous studies, by not allowing for passive smokers in the reference category, were biased by misclassification of never smokers.

It is also possible that tobacco smoke has multiple effects. Cigarettes contain about 3600 chemicals, some of which may affect the metabolism and/or mutagenicity of hormones and/or other carcinogens in breast cancer tissue (Office on Smoking and Health, 1996). Other agents in tobacco smoke have anti-estrogenic effects, which would preclude the efficacy of chemical carcinogens in breast carcinogenesis (MacMahon et al., 1982). For example, cigarette smoking induces *CYP1A2*, which decreases the level of circulating estradiol.

Finally, the assessment of a heterogeneous group of breast cancer patients may be clouding the effects of tobacco smoking if genetic differences in metabolism and detoxification may make some women more susceptible than others to the cigarette carcinogens. It may be that when women are categorized by metabolic genotypes, an association will be observed between those with "at risk" polymorphisms which we were unable to detect within the larger, genetically heterogeneous, group of cases. We suggest that genetic variability in metabolism of aromatic and heterocyclic amines, PAHs, and *N*-nitroso compounds may make some women more susceptible to their carcinogenic effects from ubiquitous exposure, from dietary sources, and from exposure through active and passive cigarette smoking. Specifically, we propose that women who have genetic polymorphisms that may result in greater activation or lesser detoxification of aromatic and heterocyclic amines (*NAT1, NAT2, CYP1A2*), PAHs (*GSTM1, CYP1A1*) and *N*-nitroso compounds (*CYP2E1*) may be at greater risk for breast cancer, if they have exposure to the substrates for these enzymes. Among women with wild-type alleles for these genes, the suspected anti-estrogenic effects of tobacco smoke may overwhelm their carcinogenic potential.

POLYCYCLIC AROMATIC HYDROCARBONS

PAHs are products of incomplete combustion in the burning of fossil fuels, and are emitted in automobile exhaust and from industrial aromatic waste output. They contaminate air, water and foods. Human exposure also includes PAHs produced by the grilling of meats, fish and poultry. PAHs are known to be powerful mammary carcinogens in murine models (Yuspa, Poirier, 1988), and PAHs are mutagenic to breast cell lines (Reddy,

Rivenson, 1993). PAHs are lipophilic and are stored in adipose tissue, including that of the breast (Morris, Seifter, 1992). In experimental models, mammary tumors have been induced in rodents by various routes of administration, including gavage, intravenous injection and application to the organ itself (Cavalieri et al., 1988; Tonelli et al., 1979; Chatterjee, Banerjee, 1982). Metabolism of PAHs by mammary epithelial cells (MEC) has been noted in cell lines derived from rats, and these cells were found to activate 7,12-dimethylbenz[a]anthracene (DMBA) to mutagenic metabolites in a dose-response fashion (Gould, 1982).

Studies with human mammary epithelial cells (HMEC) have shown that PAHs are metabolized and activated by these cells also (MacNicoll et al., 1980), and cells treated with benzo(a)pyrene, a common PAH, have a high capacity for adduct formation (Stampfer et al., 1981). When compared with human fibroblasts from the same breast specimens, HMEC showed adduct formation more quickly, and at lower concentrations of PAHs. Thus, the metabolic events leading to formation of adducts can take place entirely within the mammary epithelial cells, where 99% of all human breast cancers occur.

PAHs may also affect breast cancer risk because of the similarity in the properties of PAHs to steroid hormones. There is strong epidemiologic evidence for the role of estrogens in breast cancer etiology (Kelsey, Gammon, 1990; Harris et al., 1992). PAHs are structurally similar, transported by similar proteins, metabolized through similar pathways, and stored in adipose (Morris, Seifter, 1992). PAHs may act by affecting estrogen metabolism or by binding to the estrogen receptor.

Morris and Seifter (Morris, Seifter, 1992) plotted the geographic distribution of hydrocarbon residues, in relation to the geographic distribution of breast cancer in the United States. Hydrocarbon combustion by-products, not surprisingly, are at consistently higher levels in urban than in rural areas, clustering with the distribution of breast cancer cases, and suggesting that the higher risk ratio for urban to rural women with breast cancer may be, in part, due to exposure to higher levels of hydrocarbons.

PAHs are metabolized to reactive intermediates by polymorphic cytochrome P4501A1 (*CYP1A1*) and detoxified by phase II enzymes, including glutathione S-transferase (*GSTM1*) (Nebert, 1991; Mannervik, Danielson, 1988). Polymorphisms in these genes are known to affect levels of activity. An amino acid exchange (isoleucine to valine) in exon 7 of *CYP1A1* has been linked to increased inducible activity of the enzyme (Rose, Connolly, 1993; Gonzalez et al., 1993), and individuals who inherit the null allele for *GSTM1* are deficient for glutathione S-transferase (Alexandrie et al., 1994). Some research has indicated that polymorphisms in *CYP1A1* and *GSTM1* are associated with increased lung, bladder and colon cancer risk (Alexandrie et al., 1994; Bell et al., 1993b; Hirvonen et al., 1993b; Hamada et al., 1995). In our case-control study of postmenopausal breast cancer (Ambrosone et al., 1995a), we found that the *GSTM1* null genotype did not increase overall breast cancer risk. Among younger women, however, the null genotype appeared to be associated with increased risk. Evaluation of the *CYP1A1* exon 7 substitution indicated that the polymorphism was weakly associated with increased breast cancer risk, and that this risk was highest among light smokers. Clearly, this area of genetic susceptibility to chemical carcinogenesis in the breast requires further elucidation.

ARYL AROMATIC AND HETEROCYCLIC AMINES, AND NITROAROMATIC HYDROCARBONS

The role aromatic amines in carcinogenesis has been suspected since the nineteenth century, when an association was observed between exposure in aniline dye workers and bladder cancer risk (Hein, 1988). Occupational studies have since consistently shown an association between exposure to arylamine chemicals and incidence of bladder cancer (Hein, 1988). Environmental exposure to aromatic amines may be due to their presence in mainstream and sidestream tobacco smoke and synthetic fuels or as the result of metabolic reduction of polycyclic nitroaromatic hydrocarbons ubiquitous in diesel exhaust and in airborne particulates (Hein, 1988). Experimental evidence indicates that some aromatic amines, such as 4-aminobiphenyl and β-naphthylamine are potentially mutagenic and carcinogenic to human breast cells. *In vitro*, some aromatic amines form DNA adducts in cultured human mammary epithelial cells (Swaminathan et al., 1994), and cause unscheduled DNA synthesis (Eldridge et al., 1992), indicating a capacity of breast epithelial cells to bioactivate these compounds. Further, *in vivo*, activated aromatic amine metabolites have been shown to cause DNA damage in rodents (King et al., 1979; Allaben et al., 1983; Wang et al., 1988), to transform mouse mammary glands (Tonelli et al., 1979), and to induce rodent mammary tumors (Shirai et al., 1981; Allaben et al., 1982). Some amines and nitroaromatic hydrocarbons demonstrate organotropism, and mammary tissue is a target in female rats for several such compounds. Certain dinitropyrenes found in diesel exhaust have been shown to target the mammary gland in rodent carcinogenicity studies (King et al., 1979).

Mutagenic heterocyclic amines (HAs) are formed when meat is cooked, particularly at high temperatures or for a long period of time (Sugimura, 1986). Identified as risk factors for colon cancer (Lang et al., 1994), some HAs are powerful mammary carcinogens in rodents and may be breast cancer risk factors in humans. Certain HAs are distributed to the mammary gland and form DNA adducts in rats (Snyderwine, 1994). Specifically, 2-amino-1-methyl-6-phenylimidazo[4,5]pyridine (PhIP), 2-amino-3-methylimidazo[4,5-f]quinoline (IQ), and 2-amino-3,8-dimethylimidazo[4,5-f]quinoxaline (MeIQx), cause mammary cancer in rodents (Kato et al., 1989; Tanaka et al., 1985). In male rats, administration of both PhIP and another heterocyclic amine, 2-amino-3-methylimidazo[4,5-f]quinoline (IQ), resulted in colon cancer, but females fed IQ and PhIP supplements developed mammary, rather than colon cancer (Ito et al., 1991; Reddy, Rivenson, 1993; Hasegawa et al., 1993). Importantly, HAs are activated and form DNA adducts in cultured human mammary epithelial cells (HMEC) (Pfau et al., 1992); PhIP has been demonstrated to be more mutagenic than other heterocyclic amines in cultured mammalian cells (Thompson et al., 1987; Holme et al., 1989). For the mutagenic potential of HAs to be realized, the parent compounds must undergo metabolic activation. This appears to be a two-step process, catalyzed by hepatic cytochrome P4501A2 and extrahepatic *N*-acetyltransferases (*NAT1 and NAT2*) (Kadlubar, 1994).

Metabolism of heterocyclic and aromatic amines varies among individuals, depending, in part, on polymorphisms in genes involved in xenobiotic metabolism, including *N*-acetyltransferases 1 and 2, and cytochrome P4501A2 (*CYP1A2*) (Lang et al., 1994). Several polymorphic sites at the *NAT2* locus result in decreased *N*-acetyltransferase activity (Bell et al., 1993a; Blum et al., 1991). Slow NAT2-dependent acetylation of aromatic amines is associated with increased risk for bladder cancer (Hanssen et al., 1985; Cartwright, 1984) and may increase breast cancer risk associated with cigarette smoking (Ambrosone et al., 1995b). HAs appear to be poor substrates for *N*-acetylation at the liver, however, and may, instead, be activated by an hepatic oxidative process by CYP1A2. These metabolites may then circulate and be further activated in the target tissue (Kadlubar et al., 1992).

A relationship of aromatic amines, *NAT*, and breast cancer may be similar to that reported for bladder cancer. *NAT2* slow acetylators have been found to be at increased risk for bladder cancer, presumably because of poor detoxification of aromatic amines by hepatic N-acetylation (Hein, 1988; Hanssen et al., 1985; Cartwright, 1984). Cigarette smoking has been found to be a major risk factor for bladder cancer (Mommsen, Aagard, 1983), and studies have shown that smokers with the slow acetylator phenotype have higher circulating levels of 4-aminobiphenyl-hemoglobin adducts, reflecting delayed clearance of reactive arylamine metabolites (Vineis et al., 1994; Vineis et al., 1990; Yu et al., 1994). This mechanism for bladder carcinogenesis by aromatic amines may also be applicable to breast cancer, since comparative laboratory animal studies indicate that mammary and bladder tissues have similar sensitivities to reactive intermediates (Wang et al., 1988). Thus, women who are slow acetylators may have a decreased capacity to detoxify aromatic amines at the liver, leading to an increased number of reactive intermediates in the circulation and ultimately, promutagenic carcinogen-DNA adducts and carcinogenesis in the target organ.

While *NAT2* has high hepatic activity, *NAT1* is not expressed in the liver. *NAT1* appears to bioactivate aromatic amine metabolites by O-acetylation in the target tissue. A recently identified polymorphism in *NAT1* has been shown to result in a two to three fold increase in NAT1 activity in the bladder (Taylor et al., 1995). Additionally, there is a linear correlation between *NAT1* phenotype and adduct levels in the bladder (Badawi et al., 1995). The genetic polymorphism matches the rapid phenotype in activity, and individuals with the rapid genotype have NAT1 tissue activity and adduct levels that are two to three times higher than those with the NAT1 slow genotype. Individuals with slow *NAT2* and rapid *NAT1* polymorphisms have been found to have highest adduct levels (Badawi et al., 1995). Two recent studies have identified both *NAT1* and *NAT2* in the human breast, with *NAT1* activity present in higher levels than *NAT2* (Sadrieh et al., 1996).

As previously mentioned, heterocyclic amines are poor substrates for hepatic detoxification by *NAT2* and may instead be activated by *CYP1A2*. Further activation by O-acetylation by *NAT2* or *NAT1* in the target tissue may also occur, resulting in highly reactive intermediates that may bind to DNA and result in adduct formation. Rapid acetylation by *NAT2* appears to be related to colon cancer risk (Lang et al., 1994; Ilett et al., 1987). *NAT1* may also be implicated (Bell et al., 1995). A pilot study of colon cancer found that individuals with rapid *N*-oxidation by *CYP1A2* and rapid *O*-acetylation by *NAT2* had almost 3 times the colon cancer risk of persons with the slow phenotype (Lang et al., 1994). Because HAs also appear to be mammary carcinogens, it is possible that rapid activation by *CYP1A2, NAT1* and *NAT2* may be related to breast cancer risk. *NAT1* and *NAT2* activity has been detected in the breast (Sadrieh et al., 1996)and studies in rats and in HMEC have confirmed that PhIP, IQ, and MeIQx are activated in the mammary gland (Snyderwine, 1994; Pfau et al., 1992; Davis et al., 1994). It is possible that activated *N*-hydroxy amines are converted to their reactive N-acetoxy forms through *O*-acetylation by *NAT1* and *NAT2* in breast tissue.

N-NITROSOCOMPOUNDS

Human exposure to *N*-nitrosamines occurs through diet, endogenous formation in the stomach, tobacco smoke, occupation and medical therapies (Bartsch, Montesano, 1984). *N*-nitrosamines cause DNA damage (Delp et al., 1990)such as the promutagenic O^6-methyldeoxyguanosine adducts (Fong et al., 1990). Exposure to these compounds results in decreasing levels of the repair enzyme O^6-alkylguanine-DNA alkyl transferase (Fong et al., 1990), perhaps increasing the susceptibility to nitrosocompounds. *N*-nitrosamines also have been shown to cause rodent mammary tumors (Rivera et al., 1994; Zarbl et al., 1985; Huggins et al., 1981; el-Bayoumy, 1992), which are histologically similar to human cancers (Thompson et al., 1992; Delp et al., 1990) and can metastasize (Thompson et al., 1992; Rivera et al., 1994). *N*-nitrosamines also can transform cultured mouse mammary cells (Miyamoto et al., 1988; Delp et al., 1990) and cultured human mammary epithelial cells undergo unscheduled DNA synthesis (Eldridge et al., 1992). While it was originally believed that *N*-nitrosamine exposure induced a specific GGA→GAA transition in the 12th codon of the *HRAS1* oncogene (Sukumar et al., 1983; Zarbl et al., 1985), it is more likely that the observed mutation is a result of cell selection for pre-existing mutations (Cha et al., 1994).

Cytochrome P450IIE1 is one of several enzymes responsible for the metabolic activation of *N*-nitrosamines (including tobacco-specific nitrosamines) and other low molecular weight compounds (Yamazaki et al., 1995; Guengerich et al., 1991; Yang et al., 1990; Nouso et al., 1992). The activity of this enzyme varies widely among individuals (Hayashi et al., 1991; Uematsu et al., 1991; Peter et al., 1990). One specific genetic polymorphism is revealed through a *Dra*I restriction enzyme digestion (Uematsu et al., 1991). While clear in vitro data are lacking for evidence that the polymorphic alleles affect function, this polymorphism has been associated with altered protein levels in human liver samples (Uematsu et al., 1994) and increased 7-methyl-2'-deoxyguanosine adduct levels in human lung (Kato et al., 1995). Moreover, this polymorphism has been associated with lung cancer in a Japanese study (Uematsu et al., 1991), including a modification of smoking-related risk (Uematsu et al., 1994), although no effect has been observed in studies of Caucasians in Europe (Persson et al., 1993; Hirvonen et al., 1993a; Kato et al., 1994) and the United States (Kato et al., 1994), or African Americans in the United States (Kato et al., 1994). The polymorphism, however, has not been shown to be associated with either gastric (Uematsu et al., 1994) or nasopharyngeal carcinoma (Hildesheim et al., 1995). In our case-control study of breast cancer (Shields et al., 1996), there was no statistically significant association for the *CYP2E1* and breast cancer risk for pre- or postmenopausal women. However, when women were categorized as non-smokers versus smokers, premenopausal women with one or two C alleles, who had a history of smoking, were found be at increased risk, although the number of study subjects with this genotype was small. Similar findings were not revealed for postmenopausal women.

Cytochrome P450 2D6 is another metabolizing enzyme that might be related to breast cancer, through a tobacco smoking etiology. This enzyme metabolically activates a tobacco-specific *N*-nitrosamine (NNK) (Crespi et al., 1991; Penman et al., 1993), and a relationship to lung cancer and smoking for extensive metabolizers has been reported (Caporaso et al., 1990; Ayesh et al., 1984; Bouchardy et al., 1996). *CYP2D6* activity has been measured phenotypically in breast cancer case control studies. Some studies suggest a risk for poor metabolizer postmenopausal women (Ladero et al., 1991), and in one study when compared to women with benign breast lesions (Pontin et al., 1990). Although one study that used control subjects with benign breast lesions (Huober et al., 1991) did not find an association. *CYP2D6* polymorphisms predicting the poor metabolizer phenotype, measured by PCR, have also been found to be related to breast cancer risk in one study (Ladona et al., 1996) , although not in another (Wolf et al., 1992) that had a poorly defined control group, and another that used volunteers responding to posters (Buchert et al., 1993).

CONCLUSIONS

There is substantial experimental data to suggest that specific environmental carcinogens may be human breast cancer risk factors. The hypothesis that new etiological factors might be identified when studying women as subgroups remains to be proven. However, given that current epidemiological estimates only account for a fraction of breast cancer risk factors, utilization of molecular epidemiological approaches is currently one of the most promising methods. There are already data to implicate exposures such as tobacco smoking in breast cancer etiology, and more will undoubtedly follow.

REFERENCE LIST

Alexandrie A-K, Sundberg MI, Seidegard J, Tornling G, Rannug A (1994): Genetic susceptibility to lung cancer with special emphasis on CYP1A1 and GSTM1: A study on host factors in relation to age at onset, gender and histological cancer types. Carcinogenesis 15:1785-1790.

Allaben WT, Weeks CE, Weis CC, Burger GT, King CM (1982): Rat mammary gland carcinogenesis after local injection of N-hydroxy-N-acyl-2-aminofluorenes: relationship to metabolic activation. Carcinogenesis 3:233-240.

Allaben WT, Weis CC, Fullerton NF, Beland FA (1983): Formation and persistence of DNA adducts from the carcinogen N-hydroxy-2-acetylaminofluorene in rat mammary gland in vivo. Carcinogenesis 4:1067-1070.

Ambrosone CB, Freudenheim JL, Graham S, Marshall JR, Vena JE, Brasure JR, Laughlin R, Nemoto T, Michalek AM, Harrington A, Ford TD, Shields PG (1995a): Cytochrome P4501A1 and glutathione S-transferase (M1) genetic polymorphisms and postmenopausal breast cancer risk. Cancer Res 55:3483-3485.

Ambrosone CB, Freudenheim JL, Marshall JR, Graham S, Vena JE, Brasure JR, Michalek AM, Laughlin R, Nemoto T, Shields PG (1995b): The association of polymorphic N-acetyltransferase (NAT2) with breast cancer risk. Ann N Y Acad Sci 768:250-252.

Ayesh R, Idle JR, Ritchie JC, Crothers MJ, Hetzel MR (1984): Metabolic oxidation phenotypes as markers for susceptibility to lung cancer. Nature 312:169-170.

Badawi AF, Hirvonen A, Bell DA, Lang NP, Kadlubar FF (1995): Role of aromatic amine acetyltransferases, NAT1 and NAT2, in carcinogen-DNA adduct formation in the human urinary bladder. Cancer Res 55:5230-5237.

Bartsch H, Montesano R (1984): Relevance of nitrosamines to human cancer. Carcinogenesis 5:1381-1393.

Bell DA, Taylor JA, Butler MA, Stephens EA, Wiest J, Brubaker LH, Kadlubar FF, Lucier GW (1993a): Genotype/phenotype discordance for human arylamine N-acetyltransferase (NAT2) reveals a new slow-acetylator allele common in African-Americans. Carcinogenesis 14:1689-1692.

Bell DA, Taylor JA, Paulson DF, Robertson CN, Mohler JL, Lucier GW (1993b): Genetic risk and carcinogen exposure: a common inherited defect of the carcinogen-metabolism gene glutathione S-transferase M1 (GSTM1) that increases susceptibility to bladder cancer. J Natl Cancer Inst 85:1159-1164.

Bell DA, Stephens EA, Castranio T, Umbach DM, Watson M, Deakin M, Elder J, Hendrickse C, Duncan H, Strange RC (1995): Polyadenylation polymorphism in the acetyltransferase 1 gene (NAT1) increases risk of colorectal cancer. Cancer Res 55:3537-3542.

Biggs PJ, Warren W, Venitt S, Stratton MR (1993): Does a genotoxic carcinogen contribute to human breast cancer? The value of mutational spectra in unravelling the aetiology of cancer. Mutagenesis 8:275-283.

Blum M, Demierre A, Grant DM, Heim M, Meyer UA (1991): Molecular mechanism of slow acetylation of drugs and carcinogens in humans. Proc Natl Acad Sci U S A 88:5237-5241.

Boring CC, Squires TS, Tong T (1992): Cancer statistics, 1992 [published erratum appears in CA Cancer J Clin 1992 Mar-Apr;42(2):127-8]. CA Cancer J Clin 42:19-38.

Bouchardy C, Benhamou S, Dayer P (1996): The effect of tobacco on lung cancer risk depends on CYP2D6 activity. Cancer Res 56:251-253.

Boyle P, Leake R (1988). Progress in understanding breast cancer: epidemiological and biological interactions. Br Canc Res Trt 11:91-112

Buchert ET, Woosley RL, Swain SM, Oliver SJ, Coughlin SS, Pickle L, Trock B, Riegel AT(1993): Relationship of CYP2D6 (debrisoquine hydroxylase) genotype to breast cancer susceptibility. Pharmacogenetics 3:322-327.

Buell P (1973): Changing incidence of breast cancer in Japanese-American women. J Natl Cancer Inst 51:1479-1483.

Caporaso NE, Tucker MA, Hoover R, Hayes RB, Pickle LW, Issaq H, Muschik G, Green-Gallo L, Buivys D, Aisner S, Resau J, Trump BF, Tollerud D, Weston A, Harris CC (1990): Lung cancer and the debrisoquine metabolic phenotype. J Natl Cancer Inst 85:1264-1272.

Cartwright RA(1984), Epidemiological studies on N-acetylation and C-center ring oxidation in neoplasia. In (eds): Omenn GS, Gelboin HV Genetic Variability in Responses to Chemical Exposure. Cold Spring Harbor, NY: Cold Spring Harbor Press, pp 359-368.

Cavalieri E, Rogan E, Sinha D (1988): Carcinogenicity of aromatic hydrocarbons directly applied to rat mammary gland. J Cancer Res Clin Oncol 114:3-9.

Cha RS, Thilly WG, Zarbl H (1994): N-nitroso-N-methylurea-induced rat mammary tumors arise from cells with pre-existing oncogenic Ha-ras-1 gene mutations. Proc Natl Acad Sci USA 91:3749-3753.

Chatterjee M, Banerjee MR (1982): Selenium mediated dose-inhibition of 7,12-dimethylbenz[a] anthracene-induced transformation of mammary cells in organ culture. Cancer Lett 17:187-195.

Crespi CL, Penman BW, Gelboin HV, Gonzalez FJ (1991): A tobacco smoke-derived nitrosamine, 4-(methylnitrosamino)-1-(3-pyridyl)-1-butanone, is activated by multiple human cytochrome P450s including the polymorphic human cytochrome P4502D6. Carcinogenesis 12:1197-1201.

Davis CD, Ghoshal A, Schut HA, Snyderwine EG (1994): Metabolic activation of heterocyclic amine food mutagens in the mammary gland of lactating Fischer 344 rats. Cancer Lett 84:67-73.

Delp CR, Treves JS, Banerjee MR (1990): Neoplastic transformation and DNA damage of mouse mammary epithelial cells by N-methyl-N'-nitrosourea in organ culture. Cancer Let 55:31-37.

el-Bayoumy K (1992): Environmental carcinogens that may be involved in human breast cancer etiology. Chem Res Toxicol 5:585-590.

Eldridge SR, Gould MN, Butterworth BE (1992): Genotoxicity of environmental agents in human mammary epithelial cells. Chemical Industry Institute of Toxicology, Research Triangle Park, North Carolina 27709. Cancer Res 52:5617-5620.

Feuer EJ, Wun LM, Boring CC, Flanders WD, Timmel MJ, Tong T (1993): The lifetime risk of developing breast cancer [see comments]. J Natl Cancer Inst 85:892-897.

Fong LY, Jensen DE, Magee PN (1990): DNA methyl-adduct dosimetry and O6-alkylguanine-DNA alkyl transferase activity determinations in rat mammary carcinogenesis by procarbazine and N-methylnitrosourea. Carcinogenesis 11:411-417.

Ghoshal A, Snyderwine EG (1993): Excretion of food-derived heterocyclic amine carcinogens into breast milk of lactating rats and formation of DNA adducts in the newborn. Carcinogenesis 14:2199-2203.

Gonzalez MJ, Schemmel RA, Dugan L, Jr., Gray JI, Welsch CW (1993): Dietary fish oil inhibits human breast carcinoma growth: a function of increased lipid peroxidation. Lipids 28:827-832.

Gould MN (1982): Chemical carcinogen activation in the rat mammary gland: intra-organ cell specificity. Carcinogenesis 3:667-669.

Guengerich FP, Kim DH, Iwasaki M (1991): Role of human cytochrome P-450 IIE1 in the oxidation of many low molecular weight cancer suspects. Chem Res Toxicol 4:168-179.

Hamada GS, Sugimura H, Suzuki I, Nagura K, Kiyokawa E, Iwase T, Tanaka M, Takahashi T, Watanabe S, Kino I (1995): The heme-binding region polymorphism of cytochrome P450IA1 (CypIA1), rather than the RsaI polymorphism of IIE1 (CypIIE1), is associated with lung cancer in Rio de Janeiro. Cancer Epidemiol Biomarkers Prev 4:63-67.

Hanssen HP, Agarwal DP, Goedde HW, Bucher H, Huland H, Brachmann W, Ovenbeck R (1985): Association of N-acetyltransferase polymorphism and environmental factors with bladder carcinogenesis. Study in a north German population. Eur Urol 11:263-266.

Harris CC (1989): Interindividual variation among humans in carcinogen metabolism, DNA adduct formation and DNA repair. Carcinogenesis 10:1563-1566.

Harris JR, Lippman ME, Veronesi U, Willett W (1992): Breast cancer (1). N Engl J Med 327:319-328.

Hasegawa R, Sano M, Tamano S, Imaida K, Shirai T, Nagao M, Sugimura T, Ito N (1993): Dose-dependence of 2-amino-1-methyl-6-phenylimidazo[4,5-b]-pyridine (PhIP) carcinogenicity in rats. Carcinogenesis 14:2553-2557.

Hayashi S, Watanabe J, Kawajiri K (1991): Genetic polymorphisms in the 5'-flanking region change transcriptional regulation of the human cytochrome P450IIE1 gene. J Biochem (Tokyo) 110:559-565.

Hein DW (1988): Acetylator genotype and arylamine-induced carcinogenesis. Biochim Biophys Acta 948:37-66.

Hildesheim A, Chen C-J, Caporaso NE, Cheng Y-J, Hoover RN, Hsu M-M, Levine PH, Chen I-H, Chen J-Y, Yang C-S, Daly AK, Idle JR (1995): Cytochrome P4502E1 genetic polymorphisms and risk of nasopharyngeal carcinoma: results from a case-control study conducted in Taiwan. CEBP 4:607-610.

Hirvonen A, Husgafvel-Pursiainen K, Anttila S, Karjalainen A, Vainio H (1993a): The human CYP2E1 gene and lung cancer: DraI and RsaI restriction fragment length polymorphisms in a Finnish study population. Carcinogenesis 14:85-88.

Hirvonen A, Husgafvel-Pursiainen K, Anttila S, Vainio H (1993b): The GSTM1 null genotype as a potential risk modifier for squamous cell carcinoma of the lung. Carcinogenesis 14:1479-1481.

Holme JA, Wallin H, Brunborg G, Soderlund EJ, Hongslo JK, Alexander J (1989): Genotoxicity of the food mutagen 2-amino-1-methyl-6-phenylimidazo[4,5-b]pyridine (PhIP): formation of 2-hydroxamino-PhIP, a directly acting genotoxic metabolite. Carcinogenesis 10:1389-1396.

Huggins CB, Ueda N, Wiessler M (1981): N-Nitroso-N-methylurea elicits mammary cancer in resistant and sensitive rat strains. Proc Natl Acad Sci U S A 78:1185-1188.

Huober J, Bertram B, Petru E, Kaufmann M, Schm:ahl D (1991): Metabolism of debrisoquine and susceptibility to breast cancer. Breast Cancer Res Treat 18:43-48.

Ilett KF, David BM, Detchon P, Castleden WM, Kwa R (1987): Acetylation phenotype in colorectal carcinoma. Cancer Res 47:1466-1469.

Ito N, Hasegawa R, Sano M, Tamano S, Esumi H, Takayama S, Sugimura T (1991): A new colon and mammary carcinogen in cooked food, 2-amino-1-methyl 6-phenylimidazo[4,5-b]pyridine (PhIP). Carcinogenesis 12:1503-1506.

Kadlubar FF, Butler MA, Kaderlik KR, Chou HC, Lang NP (1992): Polymorphisms for aromatic amine metabolism in humans: relevance for human carcinogenesis. Environ Health Perspect 98:69-74.

Kadlubar FF (1994): Biochemical individuality and its implications for drug and carcinogen metabolism: recent insights from acetyltransferase and cytochrome P4501A2 phenotyping and genotyping in humans. Drug Metab Rev 26:37-46.

Kato S, Shields PG, Caporaso NE, Sugimura H, Trivers GE, Tucker MA, Trump BF, Weston A, Harris CC (1994): Analysis of cytochrome P450 2E1 genetic polymorphisms in relation to human lung cancer. Cancer Epidemiol Biomarkers & Prev 3:515-518.

Kato S, Bowman ED, Harrington AM, Blomeke B, Shields PG (1995): Human lung carcinogen-DNA adduct levels mediated by genetic polymorphisms in vivo. JNCI 87:902-907.

Kato T, Migita H, Ohgaki H, Sato S, Takayama S, Sugimura T (1989): Induction of tumors in the Zymbal gland, oral cavity, colon, skin and mammary gland of F344 rats by a mutagenic compound, 2-amino-3,4-dimethylimidazo[4,5-f]quinoline. Carcinogenesis 10:601-603.

Kelsey JL, Gammon MD (1990): Epidemiology of breast cancer. Epidemiol Rev 12:228-240.

King CM, Traub NR, Lortz ZM, Thissen MR (1979): Metabolic activation of arylhydroxamic acids by N-O-acyltransferase of rat mammary gland. Cancer Res 39:3369-3372.

Ladero JM, Benitez J, Jara C, Llerena A, Valdivielso MJ, Munoz JJ, Vargas E (1991): Polymorphic oxidation of debrisoquine in women with breast cancer. Oncology 48:107-110.

Ladona MG, Abildua RE, Ladero JM, Roman JM, Plaza MA, Agundez JA, Munoz JJ, Benitez J (1996): CYP2D6 genotypes in Spanish women with breast cancer. Cancer Lett 99:23-28.

Lang NP, Butler MA, Massengill J, Lawson M, Stotts RC, Hauer-Jensen M, Kadlubar FF (1994): Rapid metabolic phenotypes for acetyltransferase and cytochrome P4501A2 and putative exposure to food-borne heterocyclic amines increase the risk for colorectal cancer or polyps. Cancer Epidemiol Biomarkers Prev 3:675-682.

Li D, Wang M, Dhingra K, Hittelman WN (1996): Aromatic DNA adducts in adjacent t tissues of breast cancer patients: clues to breast cancer etiology. Cancer Res 56:287-293.

MacMahon B, Trichopoulos D, Cole P, Brown J (1982): Cigarette smoking and urinary estrogens. N Engl J Med 307:1062-1065.

MacNicoll AD, Easty GC, Neville AM, Grover PL, Sims P (1980): Metabolism and activation of carcinogenic polycyclic hydrocarbons by human mammary cells. Biochem Biophys Res Commun 95:1599-1606.

Madigan MP, Ziegler RG, Benichou J, Byrne C, Hoover RN (1996): Proportion of breast cancer cases in the United States explained by well-established risk factors. JNCI 87:1681-1685.

Mannervik B, Danielson UH (1988): Glutathione transferases--structure and catalytic activity. CRC Crit Rev Biochem 23:283-337.

Marshall E (1993): The politics of breast cancer [news]. Science 259:616-617.

Miyamoto S, Guzman RC, Osborn RC, Nandi S (1988): Neoplastic transformation of mouse mammary epithelial cells by in vitro exposure to N-methyl-N-nitrosourea. Proc Natl Acad Sci USA 85:477-481.

Mommsen S, Aagard J (1983): Tobacco as a risk factor in bladder cancer. Carcinogenesis 4:335-338.

Morris JJ, Seifter E (1992): The role of aromatic hydrocarbons in the genesis of breast cancer. Med Hypotheses 38:177-184.

Nebert DW (1991): Role of genetics and drug metabolism in human cancer risk. Mutat Res 247:267-281.

Nouso K, Thorgeirsson SS, Battula N (1992): Stable expression of human cytochrome P450IIE1 in mammalian cells: metabolic activation of nitrosodimethylamine and formation of adducts with cellular DNA. Cancer Res 52:1796-1800.

Obana H, Hori S, Kashimoto T, Kunita N (1981): Polycyclic aromatic hydrocarbons in human fat and liver. Bull Environ Contam Toxicol 27:23-27.

Office on Smoking and Health (1996): Smoking and Health. A report to the Surgeon General of the Public Health Services. (Abstract)

Palmer JR, Rosenberg L (1993): Cigarette smoking and the risk of breast cancer. Epidemiologic Rev 15:145-156.

Penman BW, Reece J, Smith T, Yang CS, Gelboin HV, Gonzalez FJ, Crespi CL (1993): Characterization of a human cell line expressing high levels of cDNA-derived CYP2D6. Pharmacogenetics 3:28-39.

Perera FP, Estabrook A, Hewer A, Channing K, Rundle A, Mooney LA, Whyatt R, Phillips DH (1995): Carcinogen-DNA adducts in human breast tissue. Cancer Epidemiol Biomarkers Prev 4:233-238.

Persson I, Johansson I, Bergling H, Dahl ML, Seidegard J, Rylander R, Rannug A, Hogberg J, Sundberg MI (1993): Genetic polymorphism of cytochrome P4502E1 in a Swedish population. Relationship to incidence of lung cancer. FEBS Lett 319:207-211.

Peter R, Bocker R, Beaune PH, Iwasaki M, Guengerich FP, Yang CS (1990): Hydroxylation of chlorzoxazone as a specific probe for human liver cytochrome P-450IIE1. Chem Res Toxicol 3:566-573.

Petrakis NL, Gruenke LD, Beelen TC, Castagnoli N, Jr., Craig JC (1978): Nicotine in breast fluid of nonlactating women. Science 199:303-305.

Petrakis NL, Maack CA, Lee RE, Lyon M (1980): Mutagenic activity in nipple aspirates of human breast fluid [letter]. Cancer Res 40:188-189.

Pfau W, O'Hare MJ, Grover PL, Phillips DH (1992): Metabolic activation of the food mutagens 2-amino-3-methylimidazo[4,5-f]quinoline (IQ) and 2-amino-3,4-dimethylimidazo[4,5-f]quinoline (MeIQ) to DNA binding species in human mammary epithelial cells. Carcinogenesis 13:907-909.

Pontin JE, Hamed H, Fentiman IS, Idle JR (1990): Cytochrome P450dbl phenotypes in malignant and benign breast disease. Eur J Cancer 26:790-792.

Reddy BS, Rivenson A (1993): Inhibitory effect of Bifidobacterium longum on colon, mammary, and liver carcinogenesis induced by 2-amino-3-methylimidazo[4,5-f]quinoline, a food mutagen. Cancer Res 53:3914-3918.

Rivera ES, Andrade N, Martin G, Melito G, Cricco G, Mohamad N, Davio C, Caro R, Bergoc RM (1994): Induction of mammary tumors in rat by intraperitoneal injection of NMU: histopathology and estral cycle influence. Cancer Let 86:223-228.

Rose DP, Connolly JM (1993): Effects of dietary omega-3 fatty acids on human breast cancer growth and metastases in nude mice. J Natl Cancer Inst 85:1743-1747.

Sadrieh N, Davis CD, Snyderwine EG (1996): N-Acetyltransferase expression and metabolic activation of the food-derived heterocyclic amines in the human mammary gland. Cancer Res 56:2683-2687.

Shields PG, Ambrosone CB, Graham S, Bowman ED, Harrington AM, Gillenwater KA, Marshall JR, Vena JE, Laughlin R, Nemoto T, Freudenheim JL (1996): A cytochrome P450IIE1 genetic polymorphism (CYP2E1) and tobacco smoking in breast cancer. Mol.Carcinogenesis (In press)

Shirai T, Fysh JM, Lee MS, Vaught JB, King CM (1981): Relationship of metabolic activation of N-hydroxy-N-acylarylamines to biological response in the liver and mammary gland of the female CD rat. Cancer Res 41:4346-4353.

Snyderwine EG (1994): Some perspectives on the nutritional aspects of breast cancer research. Food-derived heterocyclic amines as etiologic agents in human mammary cancer. Cancer 74:1070-1077.

Stampfer MR, Bartholomew JC, Smith HS, Bartley JC (1981): Metabolism of benzo[a] pyrene by human mammary epithelial cells: toxicity and DNA adduct formation. Proc Natl Acad Sci U S A 78:6251-6255.

Sugimura T (1986): Past, present, and future of mutagens in cooked foods. Environ Health Perspect 67:5-10.

Sukumar S, Notario V, Martin-Zanca D, Barbacid M (1983): Induction of mammary carcinomas in rats by nitroso-methylurea involves malignant activation of H-ras-1 locus by single point mutations. Nature 306:658-661.

Swaminathan S, Frederickson SM, Hatcher JF (1994): Metabolic activation of N-hydroxy-4-acetylaminobiphenyl by cultured human breast epithelial cell line MCF 10A. Carcinogenesis 15:611-617.

Tanaka T, Barnes WS, Williams GM, Weisburger JH (1985): Multipotential carcinogenicity of the fried food mutagen 2-amino-3-methylimidazo[4,5-f]quinoline in rats. Jpn J Cancer   Res 76:570-576.

Taylor JA, Umbach DM, Stephens E, Paulson D, Robertson C, Mohler JL, Bell DA (1995): The role of N-acetylation polymorphisms at NAT1 and NAT2 in smoking-associated bladder cancer. Proc Am Assoc Cancer Res 36:282(Abstract)

Thompson HJ, Adlakha H, Singh M (1992): Effect of carcinogen dose and age at administration on induction of mammary carcinogenesis by 1-methyl-1-nitrosourea. Carcinogenesis 13:1535-1539.

Thompson LH, Tucker JD, Stewart SA, Christensen ML, Salazar EP, Carrano AV, Felton JS (1987): Genotoxicity of compounds from cooked beef in repair-deficient CHO cells versus Salmonella mutagenicity. Mutagenesis 2:483-487.

Tonelli QJ, Custer RP, Sorof S (1979): Transformation of cultured mouse mammary glands by aromatic amines and amides and their derivatives. Cancer Res 39:1784-1792.

Uematsu F, Kikuchi H, Motomiya M, Abe T, Sagami I, Ohmachi T, Wakui A, Kanamaru R, Watanabe M (1991): Association between restriction fragment length polymorphism of the human cytochrome P450IIE1 gene and susceptibility to lung cancer. Jpn J Cancer Res 82:254-256.

Uematsu F, Ikawa S, Kikuchi H, Sagami I, Kanamaru R, Abe T, Satoh K, Motomiya M, Watanabe M (1994): Restriction fragment length polymorphism of the human CYP2E1 (cytochrome P450IIE1) gene and susceptibility to lung cancer: possible relevance to low smoking exposure. Pharmacogenetics 4:58-63.

Vineis P, Caporaso N, Tannenbaum SR, Skipper PL, Glogowski J, Bartsch H, Coda M, Talaska G, Kadlubar F (1990): Acetylation phenotype, carcinogen-hemoglobin adducts, and cigarette smoking. Cancer Res 50:3002-3004.

Vineis P, Bartsch H, Caporaso N, Harrington AM, Kadlubar FF, Landi MT, Malaveille C, Shields PG, Skipper P, Talaska G, et al (1994): Genetically based N-acetyltransferase metabolic polymorphism and low-level environmental exposure to carcinogens. Nature 369:154-156.

Wang CY, Yamada H, Morton KC, Zukowski K, Lee MS, King CM (1988): Induction of repair synthesis of DNA in mammary and urinary bladder epithelial cells by N-hydroxy derivatives of carcinogenic arylamines. Cancer Res 48:4227-4232.

Willett W (1989): The search for the causes of breast and colon cancer. Nature 338:389-394.

Wolf CR, Smith CA, Gough AC, Moss JE, Vallis KA, Howard G, Carey FJ, Mills K, McNeeW, Carmichael J, et al (1992): Relationship between the debrisoquine hydroxylase polymorphism and cancer susceptibility. Carcinogenesis 13:1035-1038.

Yamazaki H, Inui Y, Yun CH, Guengerich FP, Shimada T (1995): Cytochrome P450 2E1 and 2A6 enzymes as major catalysts for metabolic activation of N-nitrosodialkylamines and tobacco-related nitrosamines in human liver microsomes. Carcinogenesis 13:1789-1794.

Yang CS, Yoo JS, Ishizaki H, Hong JY (1990): Cytochrome P450IIE1: roles in nitrosamine metabolism and mechanisms of regulation. Drug Metab Rev 22:147-159.

Yu MC, Skipper PL, Taghizadeh K, Tannenbaum SR, Chan KK, Henderson BE, Ross RK (1994): Acetylator phenotype, aminobiphenyl-hemoglobin adduct levels, and bladder cancer risk in white, black, and Asian men in Los Angeles, California. J Natl Cancer Inst 86:712-716.

Yuspa SH, Poirier MC (1988): Chemical carcinogenesis: from animal models to molecular models in one decade. Adv Cancer Res 50:25-70.

Zarbl H, Sukumar S, Arthur AV, Martin-Zanca D, Barbacid M (1985): Direct mutagenesis of Ha-ras-1 oncogenes by N-nitroso-N-methylurea during initiation of mammary carcinogenesis in rats. Nature 315:382-385.

Etiology of Breast and
Gynecological Cancers, pages 101–113
© 1997 Wiley-Liss, Inc.

MOLECULAR PERSPECTIVES ON CANCER, THE CELL CYCLE AND THE INHERITED DISORDER *ATAXIA-TELANGIECTASIA*

Kevin D. Brown, Ph.D. and Danilo A. Tagle, Ph.D.

Laboratory of Gene Transfer, National Center for Human Genome Research, National Institutes of Health, Bethesda, MD 20892.

ABSTRACT

Ataxia-Telangiectasia (A-T) is an autosomal recessive disorder which presents a wide array of clinical symptoms including enhanced cancer predisposition and progressive cerebellar degeneration leading to general neuromotor dysfunction. The A-T cellular phenotype consists of higher levels of chromosome breakage, increased sensitivity to ionizing radiation and radiomimetic drugs, and defective cell cycle checkpoints in response to genome damage. Positional-cloning of the gene mutated in A-T, designated ATM, identified a 13 kb transcript encoding a 3056 amino acid protein which possesses a carboxy-terminal domain with distinct homology to phosphatidylinositol-3 kinase. Furthermore, ATM related proteins have been identified in yeast, *Drosophila* and other mammalian species which are involved in cell cycle control and cellular responses to DNA damage. Development of cellular and animal models for A-T can serve to better dissect the role and involvement of ATM in cell cycle regulation, cancer development, neuronal cell death and other hallmark symptoms of this disorder.

INTRODUCTION

Ataxia-telangiectasia (A-T) is a human autosomal recessive disorder which occurs with a frequency of 1:40,000 to 1:100,000 births in the United States. Patients afflicted with A-T present a wide range of clinical symptoms, chief among these are the development of oculocutaneous telangiectasias and progressive cerebellar degeneration. Other symptoms include extreme radiosensitivity, immunodeficiency, endocrine disorders, progeric changes to the skin, gonadal abnormalities, and marked cancer predisposition (reviewed in Sedgwick and Boder 1991, Shiloh 1995). Cerebellar ataxia first appears in early childhood and progressively worsens, generally confining patients to a wheelchair by the second decade of life. Owing to reduced immune function, many A-T patients show recurrent sinopulmonary infections and succumb to respiratory failure or cancer during the second or third decade of life.

In this chapter we will highlight recent advances which serve to create a framework of understanding concerning the molecular basis for the hereditary disease ataxia-telangiectasia. This body of evidence not only advances our knowledge of the underlying causes of A-T and the basis for the high rates of cancer observed in this disorder, but also strengthens our insights into the more general molecular mechanisms governing cancer formation.

Clinical Features of A-T

A-T patients show signs of ataxia in early childhood and later develop conjunctival telangiectases, sinopulmonary infections, and malignancies. Telangiectases typically develop between 3 and 5 years of age. Neurologic dysfunction is a clinically invariable feature with choreoathetosis and/or dystonia occurring in 90% of patients (Woods and Taylor, 1992). A-T patients show immune deficiencies and hypoplasia of the thymus gland. Serum IgG2 or IgA levels are diminished or absent in 80% and 60% of patients, respectively (Gatti et al., 1991). Waldmann and McIntire (1972) showed elevated levels of alpha-fetoprotein in the blood of A-T patients and suggested that this may be due to immaturity of the liver which is consistent with the view of a primary defect in tissue differentiation. Consistent with this is the observation by Carbonari et al. (1990) that A-T patients have more circulating T cells bearing gamma/delta receptors characteristic of immature cells than the alpha/beta receptors typical of mature cells.

Patients with A-T have a strong predisposition to malignancy, predominantly of lymphomas and lymphocytic leukemias (Taylor et al., 1996). In general, lymphomas in A-T patients tend to be of B-cell origin, whereas the leukemias tend to be of the T-cell type. Bigbee et al. (1989) demonstrated an increased frequency of somatic cell mutation in vivo in individuals with A-T. Obligate heterozygotes for the disease showed significantly higher cancer incidence rates than spouse controls (Swift et al., 1987; 1991) with breast cancer in women clearly associated with heterozygosity for A-T. A synopsis (Easton, 1994) of similar studies (Swift et al. 1987, 1991; Pippard et al, 1988; Borresen et al., 1990) gave an overall 3.9 fold estimated relative risk of breast cancer in A-T heterozygotes. Although this risk is much lower than other breast cancer susceptibility genes (i.e., p53, BRCA1 and BRCA2--Szabo and King, 1995), mutations in the A-T gene may account for a higher proportion of breast cancer cases given the relatively higher carrier frequency of A-T.

IDENTIFICATION OF THE A-T GENE: CLUES AS TO FUNCTION

After a long and arduous process involving complementation cloning and positional cloning (summarized in Shiloh, 1995 and references therein), the defective gene for A-T was recently cloned and sequenced (Savitsky et al, 1995a, b). This gene, designated ATM (for A-T mutated), resides on human chromosome 11, region q22-23. The transcript is 13 kb long and is encoded in 66 exons distributed in a genomic interval of roughly 150 kb (Uziel et al., in press). Furthermore, this gene was found to be mutated in A-T patients from the 4 complementation groups (Jaspers et al., 1988), implying that the identified gene is solely responsible for the disease. Analysis of ATM cDNA shows it to possess a ~9.2 kb open reading frame which encodes a putative protein of ~350 kD (Savitsky et al., 1995b). The carboxy-terminal region of the ATM gene product displays high sequence homology to the catalytic domain of phosphatidylinositol-3 kinases (PI-3 K). Interestingly, mutations in A-T are not clustered in the PI-3K domain but show heterogeneity throughout the entire gene (Savitsky *et al.*, 1995b; Byrd *et al.*, 1996; Gilad *et al.*, in press). Regardless, the majority (80%) of the mutations identified in A-T patients contained frameshift mutations which lead to premature termination of the ATM gene product prior to or within the carboxy-terminally located PI-3 kinase domain (Gilad *et al.*, in press). Additionally, these workers also found a patient with a missense mutation which leads to a glutamine to glycine substitution within a highly conserved portion of the predicted PI-3 kinase domain. Taken together, these results directly implicate the importance of the predicted catalytic activity of ATM in its function.

The PI-3 Kinase-Like Protein Family

Sequence comparisons of the predicted ATM gene product shows it to be a member of a growing family of large proteins which share within their primary structure sequence homology to the catalytic domain of phosphotidylinositol-3 kinase (Table I). Owing to this structural similarity to lipid kinases, these proteins have been designated PI-3 kinase (PI3K)-like proteins. In the budding yeast *Saccharomyces cerevisiae* four such PI3K-like proteins have been identified to date. The TEL1 gene is involved in monitoring and controlling telomere length (Lustig and Petes, 1986; Greenwell *et al.*, 1995). MEC1 (a.k.a. ESR1) is an essential gene required for G2 arrest following DNA damage and incomplete DNA replication in *S. cerevisiae* (Weinert *et al.*, 1994; Kato and Ogawa, 1994). Interestingly, while TEL1 activity is itself non-essential, TEL1 can rescue viability of MEC1 mutants, indicating that the products of these two genes are functionally related (Morrow *et al.*, 1995). In the fission yeast *Schizosaccharomyces pombe* the rad3 gene is required for S and G2 cell cycle checkpoint control following DNA damage (Al-Khodairy and Carr, 1992; Jiminez *et al.*, 1992; Enoch *et al.*, 1992; Seaton *et al.*, 1992) and is currently viewed as the functional homolog of the *S. cerevisiae* gene MEC1 in this organism.

The TOR proteins (TOR1, TOR2) of *S. cerevisiae* and their mammalian homologs mTOR and FRAP were identified as targets of the immunosuppresant drug rapamycin (Heitman *et al.*, 1991; Cafferkey, *et al.*, 1993; Kunz *et al.*, 1993; Brown *et al.*, 1994; Sabatini *et al.*, 1994; Sabers *et al.*, 1995). Rapamycin has been shown to block cellular events which lead to transition from G1 to S-phase (Morice *et al.*, 1993; Terada *et al.*, 1993), suggesting that these proteins play a role in this process. Consistent with this, disruption of both TOR1 and TOR2 lead to G1-phase arrest (Kunz *et al.*, 1993; Helliwell *et al.*, 1994).

Mutants of the MEI-41 gene in *D. melanogaster* were first identified as having a defect in meiotic recombination (Baker and Carpenter, 1972). Subsequently, these mutants were found to display marked sensitivity to a wide range of mutagens and high levels of chromosome breakage in mitotic cells (Boyd *et al.*, 1976; Gatti, 1979; Banga *et al.*, 1986). More recently, somatic cells from MEI-41 mutants were shown to be deficient in radiation-induced cell cycle arrest (Hari *et al.*, 1995).

The catalytic subunit of DNA-dependent protein kinase (DNA-PK$_{cs}$) was first characterized in humans but has subsequently been identified in a wide rage of eukaryotic species (for review see Anderson and Lees-Miller, 1992) and has recently been shown to be member of the PI3K-like family (Hartley *et al.*, 1995). This protein,

Table 1: The PI-3 Kinase-Like Family

Gene Product	Organism	M_r	Carboxy-terminal domain* % identity / similarity
ATM	Human	~ 350 kD	100 / 100
TEL 1	S. cerevisiae	~ 300 kD	45 / 67
MEC1	S. cerevisiae	~ 260 kD	37 / 63
rad3	S. pombe	~ 260 kD	38 / 59
MEI-41	D. melanogaster	~ 260 kD	37 / 59
TOR1	S. cerevisiae	~ 270 kD	33 / 58
TOR2	S. cerevisiae	~ 270 kD	35 / 60
mTOR	Rat	~ 280 kD	32 / 59
DNA-PK$_{cs}$	Human	~ 450 kD	28 / 51

* Comparison of the homologous carboxy-terminal 350 residues including the kinase domain to the ATM protein.

when complexed to the autoantigen Ku, is catalytically activated by binding to single and double strand breaks in DNA (Gottleib and Jackson, 1993; Morozov *et al.*, 1994) and plays a crucial role in V(D)J recombination and DNA double strand break repair (see Jeggo *et al.*, 1995). Furthermore, mutations in DNA-PK$_{cs}$ are responsible for the marked sensitivity to ionizing radiation, immune deficiency, and impaired DNA strand break repair characteristics of severe immunodeficiency (scid) mice (Blunt *et al.*, 1995). While the physiologic actions of DNA-PK are not fully elucidated, the observations that it phosphorylates several transcription factors *in vitro* (see Anderson and Lees-Miller, 1992) and is a potent inhibitor of RNA polymerase I (Kuhn *et al.*, 1995; Labhart, 1995) suggests it may modulate transcription.

While the homology of ATM and its family members to PI-3 kinase is unequivocal, the ability of many of these proteins to phosphorylate phosphoinositol (or any other lipid) is currently debatable (see Hunter, 1995). For instance, DNA-PK has been shown to phosphorylate proteins, but no detectable lipid kinase activity was detected (Hartley *et al.*, 1995), and the TOR2 gene product fails to show an intrinsic ability to phosphorylate lipid (Brown *et al.*, 1995). Further studies will be required to understand the substrate specificities of the PI3K-like family members. While elucidation of the substrate targets for these proteins is of keen interest in fully understanding their functions, a clear picture of functional relatedness has begun to emerge. Each these family members, with the possible exception of the TEL1 gene product, plays an important role in either sensing genome damage or controlling cell cycle advance.

ROLE OF THE ATM GENE PRODUCT IN CELL CYCLE CONTROL

Cells posses the ability to delay the cell cycle following damage to their DNA as a result of exposure to DNA damaging events, such as ionizing radiation (IR) or drugs which mimic the effects of IR (*i.e.*, radiomimetic drugs). There appear to be two distinct points of cell cycle arrest; one, during G1 prior to entry into S-phase and two, during G2 prior to mitosis (see Hartwell and Weinert, 1989; Murray, 1992). The former of these arrest points (termed checkpoints) presumably exists to prevent replication of damaged DNA while the latter checkpoint serves to prevent the segregation of damaged DNA into subsequent daughter cells. The widely accepted view is that these cell cycle delays allow DNA repair mechanisms time to correct genomic damage and thus limit heritable genetic errors.

It has long been established that DNA damage due to IR exposure strongly inhibits DNA synthesis in normal cells (Painter and Young, 1975). However, A-T cells continue to undergo DNA synthesis following radiation-induced DNA damage (Painter and Young, 1980; Houldsworth and Lavin, 1980; Painter, 1981), a phenomenon referred to as radioresistant DNA synthesis (RDS). The fact that A-T cells display RDS indicates that these cells possess a faulty checkpoint within S-phase which delays replication after irradiation (a phenotype shared with *S. cerevisiae* MEC1 mutants-- Paulovich and Hartwell, 1995). Furthermore, when assayed directly, A-T cells were found to show no delay in G1 to S-phase progression following DNA damage (Little and Nagasawa, 1985; Rudoph and Latt, 1989; Beamish *et al.*, 1994) indicating that A-T cells are also defective in the G1 checkpoint which normally delays cell cycle advance in response to DNA damage.

While overwhelming evidence supports the view that A-T cells possess both a defective G1 and S-phase checkpoint mechanism, characterization of a similar lesion in A-T cells at the G2 checkpoint has not been quite as straightforward. For instance, studies on the progression of A-T cells into mitosis following IR showed that these cells exhibit no delay in entry into mitosis following IR when compared to normal cells (Zampetti-Bosseler and Scott, 1981; Scott and Zampetti-Bosseler, 1982; Paules *et al.*, 1995) while other groups have shown that, post-irradiation, A-T cells show a prolonged G2 arrest (Ford *et al.*, 1984; Bates and Lavin, 1989; Beamish and Lavin, 1994; Hong *et al.*, 1994; Lavin *et al.*, 1994; Beamish *et al.*, 1994). The apparent discrepancies in these observations stem from differences in the cell cycle stage of the cells at the time of irradiation. Cells in G2 at the time of irradiation enter mitosis while normal cells arrest prior to entering mitosis. Conversely, when A-T cells are irradiated prior to entry into G2 they are subjected to G2 arrest. These observations suggest two possibilities: *a*) as previously suggested (Paules *et al.*, 1995), A-T cells irradiated prior to G2 suffer such massive genomic damage that they are rendered incapable of entering cell division, or *b*) there exists two checkpoints during G2, one early in G2 that is functional in A-T cells and one that functions later in G2 to delay entry into mitosis which is defective in A-T cells. Further experiments are required to adequately delineate among these possibilities. Nevertheless, it is clear that A-T cells lack cell cycle checkpoints which normally function during G1, S and G2 in response to DNA damage.

The molecular basis behind the cell cycle defects in A-T cells is largely unknown, however, a few key facts have come to light. For instance, Kastan *et al.* (1992), Khanna and Lavin (1993), and Canman *et al.*, (1994) observed that following IR exposure A-T cells show a clear defect in their ability to upregulate their cellular pools of p53. p53 has been shown to be required for the G1 checkpoint in mammalian cells (Kuerbitz *et al.*, 1992) presumably by acting as a transcription factor (Fields and Yang, 1990; Raycroft *et al.*, 1990; Kern *et al.*, 1991) responsible for initiating the transcription of, among others, the cell growth suppressor GADD45 (Zhan *et al.*, 1994) and p21[WAF1/CIP1], a potent inhibitor of cyclin dependent kinase activity (Harper *et al.*, 1993; El-Deiry *et al.*, 1993). Moreover, elevation of cellular p21$^{WAF1/CIP1}$ levels has been shown to result in a delay in the cyclin E-cdk2 mediated advance into S phase (Dulic *et al.*, 1994).

While these observations form a framework for understanding the nature of the defect in the G1 and S-phase checkpoints in A-T cells, they fail to address the basis for the observed lack of an irradiation-induced G2 checkpoint in A-T cells. For instance, low passage embryonic cells from mice in which both copies of their p53 alleles have been disrupted by homologous recombination show a normal G2 delay following exposure to IR (Paules *et al.*, 1995) indicating that p53 does not play a direct role, *per se*, in the establishment of the G2 checkpoint. Interestingly, these workers did find that high passage fibroblasts from p53 null mice displayed a greatly reduced G2 checkpoint function. This observation led to the suggestion that cells which suffer loss of the G1 checkpoint (as a consequence of lost p53 function) may, over time, lose certain aspects of their G2 checkpoint control. Since A-T cells have an impaired ability to upregulate their cellular levels of p53 following irradiation, it is certainly consistent with this possibility that the loss of G2 checkpoint function in cultured A-T cells may be an indirect result of their impaired G1 checkpoint control. Clearly, testing this possibility will require development of an A-T model in laboratory animals where cells can be cultured under the most stringent conditions.

What is the function of the ATM gene product? As discussed above, cells derived from patients afflicted with A-T show an impaired ability to delay cell cycle advance following DNA damage as a result of exposure to ionizing radiation. Interestingly, A-T cells show no sensitivity to other potentially DNA damaging events such as UV radiation or the alkylating carcinogen methylmethane sulfonate (MMS) since p53 upregulation in A-T cells following exposure to these agents was normal (Khanna and Lavin 1993; Artuso *et al.*, 1995). Furthermore, A-T cells do not appear to be defective in DNA repair mechanisms since these cells show normal rates of break repair (see McKinnon, 1987). Taken together, these observations have lead to the view that the ATM gene product functions in a signal transduction mechanism which retards cell cycle advance following DNA damaging events which result in strand breaks (Fig. 1). While the exact role of the ATM gene product in such a signal transduction pathway awaits further elucidation, the ATM gene product functions, either directly or indirectly, to upregulate the cellular pool of p53 and, consequently, delay cell cycle progression following genome damage.

The A-T - Cancer Connection

It is a widely accepted view that tumors arise from single cells which have acquired abnormal proliferative capability (Nowell, 1976). This is a multistep progression during which the activity of cellular growth-promoting genes, termed oncogenes, is increased and the activity of genes which normally serve to constrain growth, termed tumor suppressors, is lost or diminished (Fearon and Vogelstein, 1990). Consequently, such relaxation of cellular controls over both positive and negative regulators of growth may act to propel the cell toward an increasingly malignant form of cellular growth. Mutations responsible leading to such events can arise via a litany of mechanisms such as point mutations, gene amplifications, chromosomal aberrations, translocations, and aneuploidy.

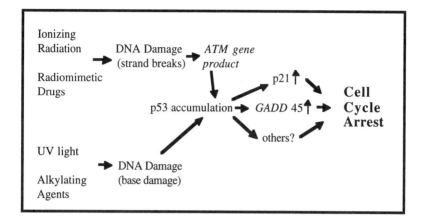

Figure 1: Role of ATM gene product in cell cycle control.

p53 has been shown to play a crucial role in delaying cell growth in response to genome damage (Lane, 1992) and, in this capacity, has been designated as a tumor-suppressor gene. Not surprisingly, p53 mutations have been found in a wide variety of cancer cells (see Levine *et al.*, 1991; Smith and Fornace, 1995). As discussed above, cells from individuals with A-T display an inability to delay cell cycle advance as a consequence of genome damage; this feature stemming from their inability to properly upregulate their cellular pools of p53. Thus, A-T cells can suffer damage to their genome without halting cell growth and subsequent cell divisions and, moreover, this unchecked damage will be passed on to all daughter cells. Clearly, the A-T cells inability to appropriately respond to genome damage is responsible for the high rate of chromosomal aberrations observed in this disorder (see Shiloh, 1995) and the increased frequency of somatic cell mutations in individuals with A-T (Bigbee *et al*, 1989). Furthermore, the effect of unchecked genome damage and consequent mutation is undoubtedly the (or one of the) underlying cause(s) of the high rate of cancer observed among individuals afflicted with A-T.

FUTURE DIRECTIONS

The discovery and cloning of the ATM gene has opened a new chapter in the understanding of the molecular basis of this disorder. The development of ATM antibodies in the near future will lead to basic investigations of the ATM gene product itself. For instance, development of such reagents, as well as yeast models, should make it possible to identify proteins which interact with the ATM gene product and identify potential substrates for the currently putative ATM kinase function. Furthermore, development of animal models will allow for a more in depth understanding of the course of the disease process in A-T as well as broaden our understanding of the occurance of cancer and other symptoms of A-T such as the neuronal cell death which is the underlying cause of the hallmark neurologic dysfunction in these patients. Perhaps these studies may also shed light on the nature of the heterogeneity of presentation of symptoms noted among various A-T individuals. Undoubtedly, the next few years promise to be an exciting time in the investigation of ataxia-telangiectasia.

REFERENCES

Al-Khodairy F, Carr AM (1992): DNA repair mutants defining G2 checkpoint pathways in Schizosaccharomyces pombe. EMBO J. 11:1343-1350.

Anderson CW, Lees-Miller SP (1992): The nuclear serine/threonine protein kinase DNA-PK. Crit. Rev. Eukary. Gene Expr. 2:283-314.

Artuso M, Esteve A, Bresil H, Vuillaume M, Hall J (1995): The role of ataxia telangiectasia gene in the p53, WAF1/CIP1 (p21)-and GADD45-mediated response to DNA damage produced by ionising radiation. Oncogene 11:1427-1436.

Baker BS, Carpenter ATC (1972): Genetic analysis of sex chromosomal meiotic mutants in Drosophila melanogaster. Genetics 71:255-286.

Banga SS, Shenkar R, Boyd JB (1986): Hypersensitivity of Drosophila mei-41 mutants to hydroxyurea is associated with reduced mitotic chromosome stability. Mutat. Res. 163:157-165.

Beamish H, Khanna KK, Lavin MF (1994): Ionizing radiation and cell cycle progression in ataxia telangiectasia. Radiat. Res. S138:S130-S133.

Beamish H, Lavin MF (1994): Radiosensitivity in ataxia-telangiectasia: anomalies in radiation-induced cell cycle delay. Int. J. Radiat. Biol. 65:175-184.

Blunt T, Finnie NJ, Taccioli GE, Smith GCM, Demengeot J, Gottlieb TM, Mizuta R, Varghese AJ, Alt FW, Jeggo PA, Jackson SP (1995): Defective DNA-dependent protein kinase activity is linked to V(D)J recombination and DNA repair defects associated with murine scid mutation. Cell 80:813-823.

Bigbee WL, Langlois RG, Swift M, Jensen RH (1989): Evidence for an elevated frequency of in vivo somatic cell mutations in ataxia telangiectasia. Am. J. Hum. Genet. 44:402-408.

Brown EJ, Albers MW, Shin TB, Ichikawa K, Keith CT, Lane WS, Schreiber SL (1994): A mammalian protein targeted by G1-arresting rapamycin-receptor complex. Nature 369:756-758.

Brown EJ, Beal PA, Keith CT, Chen J, Shin TB, Schreiber SL (1995): Control of p70 s6 kinase by kinase activity of FRAP in vivo. Nature. 377:441-446.

Borresen AL, Anderson, TI, Treti S, Heiberg A, Moller P (1990): Breast cancer and other cancers in Norwegian families with ataxia-telangiectasia. Genes Chrom. Cancer 2:339-340.

Boyd JB, Golino MD, Nguyen TD, Green MM (1976): Isolation and characterization of X-linked mutants of Drosophila melanogaster which are sensitive to mutagens. Genetics 84:485-506.

Byrd PJ, McConville CM, Cooper P, Parkhill J, Stankovic T, McGuire GM, Thick JA, Taylor AMR (1996): Mutations revealed by sequencing the 5-prime half of the gene for ataxia telangiectasia. Hum. Molec. Genet. 5:145-149.

Cafferkey R, Young P, McLaughlin MM, Bergsma DJ, Kotlin Y, Sathe GM, Faucette L, Eng WK, Johnson RK, Livi GP (1993): Dominant missense mutations in a novel yeast protein related to mammalian phosphotidylinositol 3-kinase and VSP34 abrogate rapamycin toxicity. Mol. Cell Biol. 6012-6023.

Canman CE, Wolff AC, Chen C-Y, Fornace AJ, Kastan MB (1994): The p53-dependent G1 cell cycle checkpoint patway and ataxia-telangiectasia. Cancer Res 54:5054-5058.

Carbonari M, Cherchi M, Paganelli R, Giannini G, Galli E, Gaetano C, Papetti C, Fiorilli M (1990): Relative increase of T cells expressing the gamma/delta rather than the alpha/beta receptor in ataxia-telangiectasia. New Eng. J. Med. 322:73-76.

Dulic V, Kauffmann WK, Wilson SJ, Tlsty, TD, Lees E, Harper JW, Elledge SJ, Reed SI (1994) p53-dependent inhibition of cyclin-dependent kinase activities in human fibroblasts during radiation-induced G1 arrest. Cell 76:1013-1023.

Easton DF (1994): Cancer risks in A-T heterozygotes. Int. J. Radiat. Biol. 66:S187-S182

El-Deiry WS, Tokino T, Velculescu VE, Levy DB, Parsons R, Trent JM, Lin D, Mercer WE, Kinzler KW, Vogelstein B (1993): WAF1, a potential mediator of p53 tumor suppresion. Cell 75:817-825.

Enoch T, Carr AM, Nurse P (1992): Fission yeast genes involved in coupling mitosis to completion of DNA replication. Genes Dev. 6:2035-2046.

Fearon ER, Vogelstein B (1990): A genetic model foe colorectal tumorigenesis. Cell 61:759-767.

Fields S, Yang SK (1990): Presence of a potent transcription activating sequence in the p53 protein. Science 249:1046-1049.

Gatti M (1979): Genetic control of chromosome breakage and rejoining in Drosophila melanogaster: spontaneuos chromosome abberations in X-linked mutants defective in DNA metabolism. Proc. Natl. Acad. Sci. 76:1377-1381.

Gatti RA, Boder E, Vinters HV, Sparkes RS, Norman A, Lange K (1991): Ataxia-telangiectasia: an interdisciplinary approach to pathogenesis. Medicine 70:99-117

Gilad S, Khosravi R, Uzeil T, Ziv Y, Rotman G, Savitsky K, Smith S, Harnik R, Shkedi D, Frydman M, Chessa L, Sanal O, Portnoi S, Goldwicz Z, Jaspers NGJ, Gatti RA, Lenoir G, Lavin MF, Tatsumi K, Wegner RD, Shiloh Y, Bar-Shira A. Ataxia-telangiectasia: predominance of mutations that inactivate the ATM protein by truncations or large deletions. Hum Mol. Genet. (in press).

Gottlieb TM, Jackson SP (1993): The DNA-dependent protein kinase: requirement for DNA ends and association with Ku antigen. Cell 72:131-142.

Greenwell PW, Kronmal SL, Porter SE, Gassenhuber J, Obermaier B, Petes TD (1995): TEL1, a gene involved in controlling telomere length in S. cerevisiae, is homologous to the human ataxia telangiectasia gene. Cell 82:823-829.

Hari KL, Santerre A, Sekelsky JJ, McKim KS, Boyd JB, Hawley RS (1995): The mei-41 gene of D. melanogaster is a structural and functional homolog of the human ataxia telangiectasia gene. Cell 82:815-821.

Harper JW, Adami GR, Wei N, Keyomarsi K, Elledge SJ (1993): The p21 Cdk-interacting protein Cip1 is a potent inhibitor of G1 cyclin-dependent kinases. Cell 75:805-816.

Hartley KO, Gell D, Smaith GCM, Zhang H, Divecha N, Connelly MA, Admon A, Lees-Miller SP, Anderson CW, Jackson SP (1995): DNA-dependent protein kinase catalytic subunit: a relative of phosphatidylinositol 3-kinase and the ataxia telangiectasia gene product. Cell 82:849-856.

Hartwell LH, Weinert TA (1989): Checkpoints: controls that ensure the order of cell cycle events. Science 246:629-633.

Heitman J, Movva NR, Hall MN (1991): Targets for cell cycle arrest by the immunosuppresant drug rapamycin in yeast. Science 267:1183-1185

Helliwell SB, Wagner P, Kunz J, Deuter-Reinhard M, Henriquez R, Hall MN (1994): TOR1 and TOR2 are structuraolly and functionally similar but not identical phosphotidylinositol kinase homologues in yeast. Mol. Biol. Cell 5:105-118.

Hong J-H, Gatti RA, Huo YK, Chiang C-S, McBride WH (1994): G2/M-phase arrest and release in ataxia-telangiectasia and normal cells after exposure to ionizing radiation. Radiat. Res. 140:17-23.

Houldsworth J, Lavin MF (1980): Effect of ionizing radiation on DNA sythesis in ataxia-telangiectasia cells. Nuc. Acids Res. 8:3709-3720.

Hunter T (1995): When is a lipid kinase not a lipid kinase? When it is a protein kinase. Cell 83:1-4.

Jaspers NGJ, Gatti RA, Baan C, Linssen PCML, Bootsma D (1988): Genetic complementation analysis of ataxia telangiectasia and Nijmegen breakage syndrome. Cytogenet. Cell Genet. 49:259-263.

Jeggo PA, Taccioli GE, Jackson SP (1995): Menage a trois: double strand break repair, V(D)J recombination and DNA-PK. Bioessays 17:949-957.

Jiminez G, Yucel J, Rowley R, Subramani S (1992): The rad3+ gene of Schizosaccharomyces pombe is involved in multiple checkpoint functions and in DNA repair. Proc. Natl. Acad. Sci. 89:4952-4956.

Kastan MB, Zhan Q, El-Deiry WS, Carrier F, Jacks T, Walsh WV, Plunkett BS, Vogelsein B, Fornace AJ (1992): A mammailan cell cycle checkpoint pathway utilizing p53 and GADD45 id defective in ataia-telangiectasia. Cell 71:587-597.

Kato R, Ogawa H (1994): An essential gene, ESR1, is required for mitotic cell growth, DNA repair and meiotic recombination in Saccharomyces cerevisiae. Nucl. Acids Res. 22:3104-3112.

Kern SE, Kinzler KW, Bruskin A, Jarosz D, Friedman P, Prives C, Vogelstein B (1991): Identification of p53 as a sequence specific DNA binding protein. Science 252:1707-1711.

Khanna KK, Lavin MF (1993): Ionizing radiation and UV induction of p53 protein by different pathways in ataxia telangiectasia cells. Oncogene 8:3307-3312.

Kuhn A, Gottleib TM, Jackson SP, Grummt I (1995): DNA-dependent protein kinase: a potent inhibitor of transcription by RNA polymerase I. Genes Dev. 9:193-203.

Kunz J, Henriquez R, Schneider U, Deuter-Reinhard M, Movva NR, Hall MN (1993): Target of rapamycin in yeast, TOR2, is an essential phosphotidylinositol kinase homolog required for G1 progression. Cell 73:585-596.

Labhart P (1995): DNA-dependent protein kinase specifically represses promoter-directed transcription initiation by RNA polymerase I. Proc. Natl. Acad. Sci. 92:2934-2938.

Lane DP (1992): p53, guardian of the genome. Nature 358:15-16.

Lavin MF, Khanna KK, Beamish H, Teale B, Hobson K, Watters D (1994): Defect in radiation signal transduction in ataxia telangiectasia. Int. J. Radiat. Biol. 66:S151-S156.

Levine AJ, Momand J, Finlay CA (1991): The p53 tumour suppressor gene. Nature 351:453-456

Little JB, Nagasawa H (1985): Effect on confluent holding on potentially lethal damage repair, cell cycle progression, and chromosomal aberrations in human noral and ataxia telangiectasia fibroblasts. Radiat. Res. 101:81-93.

Lustig A, Petes TD (1986): Identification of yeast mutants with altered telomere structure. Proc. Natl. Acad. Sci. 83:1398-1402.

McKinnon PJ (1987): Ataxia-telangiectasia: an inherited disorder of ionizing radiation in man. Hum. Genet. 75:197-208.

Morice WG, Brunn GJ, Wederrecht G, Siekierka JJ, Abraham RTJ (1993): Rapamycin-induced inhibition of of p34cdc2 kinase activation is assocaited with G1/S-phase growth arrest in T lymphocytes. J. Biol. Chem. 268:3734-3738.

Morozov VE, Falzon M, Anderson CW, Kuff EL (1994): DNA-dependent protein kinase is activated by nicks and larger single-stranded gaps. J. Biol. Chem. 269:16684-16688.

Morrow DM, Tagle DA, Shiloh Y, Collins FS, Heiter P (1995): TEL1, an S. cerevisiae homolog of the human gene mutated in ataxia telangiectasia, is functionally related to the yeast checkpoint gene MEC1. Cell 82:831-840.

Murray AW (1992): Creative blocks: cell-cycle checkpoints and feedback controls. Nature 359:599-604.

Nowell PC (1976): The clonal evolution of tumor cell populations. Science 194:23-28.

Painter RB, Young BR (1975): X-ray-induced inhibition of DNA synthesis in Chinese hamster ovary, human HeLa and mouse L cells. Radiat. Res. 64:648-656.

Painter RB, Young BR (1980): Radiosensitivity in ataxia-telangiectasia: a new explanation. Proc. Natl. Acad. Sci. 77: 7315-7317.

Painter RB (1981): Radioresistant DNA synthesis: an intrinsic feature of ataxia telangiectasia. Mutat. Res. 84: 183-190.

Paules RS, Levedakou EN, Wilson SJ, Innes CL, Rhodes N, Tlsty TD, Galloway DA, Donehower LA, Tainsky MA, Kauffmann WK (1995): Defective G2 checkpoint function in cells from individuals with familial cancer syndromes. Cancer Res. 55:1763-1773.

Paulovich AG, Hartwell LH (1995): A checkpoint regulates the rate of progression through S phase in S. cerevisiae in response to DNA damage. Cell 82:841-847.

Pippard EC, Hall AJ, Barker DJP, Bridges BA (1988): Cancer in homozygotes and heterozygotes of ataxia-telangiectasia and xeroderma pigmentosum in Britain. Cancer Res. 48:2929-2932.

Raycroft L, Wu H, Lozano G (1990): Transcriptional activation by wild-type but not transforming mutants of the p53 anti-oncogene. Science 249:1049-1051.

Rudolph NS, Latt SA (1989): Flow cytometric analysis of X-ray sensitivity in ataxia telangiectasia. Mut. Res. 211:31-41.

Sabatini DM, Erdjument-Bromage H, Lui M, Tempst P, Syner SH (1994): RAFT1: A mammalian protein that binds to FKBP12 in a rapamycin-dependent fashion and is homologous to yeast TORs. Cell 78:35-43.

Sabers CJ, Martin MM, Brunn GJ, Williams JM, Dumont FJ, Wiedrrecht G, Abraham RT (1995): Isolation of a protein target of the FKBP12-rapamycin complex in mammalian cells. J. Biol. Chem. 270:815-822.

Savitsky, K, Bar-Shira A, Gilad S, Rotman G, Ziv Y, Vanagaite L, Tagle DA, Smith S, Uziel, T., Sfez S, Ashkenazi M, Pecker I, Frydman M, Harnik R, Patanjali SR, Simmons A, Clines GA, Sarteil A, Gatti RA, Chessa L, Sanal O, Lavin MF, Jaspers NGJ, Taylor AMR, Arlett CF, Miki T, Weissman SM, Lovett M, Collins FS, Shiloh Y (1995a): A single ataxia telangiectasia gene with a prduct similar to PI-3 kinase. Science 268:1749-1753.

Savitsky K, Sfez S, Tagle DA, Ziv Y, Sarteil A, Collins FS, Shiloh Y, Rotman G (1995b): The complete sequencew of the coding region of tyhe ATM gene reveals similarity to cell cycle regulators in different species. Hum. Mol. Genet. 4:2025-2032.

Scott D, Zampetti-Bosseler F (1982): Cell cycle dependence of mitotic delay in X-irradated normal and ataxia telangiectasia fibroblasts. Int. J. Radat. Biol. 42:679-683.

Seaton BL, Yucel J, Sunnerhagen P, Subramani S (1992): Isolation and characterization of the Schizosaccharomyces pombe rad3 gene, involved in the DNA damage and DNA synthesis checkpoints. Gene 119:83-89.

Sedgwick RP, Boder E (1991): Ataxia-Telangiectasia. Handbook of Clinical Neurology. 16:347-423.

Shiloh Y (1995): Ataxia-telangiectasia: Closer to unraveling the mystery. Eur. J. Hum. Genet. 3:116-138.

Smith ML, Fornace AJ (1995): Genomic instability and the role of p53 mutations in cancer cells. Curr. Opin. Oncol. 7:69-75.

Swift M, Morrell D, Massey RB, Chase CL (1991): Incidence of cancer in 161 families affected with ataxia-telangiectasia. N. Eng. J. Med. 325:1831-1836.

Swift M, Reitnauer PJ, Morrell D, Chase CL (1987): Breast and other cancers in families with ataxia-telangiectasia. New Eng. J. Med. 316: 1289-1294.

Szabo CI, King MC (1995): Inherited breast and ovarian cancer. Hum Mol Genet 4:1811-1817.

Taylor AMR, Metcalfe JA, Thick J, Mak Y-F (1996): Leukemia and lymphoma in ataxia telangiectasia. Blood. 87:423-438.

Terada N, Franklin RA, Lucas JJ, Blenis J, Gelfand EW (1993): Failure of rapamycin to block proliferation once resting cells have entered the cell cycle despite inactivation of p70 S6 kinase. J. Biol. Chem. 268:12062-12068.

Uziel T, Savitsky K, Platzer M, Ziv Y, Helbitz T, Nehls M, Boehm T, Rosenthal A, Shiloh Y, Rotman G (1996): Genomic organization of the ATM gene. Genomics (in press).

Waldmann TA, McIntire KR (1972): Serum-alpha-fetoprotein levels in patients with ataxia-telangiectasia. Lancet II:1112-1115.Weinert TA, Kiser GL, Hartwell LH (1994): Mitotic checkpoint genes in budding yeast and the dependence of mitosis on DNA replication and repair. Genes Dev. 8:652-665.

Woods CG, Taylor AMR (1992): Ataxia telangiectasia in the British Isles: the clinical and laboratory features of 70 affected individuals. Quart. J. Med. 82:169-179.Zakian VA (1995): ATM-related genes: what do they tell us about functions of the human gene? Cell 82:685-687.

Zampetti-Bosseler F, Scott D (1981): Cell death, chromosome damage and mitotic delay in normal human, ataxia telangiectasia and retioblastoma fibroblasts afetr X-irradiation. Int. J. Radiat. Biol. 39:547-558.

Zhan Q, Lord KA, Alamo I, Hollander MC, Carrier F, Ron D, Kohn KW, Hoffman B, Liebermann DA, Fornace AJ (1994): The gadd and MyD genes define a novel set of mammalian genes encoding acidic proteins that synergistically suppress cell growth. Mol Cell Biol. 14:2361-2371.

Etiology of Breast and
Gynecological Cancers, pages 115–124
© 1997 Wiley-Liss, Inc.

Radiation and Breast Cancer Risk

Charles E. Land

Radiation Epidemiology Branch, National Cancer Institute

INTRODUCTION

This year (1995) marks the hundredth anniversary of Roentgen's discovery of X radiation at the University of Würzberg in Bavaria. Radioactivity was discovered by Becquerel the following year (1896), in Paris. Thus, we have been aware of radioactivity and ionizing radiation for only a short time, although they are fundamental forces of nature. The current year also marks the fiftieth anniversaries of the first explosion of an atomic bomb, at Alamagordo, New Mexico, and their first, second, and so far only uses in war, at Hiroshima and Nagasaki, Japan.

Ionizing radiation is an established human carcinogen for many organ sites, and is probably the best understood of environmental carcinogens to which human beings are commonly exposed. We know a great deal about the relationship between ionizing radiation exposure and female breast cancer risk, possibly more than for any other site. We have reached this point partly through experimental studies using animal models, and partly through epidemiological and multidisciplinary investigations of populations exposed to substantial doses of radiation for therapeutic and diagnostic medicine and, especially, radiation from the Hiroshima and Nagasaki bombings. Paradoxically, and partly because recognition and quantification of the carcinogenic effects of exposure to ionizing radiation have motivated regulations and practices that tend to minimize such exposure, radiation normally is a very minor contributor to our overall cancer burden (National Research Council, 1990; United Nations, 1994).

BREAST CANCER INCIDENCE AMONG A-BOMB SURVIVORS

Epidemiological and multidisciplinary studies of cancer risk among A-bomb survivors constitute the largest single source of information about radiation-related cancer risk among human beings. The studies are based on a cohort of 120,000 survivors and nonexposed persons resident in Hiroshima and Nagasaki at the time of the 1950 Japanese national census. The cohort includes 70,100 women, of whom 50,900 were exposed and have been assigned individual radiation dose estimates, based on reported location at the time of the bombing and reconstructed shielding history. Most of the breast cancer results reported here were obtained from the latter subgroup.

The radiation dose response for breast cancer incidence during 1950-1985, expressed as risk relative to that among persons exposed to less than 1 mSv is shown in Figure 1 for all exposure ages combined (Tokunaga et al. , 1994). The plotted, dose-specific relative risk estimates correspond to intervals of dose, and are plotted according to the mean dose of each interval. Numbers of cases are given above or below the confidence bounds for each estimate. The estimated slope of the plotted line was highly significant statistically, and only a negligible amount of quadratic departure from a linear dose response model was consistent with the data. The inset shows that the data at very low doses, whose differences mainly reflect random variation in observations of risk at zero dose, are consistent with the linear model estimated from all the data. They suggest neither the existence of a low-dose threshold, below which there is no excess risk, nor a level of excess risk per unit dose that is higher at low doses than at high doses.

The slope of the linear dose response, expressed in excess relative risk at one sievert (Sv), decreased significantly by age at exposure. In the data through 1985, the functional form of this dependence on exposure age was fit equally well by a negative exponential function of age, or by a step function with steps at 20 and 40 years of age at exposure. More recent follow-up data through 1990 (preliminary results of an analysis in progress) conform significantly more closely to the step function model than to a simple exponential function of exposure age. The step function model, as fit to the 1950-1985 data, is shown in Figure 2. It may seem intuitively appealing that the steps in this model should correspond roughly to the beginning and end of

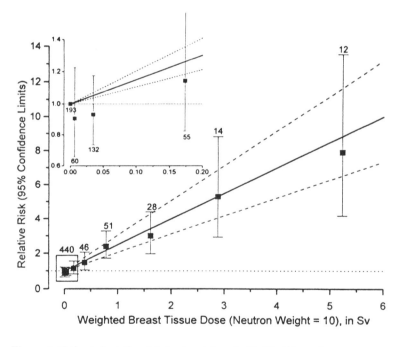

Figure 1. Estimated relative risk, by dose interval with fitted linear dose response.

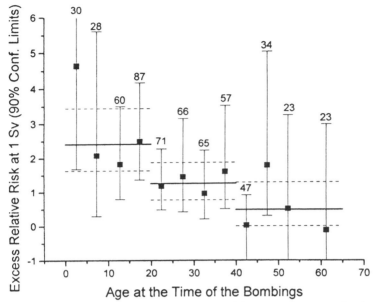

Figure 2. Linear model estimates of excess relative risk at 1 Sv, by age at the time of the bombings. The fitted step function corresponds to ages 0-19, 20-39, and 40 years or older.

childbearing, and somewhat counterintuitive that risk should have no apparent dependence upon whether exposure occurred before, after, or around the usual ages at menarche or breast budding.

In Figure 3, estimated excess relative risks at 1 Sv are shown separately for women 0-19, 20-39, and 40 years of age or older at exposure, but distributed by age at observation for risk within these broad age-at-exposure intervals. The horizontal lines are the same age-at-exposure group estimates shown in the step function in Figure 2. One interesting pattern is that, regardless of exposure age, there is little evidence of radiation-related excess risk until attained ages of 30 years or older, i.e., until the exposed women were old enough to have breast cancer, or until 10 years or so after exposure, whichever occurred later. Another pattern is that, within the three age-at-exposure intervals, and for attained ages older than 35, the horizontal lines fit the individual estimates, which are presented with 90% confidence limits, rather well. For exposure at a given age, excess relative risk, once stabilized, does not appear to vary by increasing age at observation. In other words, the *rate* of radiation-related risk tends to increase proportionally to the age-related increase in baseline risk, so that the *ratio* of excess to baseline risk has remained pretty much the same within age-at-exposure cohorts.

There is one remarkable exception to the preceding sentence, however: the dose-specific estimate of excess relative risk among women exposed before age 20 and observed at 25-34 years

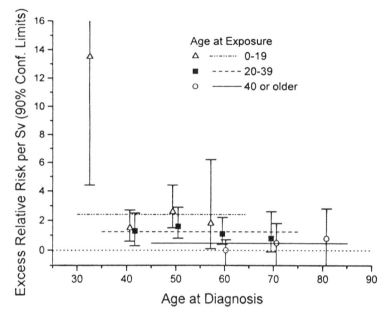

Figure 3. Linear model estimates of excess relative risk at 1 Sv, with 90% confidence limits, by 10-year interval of attained age within 20-year intervals of age at the time of the bombings. Horizontal lines correspond to zero risk and to levels of the step function shown in Figure 2, for exposure ages 0-19, 20-39, and 40 years and older, respectively.

of age (in fact, almost all these cases were diagnosed at ages 30-34) is six times as high as the summary estimate for the same women at all ages at observation combined, a statistically significant difference. The phenomenon reflects both a low baseline rate of early-onset breast cancer, and a radiation-related excess rate as high as that observed at older ages in the same birth cohort (Table 1). It does not appear to be the result of fortuitous early diagnosis of high-dose cancers that normally would have been diagnosed after age 35, although that remains a possibility.

We know that heritable mutations in certain genes, notably BRCA1 and BRCA2, p53, and perhaps ATM, predispose to breast cancer as determined from studies of familial aggregations of breast cancer, and that the first three of these are associated particularly with early-onset breast cancer. Claus et al. (1996) have estimated that about 7% of breast cancer cases in the general population are carriers of an (unidentified) breast cancer susceptibility gene, the proportion of cases attributable to the gene decreases markedly with age, from about 33% at ages 20-29 to 2% at ages 70-79. The mutant gene frequency of BRCA1 among non-Jewish, Caucasian women has been estimated to be about one in 800, and about 7.5% among breast cancer cases diagnosed before age 35 (FitzGerald et al., 1996, Langston et al., 1996). About 1% of Ashkenazi Jews are thought to have inherited a single mutation, denoted 185delAG, which is apparently derived by descent from a common ancestor (Struewing et al., 1995, Collins, 1996); in a recent study

Table 1. Comparison of observed breast-cancer rates for women less than 20 yr old at the time of the bombings with those expected, in the absence of exposure, according to age-specific rates from the Hiroshima and Nagasaki tumor registries by exposure (dose) group and attained age: cases per 10^5 PY.

Dose interval		Attained age (yr)			
(mean dose)		30-34	35-44	45-54	55-64
< 0.1 Gy	Observed	11.1	38.8	62.4	84.1
(0.01 Sv)	Expected	13.6	49.1	71.4	76.2
0.1-0.49 Gy	Observed	72.9	56.9	120.7	53.6
(0.28 Sv)	Expected	13.4	47.6	75.2	82.0
0.5-1.99 Gy	Observed	87.0	92.5	296.7	181.2
(1.19 Sv)	Expected	13.6	49.2	68.4	70.5
2.0-6.0 Gy	Observed	221.7	302.2	405.0	829.3
(4.35 Sv)	Expected	13.5	49.5	75.4	76.7

(FitzGerald et al., 1996) eight of 39 cases (21%) of female breast cancer diagnosed before age 40 among Ashkenazi Jews had this particular mutation. Relatively little is known regarding the likely prevalence of heritable gene mutations predisposing to breast cancer among Japanese. A recent study by Inoue et al. (1995) found germline mutations of the BRCA1 gene in only two of 20 Japanese breast cancer families. Both families had the same mutation, a previously unreported one. Less is known about BRCA2 mutations in any population, and germline mutations in p53 are relatively rare.

We are reasonably sure of one heritable mutation in man that increases sensitivity to radiation carcinogenesis: patients with bilateral retinoblastoma are predisposed to osteosarcoma and soft-tissue sarcoma, and those who are treated by radiation have a markedly increased risk of osteosarcoma and soft-tissue sarcoma in the radiation field (Eng et al., 1993). Women with germline mutations in BRCA1 or BRCA2 have been estimated to have lifetime breast cancer risks on the order of 80% (Ford et al., 1994; Wooster et al., 1994). If they are sensitive to radiation carcinogenesis, the effect of radiation exposure would be to shift the age distribution of breast cancer diagnosis in the population subgroup with such heritable mutations toward the younger ages following exposure. This is a commonplace phenomenon in experimental tumorigenesis studies using animal models that are both sensitive to the tested agent and that have very high lifetime risk of tumors in the absence of the agent, e.g., studies of radiation-related mammary adenoma in Sprague-Dawley rats (Shellabarger, 1976). In effect, irradiated subjects in the subgroup with heritable breast cancer gene mutations, each of whom would, with high probability, develop a breast cancer at some age in the absence of radiation exposure, should tend to develop one at an earlier age, simply because irradiation increases risk and the first of many cancers in an individual tends to occur earlier than the first of few. The effect on a mixed population should be to increase the proportion of high-dose cancer cases with germline mutations among cases with early onset, for which the population baseline rate is very low; this would coincidentally increase the radiation-related dose response for early-onset breast cancer.

An obvious next step is breast cancer gene mutation assays for the early-onset breast cancer cases among the A-bomb survivors. This will not be easy, since the youngest survivors reached 35 years of age in 1980, and unbuffered, formalin-fixed tissue in paraffin blocks, which is all that is available for many of the cases, is not easy to work with. Also, the spectrum of BRCA1 and BRCA2 mutations in the Japanese population is not well characterized, and can be expected to be somewhat different from that in the United States and Europe. However, the problems are surmountable, and answers can be expected eventually.

RISK IN IRRADIATED WESTERN POPULATIONS

The first evidence of a radiation-related risk of breast cancer in women was observed in former patients at a Nova Scotia tuberculosis sanitorium who received multiple chest fluoroscopies while being monitored during pneumothorax treatment (MacKenzie, 1969). Other evidence has come from studies of patients of tuberculosis sanitoria in the United States (Boice et al., 1990) and in Canada (Miller et al., 1989), New York patients treated by x ray for acute postpartum mastitis (Shore et al., 1986) and Swedish patients treated for that and other benign breast diseases (Mattson, 1995), patients treated for Hodgkins Disease at Stanford University Hospital (Hancock, 1993), and women treated during infancy in Rochester, New York, for enlarged thymus (Hildreth, 1989). Although none of these populations is as general and unselected as the A-bomb survivors, it is nevertheless possible to estimate radiation-related breast cancer risk for an American population, whose age-specific baseline breast cancer rates are several times higher than those for Japan, by relying only on data from American populations. When this is done, it is reasonably clear that, despite the difference in baseline rates, American women irradiated at a given age with a given dose have about the same rates of radiation-related breast cancer as Japanese women exposed under the same circumstances. Another way of putting it is that additive, rather than multiplicative, models should be used for transporting radiation-related breast cancer risk estimates between Japan (i.e., the A-bomb survivor experience) and the United States (Land et al., 1980, Dale Preston, personal communication, UNSCEAR, 1994, Land, 1995). Still another is that whatever is responsible for the marked difference in breast cancer rates between Japan and the United States interacts additively, and not multiplicatively, with radiation in the causation of breast cancer.

INTERACTIONS WITH REPRODUCTIVE HISTORY

Breast cancer risk factors have been widely studied, in many countries. The most important, and most widely confirmed, factors are (1) having already been diagnosed with a breast cancer in the contralateral breast, (2) a family history of breast cancer, and (3) reproductive history including number of births or full-term pregnancies, age at first full-term pregnancy, lactation history, age at menarche, and age at natural or surgical menopause. A case-control interview study of the LSS sample was conducted to verify the importance of these and other variables in the A-bomb survivor population, and to investigate the joint effects (interactions) of such factors in combination with radiation exposure (Land et al., 1994a, 1994b). Cases (all diagnosed before 1981) and controls were matched on radiation dose as well as on city and date of birth, making it impossible to estimate radiation effects from the case-control data. However, that information was already available from incidence studies of the entire cohort, and matching on dose improved statistical power for the interaction analysis, given the cohort dose-response data.

There was very little information about family history of breast cancer in these data; it appears that many, if not most, of the breast cancer cases themselves did not realize they had been treated for cancer. This reflects traditional medical practice in Japan, which seeks to reassure the patient and avoid emotional reactions that might interfere with treatment success. Age at menarche and age at a menopause were not strong risk factors. However, number of births, age at first full-term pregnancy, and cumulative period of lactation were strongly related to breast cancer risk, as were a number of other, highly correlated variables. These three variables were selected for the interaction analyses because of their strong relationship to risk, their importance in the scientific literature and because, although correlated, each had some independent relationship with risk after adjustment for the others. Number of births and cumulative lactation

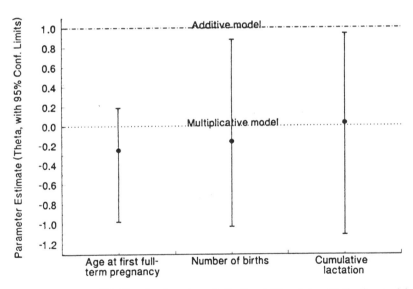

Figure 4. Summary of likelihood ratio test results for the additive and multiplicative models for the pairwise interactions with radiation dose of three reproductive history variables.

were more closely correlated than was either of them with the age at first full-term pregnancy.

The interaction analyses evaluated the additive and multiplicative, pairwise interaction models for radiation dose and one other factor, here represented by X, in the context of a more general model. The general model included each of the other two as a special case, according to the value of a single parameter, θ:

General Model $\qquad$ Relative risk = $\{1 + \alpha \text{ Dose}\} \{1 + \beta X/(1 + \alpha \text{ Dose})^{\theta}\}$

Multiplicative Model: Relative risk = $(1 + \alpha \text{ Dose}) (1 + \beta X)$ $\qquad$ (θ=0)

Additive model: $\qquad$ Relative risk = $1 + \alpha \text{ Dose} + \beta X$ $\qquad$ (θ=1)

For each factor represented by X (age at first full-term pregnancy, number of births, and cumulative lactation period), the additive model was rejected, whereas the multiplicative model was consistent with the data (Figure 4). Thus, for example, women who had a full-term pregnancy at an early age were protected against breast cancer in general, and against radiation-related breast cancer in particular.

Evidence against the additive model was at least as strong for subjects exposed before age 20, or before age 17, as it was for subjects who were older at the time of the bombings. To some extent this reflects the steeper radiation dose response associated with exposure during childhood and adolescence, i.e., the data from younger subjects are likely to be more informative about interaction because at least one of the main effects is stronger. The result, as it pertains to age at first full-term pregnancy, suggests that an effect of an early full-term pregnancy was to undo some of the cancer predisposing effects of earlier exposure to breast tissue. That is, terminal differentiation of cells for milk secretion, induced by a full-term pregnancy, may reduce the proliferative potential even of cells already initiated by radiation. This interpretation is consistent with experimental results obtained by Clifton, et al. (1975, 1978). In that work, female rats were irradiated and injected with prolactin-secreting, transplantable pituitary tumors. One group received no further treatment; another received adrenalectomy, which precluded the production of adrenal corticoids necessary for cell differentiation for milk secretion, and another received both adrenalectomy and glucocortisol replacement therapy. High levels of radiation-induced mammary cancer were experienced by the adrenalectomy-only group compared to rats with intact adrenals or adrenalectomized rats given glucocortisol replacement therapy.

CONCLUSIONS

It is of considerable interest that radiation exposure can cause breast cancer in women, and it is worthwhile to refine risk estimates so that we have a fairly good idea of just how much risk is associated with exposure to various sources of radiation, including cosmic rays, diagnostic and therapeutic medical x ray, routine and extraordinary industrial releases, and warfare. Such information is essential for devising strategies for avoiding excessive exposure without undue cost and loss of benefits from various practices that involve radiation exposure. This is the main reason for the existence of such organizations as the United Nations Subcommittee on the Effects of Ionizing Radiation, the International Commission on Radiation Protection, and the US National

Council on Radiation Protection and Measurements, among others, and the driving force behind much of the funding for radiation-related research.

But the existence of heavily exposed subsets of some irradiated populations under study has led to insights into how a single carcinogen, such as ionizing radiation, may interact with host factors and other agents in the causation of cancer. The multifactorial nature of carcinogenesis is evident, for example, from the experience of female atomic bomb survivors exposed to 0.5 Sv or more, among whom about 67 of 105 breast cancers observed since 1950 are attributable to their exposures; these risks are clearly modified by other factors, many of them known. There is much more to learn through further follow-up and study of this and other irradiated cohorts.

REFERENCES

Boice JD Jr, Preston DL, Davis FG, Monson RR (1990): Frequent chest X-ray fluoroscopy and breast cancer incidence among tuberculosis patients in Massachusetts. Radiat Res 125:214-222.

Clifton KH, Sridharan BN, Douple EB (1975): Mammary carcinogenesis-enhancing effect in irradiated rats with pituitary tumor MtT-F4. J Natl Cancer Inst 55:485-7.

Clifton KH, Crowley J (1978): Effects of radiation type and role of glucocorticoids, gonadectomy and thyroidectomy in mammary tumor induction in MtT-grafted rats. Cancer Res 38:1507-13.

Claus EB, Schildkraut JM, Thompson WD, Risch NJ (1996): The genetic attributable risk of breast and ovarian cancer. Cancer 77:2318-2324.

Collins FS (1996): BRCA1 - Lots of mutations, lots of dilemmas. NEJM 34:186-188

Eng C, Li FP, Abramson DH, et al. (1993): Mortality from second tumors among long-term survivors of retinoblastoma. J Natl Cancer Inst 85:1121-8.

FitzGerald MG, MacDonald DJ, Krainer M, et al. (1996): Germ-line BRCA1 mutations in Jewish and non-Jewish women with early-onset breast cancer. N Engl J Med 334:143-149.

Ford D, Easton DF, Bishop DT, Narod SA, Goldgar DE, and the Breast Cancer Linkage Consortium (1994): Risks of cancer in BRCA1-mutation carriers. Lancet 343:692-695

Hancock SL, Tucker MA, Hoppe RT (1993). Breast cancer after treatment of Hodgkin's disease. J Natl Cancer Inst 181:25-31.

Hildreth NG, Shore RE, Dvoretsky PM (1989): The risk of breast cancer after irradiation of the thymus in infancy. New Engl J Med 321:1281-1284.

Inoue R, Fukutomi T, Ushijima T, Matsumoto Y, et al. (1995): Germline mutation of BRCA1 in Japanese breast cancer families. Cancer Res. 55:3521-3524.

Kelsey JL, Gammon MD, John EM (1993): Reproductive factors and breast cancer. Epidemiol Rev 15:36-47.

Land CE (1995): Studies of cancer and radiation dose among atomic bomb survivors. The example of breast cancer. J Amer Med Assoc 274:402-407.

Land CE, Boice JD Jr, Shore RE, Norman JE, Tokunaga M (1980): Breast cancer risk from low-dose exposures to ionizing radiation: Results of a parallel analysis of three exposed populations of women. J Natl Cancer Inst 65:353-375.

Land CE, Hayakawa N, Machado S, et al. (1994): A case-control interview study of breast cancer among Japanese A-bomb survivors: I. Main effects. Cancer Causes and Control

5:157-165.

Land CE, Hayakawa N, Machado S, et al. (1994): A case-control interview study of breast cancer among Japanese A-bomb survivors: II. Interactions between epidemiological factors and radiation dose. Cancer Causes and Control 5:167-176.

Langston AA, Malone KE, Thompson JD, Daling JR, Ostrander EA (1996): BRCA1 mutations in a population-based sample of young women with breast cancer. New Engl J Med 34:137-142.

MacKenzie I (1965): Breast cancer following multiple fluoroscopies. Br J Cancer 19:1-8.

Mattson A, Ruden B, Hall P, Wilking N, Rutqvist LE (1993): Radiation-induced breast cancer and long term follow-up of radiotherapy for benign breast disease. J Natl Cancer Inst 85:1679-1685.

Miller AB, Howe GR, Sherman GJ, et al. (1989): Mortality from breast cancer after irradiation during fluoroscopic examinations in patients being treated for tuberculosis. N Engl J Med 321:1285-1289.

National Research Council, Committee on the Biological Effects of Ionizing Radiations. Health Effects of Exposure to Low Levels of Ionizing Radiation (BEIR V): National Academy Press, Washington, DC, 1990.

Shellabarger CJ. (1976): Radiation carcinogenesis: Laboratory studies. Cancer 37:1090-1096.

Shore RE, Hildreth N, Woodard E, Dvoretsky P, Hempelmann L, Pasternack B (1986): Breast cancer among women given x-ray therapy for acute postpartum mastitis. J Natl Cancer Inst 77:689-696.

Struewing JP, Abeliovich D, Peretz T, et al (1995): The carrier frequency of othe BRCA1 185delAG mutation is approximately 1 percent in Ashkenazi Jewish individuals. Nat Genet 11:198-200.

Tokunaga M, Land CE, Tokuoka S, Nishimori I, Soda M, Akiba S (1994): Incidence of female breast cancer among atomic bomb survivors, Hiroshima and Nagasaki, 1950-1985. Radiat Res 138:209-223.

United Nations Scientific Committee on the Effects of Atomic Radiation. 1994. Sources, Effects and Risks of Ionizing Radiation. Annex A. Epidemiological Studies of Radiation Carcinogenesis. E.94.IX.11 New York: United Nations.

Wooster R, Neuhausen SL, Mangion J, et al (1994): Localization of a breast cancer susceptibility gene, BRCA2, to chromosome 13q12-13. Science 265:2088-2090.

Etiology of Breast and
Gynecological Cancers, pages 125–131
© 1997 Wiley-Liss, Inc.

GENOTOXICITY OF ENVIRONMENTAL AGENTS IN HUMAN MAMMARY EPITHELIAL CELLS: A TRIGGER FOR HUMAN BREAST CANCER

Sandra R. Eldridge, Michael N. Gould, and Byron E. Butterworth

Pathology Associates International, Frederick, MD 21701 (SRE), University of Wisconsin Comprehensive Cancer Center, Madison, WI 27511 (MNG), and Chemical Industry Institute of Toxicology, Research Triangle Park, NC 21709 (BEB)

INTRODUCTION

Breast cancer is the most common cancer in American women, resulting in a mortality second only to the mortality caused by cigarette-induced lung cancer (American Cancer Society, 1990). Further, the incidence of breast cancer is increasing at a steady rate (American Cancer Society, 1990). Despite its prevalence, the etiology of human breast cancer is poorly understood. While many environmental variables such as diet may modulate the promotion and/or progression of breast cancer, the only environmental agent that has been proven to induce breast cancer in women is ionizing radiation (Howe, 1984, Tokunaga, et al, 1984). While no clear epidemiological link between environmental chemicals and human breast cancer has been established, it has been suggested that passive smoking may increase that risk of breast cancer (Horton, 1988). The ability of environmental xenobiotics such as polycyclic aromatic hydrocarbons (PAH) to induce mammary cancer in rodents is, however, well documented (Dao, 1969, Huggins, 1979). Furthermore, ubiquitous environmental pollutants such as PAH can be stored in human breast fat (Obana, et al, 1981), suggesting that human breast tissue might be exposed to potential carcinogens. Thus, it is important to determine if the human breast can metabolically activate carcinogens and if it may be a target for neoplastic transformation by environmental agents. The question of the relevance of rodent studies to human carcinogenesis is of major concern. One approach to this question is to develop *in vitro* models for key biological activities of environmental chemicals using human cells.

Numerous genotoxicity assays successfully identify the potential carcinogenic activity of chemical agents the primary biological activity of which is alteration of the DNA (McCann, et al, 1975, Tennant, et al, 1987). One widely used genotoxicity assay is the measurement of chemically induced DNA repair as a means of assessing the ability of a test agent to reach and alter the DNA. [³H]Thymidine incorporated into the DNA of nondividing cells during excision repair is used to quantitate DNA repair and has been termed unscheduled DNA synthesis (UDS) (Rasmussen and Painter, 1966). DNA repair assays have been described for a variety of rodent and human cell types (Rasmussen and Painter, 1966, Williams, 1976, Butterworth, et al, 1987, Doolittle and Butterworth, 1984, Working and Butterworth, 1984, Loury, et al, 1987, Sawyer, et al, 1988, Butterworth, et al, 1989). The *in vitro* UDS assay described for rat hepatocytes

(12) was modified for human mammary epithelial cells (HMEC) (Eldridge, et al., 1992). Normal HMEC were derived from residual surgical material from reduction mammoplasties of five healthy women 19 to 22 years of age (Cases B402, B499, B708, 3014, and 3085) following procedures for the isolation and cultivation of HMEC (20, 21).

Since species and tissue specificities are observed in chemical carcinogenesis (Langenbach, 1983), it is important to establish predictive tests in target cells. The measurement of chemically induced DNA repair as UDS in normal HMEC provides a qualitative indication of potential risk rather than quantitative risk assessment.

ROLE OF ENVIRONMENTAL FACTORS IN TRIGGERING BREAST CANCER

In view of the increasing incidence of human breast cancer and the possible role of environmental factors, it is important to identify environmental agents that are genotoxic in HMEC. Since carcinogens often exhibit species- and tissue-specific differences in factors such as biotransformation, the most relevant mechanistic information that is useful for risk assessment may be derived from test systems that utilize the actual human tissue at risk. Toward this end, we developed an assay for measuring DNA repair in secondary cultures of HMEC. This asssay provides a qualitative indication of potential genotoxic activity in these cells.

A wide variety of agents were examined to determine their ability to induce UDS in HMEC (Table 1). The results reflect the metabolic activation and excision-repair capabilities of the HMEC. Positive responses were observed with chemicals requiring metabolic activation: benzo(a)pyrene (BP), aflatoxin B_1 (AFB_1), 1,6-dinitropyrene (1,6-DNP) and 2-acetylaminofluorene (2-AAF). BP is a ubiquitous environmental agent of a chemical class known to induce mammary tumors in rat (Dao, 1969, Huggins, 1979). AFB_1 is a naturally occurring fungal metabolite that has been detected in human breast milk (Lamplugh, et al, 1988). 1,6-DNP is a mutagenic environmental pollutant found in diesel exhaust, effluents from coal-fired power plants, and cigarette smoke (Mermelstein, et al, 1981, Rosenkranz, 1982). It is a polycyclic aromatic nitro compound and potent inducer of DNA repair in rat and human hepatocytes (Butterworth, et al, 1983). 2-AAF, a mouse liver and bladder carcinogen, induced a positive response in the HMEC UDS assay. Thus, the positive response in HMEC for all of these agents may suggest a potential health hazard from exposure to these compounds.

Tobacco smoke condensate (TSC) produced a weak but positive response in secondary cultures of HMEC (Table 1). TSC contains numerous components and is genotoxic in a variety of test systems (DeMarini, 1983). Nicotine and its metabolite continine are detected in breast milk of mothers who smoke (Luck, et al, 1985, Woodward, et al, 1986). Epidemiology data do not support a causal relationship between smoking and breast cancer (Baron, 1984). However, these studies have considered only smokers and non-smokers. When age at start of smoking was examined, a 30% increase in relative risk was found for women who started smoking prior to age 17 years (Brinton, et al, 1986). These results are consistent with radiation-induced breast cancer, in which the greatest risk is among women under 20 years of age at the time of exposure (Committee on the Biological Effect of Ionizing Radiation, 1990). Furthermore, exposure to passive smoke is suggested to be major risk factor for breast cancer (Horton, 1988). Taken together, these data suggest an additional potential health risk to women from cigarette smoke, particularly when exposure to tobacco smoke occurs during childhood.

Comparisons of the DNA repair response in HMEC to two PAH revealed BP to be a much stronger inducer of UDS than an equimolar concentration of DMBA (Table 1). These data correlate with *in vitro* mutagenicity and DNA binding levels in HMEC (Gould, et al, 1986, Moore, et al, 1986, Moore, et al, 1987). When *in vitro* mutagenicity and DNA binding levels of BP and DMBA were compared in rat mammary epithelial cells, a pattern opposite to that of HMEC was obtained which correlates with the carcinogenic activity of DMBA in the rat mammary gland (Gould, et al, 1986, Moore, et al, 1986, Moore, et al, 1987). DMBA is a more effective mammary carcinogen than BP in rats (Meselson, 1977). When sister chromatid exchange induced by BP and DMBA was compared in human and rat mammary epithelial cells, results confirmed the notion that BP has a greater genotoxic effect than DMBA in HMEC (Mane, et al, 1990). The existence of DNA adducts in HMEC *in situ* has been demonstrated; human and rat mammary epithelial cells form different DNA adducts when exposed to BP *in vitro* (Seidman, et al, 1988). The differential UDS response observed with BP and DMBA in HMEC, together with the previous studies mentioned above, suggest that caution be applied when extrapolating rodent data to humans in the absence of mechanistic information and that the potential involvement of BP in human breast cancer should be considered.

CONCLUSIONS

Despite an increasing incidence of human breast cancer, its etiology remains unknown. Since some environmental chemicals are stored in human breast fat and are rodent mammary carcinogens, determining the carcinogenic potential of environmental agent in this key target tissue is important. Genotoxicity assays are used to identify potential carcinogens based on their ability to alter the DNA. One widely used genotoxicity assay is the measurement of DNA repair as a means to assess the ability of a test agent to reach and alter the DNA. Since species and tissue specifications are observed in chemical carcinogenesis, it is important to establish predictive tests in target cells. Therefore, the UDS assay was developed to measure genotoxic activity of environmental agents in normal HMEC. A wide variety of agents were examined to determine their ability to induce UDS in early passage cultures of normal HMEC derived from reduction mammoplasties. Of the chemicals demonstrated to be genotoxic in HMEC, some are known to cause cancer in rodents or to be contaminants in human breast tissue. The observation of genotoxic activity in the HMEC UDS assay suggests that mammary cells might be target for carcinogenic activity of some environmental agents. However, other factors such as accuracy of DNA repair processes, pharmacokinetics and epidemiology must be considered to establish a carcinogenic effect of chemicals on HMEC. These studies support the role of environmental agents in human breast cancer and aid in the validation of proposed animal models by determining whether chemicals are DNA reactive or metabolized to DNA reactive species in this critical target tissue.

Table 1: DNA Repair Responses in Human Mammary Epithelial Cells

Agent	Concentration	Case B402		Case B499		Case B708		Case 3014		Case 3085	
		NG[a]	% in repair[b]	NG[a]	% in repair[b]	NG[a]	% in repair[b]	NG[a]	% in repair[b]	NG[a]	% in repair[b]
Control		-0.4	4	0.1	2	0.1	4	0.5	7	0.8	2
BP	0.001 mM	-0.7	2	-0.3	0	26[c]	86d	16[c]	78[d]	5.7[d]	52[d]
	0.01 mM	27[c]	80[d]	32[c]	88[d]	25[c]	83d	13[c]	67[d]	16[d]	75[d]
DMBA	0.001 mM	-0.2	12[d]	0.6	4	1.0	8	1.3	5	0.8	15[d]
	0.001 mM	1.9	25[d]	0.5	3	0.4	3	-0.2	5	1.1	10[d]
AFB[1]	0.001 mM	-0.1	8	1.2	10[f]	2.4	23[d]	4.8[c]	42[d]	1.2	8
	0.01 mM	23[c]	83[d]	22[c]	87[d]	22[c]	93[d]	18[c]	72[d]	13[c]	68[d]
TSC	0.25%	0.9	3	1.0	15[f]	1.5	13[d]	2.1[c]	15[d]	2.2[c]	21[d]
	2.5%	1.6[d]	19[d]	3.9[c]	33[d]	2.3	21[d]	0.3	10	-0.4	10[d]
UV	100 J/m²	92[c]	100[d]	96[c]	100[d]	102[c]	100[d]	88[c]	100[d]	92[c]	100[d]

[a] NG for at least 30 cells counted for each 2 slides.

[b] An individual cell with ≥6 NG is considered in repair.

[c] Significantly greater than control at $P<0.01$; Student's t test.

[d] Significantly greater than control at $P<0.05$; χ^2 test.

[e] Significantly greater than control at $P<0.05$; Student's t test.

REFERENCES

American Cancer Society (1990): "Cancer Facts and Figures". New York: American Cancer Society, Inc.

Baron JA (1984): Smoking and estrogen-related disease. Am J Epidemiol 119:9-22.

Brinton LA, Schairer C, Stanford JL, Hoover RN (1986): Cigarette smoking and breast cancer. Am J. Epidemiol 123:614-622.

Butterworth BE, Ashby J, Bermudez E, Casciano D, Mirsalis J, Probst G, Williams GA (1987): A protocol and guide for the in vitro rat hepatocye DNA repair assay. Mutat Res 189:113-121.

Butterworth BE, Earle LL, Strom S, Jirtle R, Michalopoulo G (1983): Induction of DNA repair in human and rat hepatocytes by 1,6-dinitropyrene. Mutat Res 122:73-80.

Butterworth BE, Smith-Oliver T, Earle L, Loury D, White RD, Doolittle D, Working P, Cattley RC, Jirtle R, Michalopoulos G, Strom S (1989): Use of primary cultures of human hepatocytes in toxicology studies. Cancer Res 49:1075-1084.

Committee on the Biological Effects of Ionizing Radiation (1990): "Health Effects of Exposure to Low Levels of Ionizing Radiation." BEIR V. Washington DC: National Academy Press.

Dao TL (1969): Studies on mechanism of carcinogenesis in the mammary gland. Prog Exp Tumor Res 11:235-261.

DeMarini DM (1983): Genotoxicity of tobacco smoke and tobacco smoke condensate. Mutat Res 114:59-89.

Doolittle DJ, Butterworth BE (1984): Assessment of chemically-induced DNA repair in rat tracheal epithelial cells. Carcinogenesis 5:773-779.

Eldridge SR, Gould MN, Butterworth BE (1992): Genotoxicity of environmental agents in human mammary epithelial cells. Cancer Res 52:5617-5621.

Eldridge SR, Martens TW, Sattler CA, Gould MN (1989): Association of decreased intercellular communication with the immortal but not the tumorigenic phenotype in human mammary epithelial cells. Cancer Res 49:4326-4331.

Gould M, Grau DR, Seidman LA, Moore CJ (1986): Interspecies comparison of human and rat mammary epithelial cell-mediated mutagenesis by polycyclic aromatic hydrocarbons. Cancer Res 46:4942-4945.

Horton AW (1988): Indoor tobacco smoke pollution: a major risk for both breast and lung cancer? Cancer (Phila.) 62:6-14.

Howe GR (1984): Epidemiology of radiogenic breast cancer. In Boice JD Jr., Fraumeni JF (eds): ÒRadiation Carcinogenesis: Epidemiology and Biological Significance.Ó New York: Raven Press, pp 119-130.

Huggins CB (1979): Induction of mammary cancer in rats. In "Experimental Leukemia and Mammary Cancer." Chicago: University of Chicago Press, pp 73-79.

Lamplugh SM, Hendrickse RG, Apeagyei F, Mwanmut DD (1988): Aflatoxins in breast milk, neonatoal cord blood, and serum of pregnant women. Br Med J 296:968.

Langenbach R, Nesnow S, Rice JM (1983): "Organ and Species Specificity in Chemical Carcinogenesis." New York: Plenum Publishig Corp.

Loury DJ, Smith-Oliver T, Butterworth BE (1987): Assessment of unscheduled and replicative DNA synthesis in rat kidney cells exposed in vitro or in vivo to unleaded gasoline. Toxicol Appl Pharmacol 87: 127-140.

Luck W, Nau H, Hansen R, Stedlinger R (1985): Extent of nicotine and cotinine transfer to the human fetus, placenta and amniotic fluid of smoking mothers. Dev Pharmacol Ther 8:384-395.

Mane SS, Purnell DM, Hsu I-C (1990): Genotoxic effects of five polycyclic aromatic hydrocarbons in human and rat mammary epithelial cells. Environ Mol Mutage 15:78-82.

McCann J, Choi E, Yamasaki E, Ames BN (1975): Detection of carcinogens as mutagens in the Salmonella/microsome test: assay of 300 chemicals. Proc Natl Acad Sci USA 72:5135-5139.

Mermelstein R, Kiriazides DK, Butler M, McCoy EC, Rosenkranz HS (1981): The extraordinary mutagenicity of nitropyrenes in bacteria. Mutat Res 89:187-196.

Meselson M, Russell K (1977): Comparison of carcinogenic and mutagenic potency. In Hiatt HH, Watson JD, Winsten JA (eds): "Origins of Human Cancer, Vol. C." Cold Spring Harbor, NY: Cold Spring Harbor Laboratory, pp 1473-1481.

Moore CJ, Eldridge SR, Tricomi WA, Gould MN (1987): Quantitation of benzo(a)pyrene and 7,12-dimethylbenz(a)anthracene binding to nuclear macromolecules in human and rat mammary epithelial cells. Cancer Res 47:2609-2613.

Moore CJ, Tricomi WA, Gould MN (1986): Interspecies comparison of polycyclic aromatic hydrocarbon metabolism in human and rat mammary epithelial cells. Cancer Res 46:4946-4952.

Obana H, Hori S, Kahimoto L, Kunita N (1981): Polycyclic aromatic hydrocarbons in human fat and liver. Bull Environ Contam Toxicol 27:23-27.

Rasmussen RE, Painter RB (1966): Radiation-induced DNA synthesis in cultured mammalian cells. J Cell Biol 9:11-19.

Rozenkranz HS (1982): Direct-acting mutagens in diesel exhausts: magnitude of the problem. Mutat Res 101:1-10.

Sawyer TW, Gill RD, Smith-Oliver T, Butterworth BE, DiGiovanni J (1988): Measurement of unscheduled DNA synthesis (UDS) in primary cultures of adult mouse epidermal keratinocytes. Carcinogenesis 9:1197-1202.

Seidman LA, Moore CJ, Gould MN (1988): ^{32}P-postlabeling analysis of DNA adducts in human and rat mammary epithelial cells. Carcinogenesis 9:1071-1077.

Stampfer MR (1985): Isolation and growth of human mammary epithelial cells. J Tissue Culture Methods 9:107-115.

Tennant RW, Margolin BH, Shelby MD, Zeiger E, Hasema JK, Spalding J, Caspary W, Resnick M, Stasiewicz S, Anderson B, Minor R (1987): Prediction of chemical carcinogenicity in rodents from in vitro genetic toxicity assays. Science (Washington DC) 236:933-941.

Tokunage M, Land CE, Yamamoto T, Asano M, Tokuoka S, Ezaki H, Nishimori I, Fujikura T (1984): Epidemiology of radiogenic breast cancer. In Boice JD Jr., Fraumeni JF (eds): "Radiation Carcinogenesis: Epidemiology and Biological Significance." New York: Raven Press, pp 45-56.

Williams GM (1976): Carcinogen induced DNA repair in primary rat liver cell cultures: a possible screen for chemical carcinogens. Cancer Lett 1:231-236.

Woodward A, Grgurinovich N, Ryan P (1986): Nicotine and cotinine in the amniotic fluid of smokers in the second trimester of pregnancy. Am J Obstet Gynecol 120:64-44.

Etiology of Breast and
Gynecological Cancers, pages 133–145
© 1997 Wiley-Liss, Inc.

ORGANOCHLORINE EXPOSURE AND RISK FOR BREAST CANCER

Stephen H. Safe[1]* and Timothy Zacharewski[2]

Department of Veterinary Physiology and Pharmacology (S.S.)
Texas A&M University
College Station, TX 77843-4466
TEL: 409-845-5988 / FAX: 409-862-4929
and

Department of Pharmacology and Toxicology (T.Z.)
University of Western Ontario
London, Ontario N6A 5C1
Canada

ABSTRACT

Organochlorine industrial compounds, combustion products and pesticides have been widely identified in the environment and residues have been detected in extracts prepared from fish, wildlife, human tissues as well as human milk and serum. Many of these compounds possess sex steroid activities and therefore have the potential to disrupt endocrine-regulated homeostasis. Organochlorines which exhibit hormonal activity include: (i) polychlorinated biphenyls (PCBs), hydroxylated PCBs, o,p'-DDT, and other organochlorine insecticides which exhibit estrogen receptor (ER) agonist activities; (ii) p,p'-DDE, a ligand for the androgen receptor which exhibits antiandrogen activity; (iii) PCBs, 2,3,7,8-tetrachlorodibenzo-p-dioxin (TCDD), and related aromatic hydrocarbons which bind the aryl hydrocarbon (Ah) receptor and exhibit tissue-specific antiestrogenic activity; and (iv) hydroxylated aromatics which bind transthyretin, a thyroid hormone binding protein. Although, it has been suggested that the estrogenic activity of PCBs and DDE may be a contributing factor for development of breast cancer in women, levels of these compounds are not consistently elevated in breast cancer patients and there is no evidence that women occupationally-exposed to relatively high levels of PCBs or DDE exhibit an increased incidence of breast cancer. In contrast, epidemiology studies suggest that women exposed to high levels of TCDD during an industrial accident in Seveso, Italy, have a decreased incidence of both breast and endometrial cancer. Based on the dietary intake of hormone or antihormone mimics derived from natural compounds in food, the estrogenic contribution of organochlorine compounds is small and their role in development of breast cancer is questionable.

INTRODUCTION

Organochlorine compounds such as the polychlorinated biphenyls (PCBs), dibenzofurans (PCDFs), dibenzo-p-dioxins (PCDDs), and various organochlorine insecticides, such as 1,1,1-trichloro-2,2-bis(p-chlorophenyl)ethane (p,p'-DDT) and its

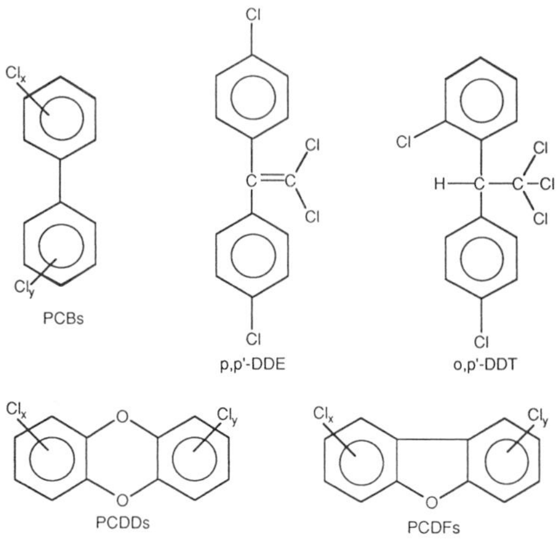

Figure 1: Structures of some organochlorine pollutants.

major metabolite, 1,1-dichloro-2,2-bis(p-chlorophenyl)ethylene (p,p'-DDE), have been identified as environmental contaminants (Fig. 1). Due to their high lipophilicity and persistence, organochlorine compounds preferentially bioaccumulate in the food chain and residues are routinely detected in fish, wildlife, human adipose tissue, serum and breast milk (Robinson et al., 1990; Schmitt et al., 1990; Safe 1994; Lake et al., 1995). p,p'-DDT and its major metabolite p,p'-DDE were initially identified in the environment during the 1960s and several studies have reported an association between DDT/DDE levels and reproductive problems in wildlife populations (Schmitt et al., 1990; Tanabe et al., 1994). PCBs and later PCDDs/PCDFs have also been routinely detected in environmental samples, and wildlife populations (particularly birds) exposed to halogenated aromatics in contaminated regions such as areas within the Great Lakes exhibited impaired reproduction (Giesy et al., 1994). Consequently, regulatory agencies have either banned or restricted the use of many environmentally-persistent organochlorine compounds which has resulted in decreased organochlorine levels in many ecosystems, and reproductive success of wildlife in these areas has recovered (Robinson et al., 1990; Schmitt et al., 1990; Turle et al., 1991; Giesy et al., 1994;).

Recent scientific concern regarding organochlorine chemicals and other industrial compounds has focused on their endocrine-disrupting properties and their activity as hormone mimics (Thomas and Colborn, 1992; Colborn et al., 1993; Davis et al., 1993; Hunter and Kelsey, 1993; Sharpe and Skakkebaek 1993). It has been hypothesized that industrial-derived compounds which exhibit estrogenic activity may contribute to the increased incidence of breast cancer in women and reproductive problems such as decreased sperm counts in males (Davis et al., 1993; Sharpe and Skakkebaek 1993). The validity of these hypotheses have been debated (Safe 1995a,b) and clearly require additional research. This paper will examine the evidence regarding the hypothesized role of environmental estrogens in development of breast cancer in women.

ROLE OF DDE AND PCBS IN BREAST CANCER

Wolff and coworkers reported that PCB residues in mammary tissue were higher in a group of 20 breast cancer patients in Connecticut compared to levels in 20 control patients with benign disease (Falck et al., 1992). Another study showed that serum DDE levels were higher in 58 New York City women with breast cancer compared to 171 control patients and it was suggested that "chemical contamination with organo-chlorine residues may be an important etiologic factor in breast cancer" (Wolff et al., 1993). In a subsequent prospective study among white, black and Asian women in California, Krieger and coworkers determined serum organochlorine levels in 150 breast cancer patients and the same number of controls (Krieger et al., 1994). Their results showed that there were no significant differences in organochlorine levels in the patients versus controls, and concluded "The data do not support the hypothesis that exposure to DDE and PCBs increases the risk of breast cancer" (Krieger et al., 1994). The role of DDE and PCBs as etiologic agents for breast cancer are also not supported by results from women more highly exposed to these chemicals. For example, the standard mortality ratios (SMRs) (observed/expected deaths x 100) for all malignant neoplasms, breast cancer and cancer of female genital organs in 1318 women employed in 2 plants which manufactured PCB-filled electrical capacitors were 78, 77 and 85, respectively (Brown, 1987). Thus, women exposed to relatively high levels of PCBs did not have an increased incidence of breast cancer. In addition, there is no evidence for an increase of breast cancer associated with exposure to DDT (Higginson, 1985). Therefore, these results suggest that lower environmental exposures to PCBs and DDT at environmental levels are unlikely to contribute significantly to development of this disease.

The analytical data which report elevated organochlorine levels in breast cancer patients from some locations (e.g. Connecticut, New York City and Quebec) (Mussalo-Rauhamaa et al., 1990; Falck et al., 1992; Wolff et al., 1993; Dewailly et al., 1994) but not others (California, Denmark) (Unger et al., 1984; Krieger et al., 1994) is intriguing. A recent nested case-control study reported that women in Michigan with higher serum polybrominated biphenyl (PBB) levels had an increased risk for developing breast cancer compared to women with lower PBB levels (Henderson et al., 1995). Like PCBs, there is no experimental evidence linking PBBs with breast cancer in women or in animal models. Nevertheless, the observations that in some locations women with breast cancer have higher levels of organohalogen compounds may provide some future insights into other factors which play a role in development of this disease. The human diet is the major source of exposure to organochlorine compounds and levels are highest in fish and wildlife products and in foods with a high fat content. It is possible that high organochlorine levels in breast cancer patients in some locations may be attributed to unusual dietary intakes and this should be further investigated.

ESTROGENIC ACTIVITIES OF ORGANOCHLORINE COMPOUNDS

o,p'-DDT and kepone were among the first organochlorine compounds which were characterized as estrogens using *in vitro* and *in vivo* bioassays (Bitman et al., 1968; Welch et al., 1969; Bitman and Cecil, 1970; Hammond et al., 1979; Robinson et al., 1984). Subsequently, several other organochlorine chemicals have been identified as estrogens and these include the pesticides endosulfan, toxaphene, dieldrin and methoxychlor, some PCB mixtures and individual congeners, as well as hydroxylated PCBs (Ecobichon and MacKenzie, 1974; Korach et al., 1988; Soto et al., 1994). o,p'-DDT and kepone are among the most well-characterized estrogenic industrial chemicals; both compounds competitively bind to the estrogen receptor (ER) and induce several estrogen regulated responses in the rodent uterus and mammalian cells in culture. For example, the results in Figure 2 illustrate the concentration-dependent induction of luciferase activity in Hela cells stably trans-fected with a Gal4:human ER chimeric receptor and a 17mer-regulated luciferase reporter gene. At a concentration of 10^{-9} M 17β-estradiol (E2) , there was maximal (100%) induction of luciferase activity which was inhibited by cotreating cells with 10^{-7} M ICI 164384, a potent antiestrogen. Both o,p'-DDT and kepone also induce luciferase activity in this bioassay; however, the EC_{50} values for this estrogenic response was 10^{-7} M and > 10^{-5} M, respectively, indicating that these estrogenic organochlorine compounds were > 1000 times less active than E2 (EC_{50} ~ 50 pM). These data are consistent with results of other studies (Soto et al., 1994) which indicate that most organochlorine environmental contaminants exhibit relatively weak estro-genic activity.

Korach and coworkers (Korach et al., 1988) previously reported that hydroxylated PCBs also bound to the. ER and exhibited estrogenic activity. The most active compounds, 2,',4',6'-trichloro-4-biphenylol and 2',3',4',5'-tetrachloro-4-biphenylol were substituted with a single para-hydroxyl group on one phenyl ring and 3 or 4

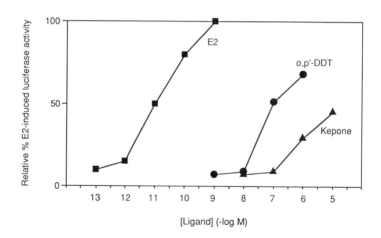

Figure 2: Estrogenic activity pf E2, o,p'DDT and kepone. HeLa cells stably-transfected with a Gal4:ER chimeric receptor and a 17mre-regulated luciferase reporter gene constructs were treated with the test compounds and induced luciferase activity was measured.

chlorine groups on the second ring. Estrogenic activity of hydroxy-PCBs was decreased by increased chloro substitution of the phenolic ring, addition of a para-hydroxyl group on the second ring or by hydroxyl substitution at meta or ortho positions. Recent studies have identified various hydroxylated PCBs in wildlife samples and in human serum (Bergman et al., 1994). The hydroxylated PCBS identified in human serum are substituted with para- or meta-hydroxy groups which are flanked by 2-ortho-chloro substituents. Many of the hydroxylated PCBs identified in human serum have been synthesized (Safe et al., 1995) and research in our laboratories have investigated the estrogenic activity of the following compounds: 2,2',3,4',5,5'-hexachloro-4-biphenylol; 2,3,3',4',5-pentachloro-4-biphenylol; 2',3,3',4',5-pentachloro-4-biphenylol; 2,2',3,3',4',5-hexachloro-4-biphenylol; 2,2',3,3',4',5,5'-heptachloro-4-biphenylol; 2,2',3,4',5,5',6-heptachloro-4-biphenylol; 2,2',3,4,4',5,5'-heptachloro-3-biphenylol. None of these compounds significantly bound to the rat uterine ER using a competitive binding displacement assay. Estrogenic activity was initially investigated in Hela cells stably-transfected with a Gal4:human ER chimeric receptor and a 17mer-regulated luciferase reporter gene. The chimeric receptor contains the ligand-binding domain of the ER and the DNA-binding domain of the Gal4 yeast protein. At concentrations as high as 10^{-5} M, the hydroxylated PCBs did not significantly induce luciferase activity whereas the significant induction was observed using 10^{-11} M E2. These results suggest that hydroxylated PCBs are unlikely to contribute to the overall estrogen burden of women.

COMPARATIVE HUMAN EXPOSURES TO ESTROGENIC ORGANOCHLORINE COMPOUNDS AND ESTROGENIC BIOFLAVONOIDS

Persistent organochlorine compounds are not only widely distributed in the environment but are also present in various foods and diet is the major source of human exposure to these compounds. Levels of various pesticides and pollutants in foods are routinely monitored by the Food and Drug Administration and the estimated consumption of estrogenic pesticides in foods by 16-17 year old individuals is approximately 2.5 µg/day. This includes DDT and related metabolites, 0.026; dieldrin, 0.0016; endosulfan, 0.0135; and p,p'-methoxychlor, 0.0005 (Winter, 1992). The total estimated exposure to these compounds (2.5 µg/day) is dominated by p,p-DDE which is the major organochlorine pollutant present in food and in human tissues (Winter, 1992). Most studies indicate that p,p'-DDE is not estrogenic (Bitman and Cecil, 1970). In contrast, humans are exposed to relatively high levels of estrogenic bioflavonoids (Kuhnau, 1976; Verdeal and Ryan, 1979) which exhibit both estrogenic and antiestrogenic activities (Markaverich et al., 1988, 1995; Mäkelä et al., 1995; Ruh et al., 1995). The results summarized in Table 1 compare human dietary intakes of estrogenic bioflavonoids, estrogenic drugs including the morning after pill, birth control pills and estrogens for postmenopausal therapy and estrogenic organochlorine pesticides. Based on mass balance estimates, the bioflavonoids in food and the estrogenic drugs dominate the overall dietary intakes of estrogenic compounds. Moreover, since the relative estrogenic potencies of bioflavonoids and organochlorine pesticides are relatively low (i.e. 10^{-4} to 10^{-6} times less active than E2) (Mäkelä et al., 1994; Soto et al., 1994), mass potency estimates [i.e. mass x potency (relative to E2)

= estrogen equivalents (EQ)] or EQs for bioflavonoids and organochlorine compounds would be exceedingly low compared to that of estrogenic drugs. The effects of postmenopausal hormone replacement therapy (HRT) on breast cancer incidence in women have been extensively investigated and these studies estimate increased risks from 1.3- to 2-fold (Hulka et al., 1994). There is evidence in some studies that the risks may increased with age, and Hulka and coworkers (Hulka et al., 1994) state that "However, one views the epidemiologic studies of HRT, it is evident that the risks incurred are modest". Thus, it seems unlikely that the relatively low levels of exposure to the weakly estrogenic organochlorine pesticides would significantly add to the overall lifetime burden of women to estrogens. Nevertheless, the potential human exposure to other industrial estrogens and other "natural" dietary estrogens should be further investigated in order to assess the potential health impacts of these compounds. While, it is unlikely that these compounds significantly contribute to overall exposure of women to estrogens, it is possible that exposure of some groups to these compounds at critical periods of development may be important (Brown and Lamartiniere, 1995).

Table 1: Estimated dietary exposures to estrogenic drugs, bioflavonoids and organochlorine pesticides (Kuhnau, 1976; Verdeal and Ryan, 1979; Winter, 1992).

Source	Intake - mass (µg/day)	EQ (µg/day)[a]
Morning after pill	333,500	333,500
Birth control pill	16,675	16,675
Post-menopausal therapy	3,350	3,350
Flavonoids in foods	100,000 - 1,000,000	?
Environmental organochlorine pesticides	2.5	?

[a] The potency of estrogenic drugs is approximately 1.0; the values for flavonoids in food and environmental estrogens vary from 10^{-4} to 10^{-6}.

ORGANOCHLORINE COMPOUNDS AS ANTIESTROGENS

TCDD and structurally-related halogenated aromatic hydrocarbons elicit a broad spectrum of tissue-, organ-, strain-, species-, sex-, and age-specific toxic and bio-chemical responses in laboratory animals and mammalian cells in culture. These effects include induction of both phase I and phase II drug-metabolizing enzyme activities, a wasting syndrome, lymphoid and thymic involution, hepatotoxicity, immunotoxicity, developmental and reproductive toxicity, chloracne and dermal toxicity, carcinogenicity and modulation of diverse endocrine response pathways (Goldstein and Safe, 1989; Safe 1995c). Although the response-specificity of TCDD is poorly understood, there is extensive evidence which supports the role of the Ah receptor as an initial cellular target for TCDD and related compounds. The proposed molecular mechanism of action of TCDD is based primarily on induction of CYP1A1 gene expression in which the Ah receptor functions as a ligand-dependent transcriptional enhancer and interacts with dioxin response elements (DREs) located in the 5'-flanking region of the gene (Swanson and Bradfield 1993; Whitlock, Jr., 1993). The nuclear Ah receptor complex is a unique heterodimeric transcription factor consisting of the Ah receptor ligand binding protein and the Ah receptor nuclear translocator (Arnt) protein. Studies support a comparable mechanism for induction of several genes, and it is hypothesized that the other biochemical and toxic effects elicited by TCDD are the result of the altered expression of other as yet unidentified genes (Swanson and Bradfield, 1993; Whitlock, Jr., 1993).

Kociba and coworkers (Kociba et al., 1978) reported that female Sprague-Dawley rats maintained on diets of 0.1, 0.01 and 0.001 μg TCDD/kg/day for 2 years developed hepatocellular carcinomas. However, in these same animals TCDD caused a dose-dependent decreased in the occurrence of spontaneous mammary and uterine tumors. Since growth of both mammary and uterine tumors can be estrogen-dependent, these data suggest that TCDD may have antiestrogenic properties. These observations have spurred considerable research activity in this and other laboratories on the characterization and mechanism of action of TCDD as an antiestrogen. Holcomb and Safe (Holcomb and Safe, 1994) also showed that TCDD (10 μg/kg) coadministered with DMBA delayed mammary tumor formation and administration of TCDD (10 μg/kg) to rats with DMBA-induced mammary tumors significantly inhibited tumor growth compared with control (corn oil) animals. Gierthy and coworkers (Gierthy et al., 1993) also reported the antitumorigenic activity of TCDD in immunosuppressed B6D2F1 mice bearing MCF-7 cell xenografts and treated with E2. Initial studies (Gallo et al., 1986) first demonstrated that TCDD caused a significant decrease in E2-induced uterine wet weight in weanling C57BL/6 and other strains of mice. Research in our laboratories has focused on the effects of TCDD on a broad spectrum of E2-induced responses in the female rat uterus and human breast cancer cells (Safe, 1995c). For example, TCDD inhibited the following E2-induced responses in the female rat uterus: the PR levels, epidermal growth factor receptor binding, uterine wet weights, and uterine peroxidase activity. TCDD also inhibited E2-induced uterine EGF receptor and c-*fos* protooncogene mRNA levels and caused a downregulation of cytosolic and nuclear ER levels.

The antiestrogenic activity of TCDD and related compounds has also been investigated using human breast cancer cell lines. Gierthy and coworkers (Gierthy et al., 1987, 1993; Gierthy and Lincoln, 1988) have reported that TCDD suppressed the E2-induced secretion of tissue plasminogen activator activity, cell proliferation and postconfluent focus production in MCF-7 cells. Research in our laboratories (Biegel and Safe, 1990; Zacharewski et al., 1991, 1994; Krishnan and Safe, 1993; Harper et al., 1994; Krishnan et al., 1995; Safe, 1995c) also focused on the antiestrogenic effects of TCDD and related compounds in human breast cancer and rodent cell lines. In cell proliferation studies, TCDD inhibited the growth of ER-positive MCF-7 cells, but did not alter the growth of ER-negative MDA-MB-231 cells. TCDD also inhibited the E2-induced secretion of the 32-, 54- and 160-kDa proteins and inhibited ER-induced PR, cathepsin D and pS2 gene expression in MCF-7 cells. TCDD also downregulated the nuclear ER in MCF-7 and in wild-type mouse Hepa 1c1c7 cells but not in Ah-nonresponsive class 2 mutant Hepa 1c1c7 indicating that a functional nuclear Ah receptor is required for this response (Zacharewski et al., 1991). Similar results have also been reported for inhibition of E2-induced pS2 gene expression in wild-type and mutant Hepa cells (Zacharewski et al., 1994).

Not surprisingly similar antiestrogenic activities have been reported for other Ah receptor agonists. For example, the 4-ring polynuclear aromatic hydrocarbons (PAHs),

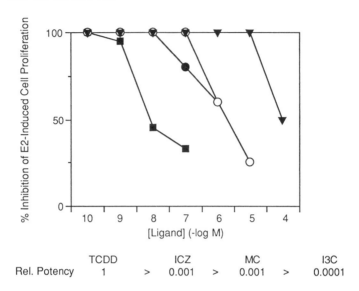

Figure 3: Comparative antiestrogenic activity of different Ah receptor agonists. MCF-7 human breast cancer cells were treated with 10^{-9} M E2 and the inhibition of E2-induced proliferation of MCF-7 cells by TCDD (■), 13C (▼), ICZ (●) and MC (○) was determined. The relative potencicies of these compounds as inhibitors of cell growth were 1, 0.0001, 0.001 and 0.001, respectively (Chaloupka et al., 1992; Tiwari et al., 1994; Liu et al., 1994).

such as benzo[a]pyrene, 3-methylcholanthrene and benz[a]anthracene, competitively bind to the Ah receptor and also inhibited E2-induced proliferation, secretion of cathepsin D and PR levels in MCF-7 cells (Chaloupka et al., 1992). Indole-3-carbinol (I3C), a natural product found in cruciferous vegetables such as cauliflower and Brussels sprouts, is a relatively weak Ah receptor agonist which inhibits growth of MCF-7 breast cancer cells (Liu et al., 1994; Tiwari et al., 1994). Indolo[3,2-b]carbazole (ICZ) is formed by the acid-catalyzed condensation of I3C and can be detected in the gut of laboratory animals (Bjeldanes et al., 1991). ICZ is a relatively potent Ah receptor agonist and not surprisingly inhibits many of the same E2-induced responses in MCF-7 cells reported for TCDD (Bjeldanes et al., 1991; Liu et al., 1994). Based on relative antiestrogenic potencies in MCF-7 cells, the antiestrogen potency factors of TCDD and related compounds (exodioxins) and naturally-occurring Ah receptor agonists which are present in food can be determined. For example, the results in Figure 3 illustrate the relative potencies of TCDD (1), ICZ (0.01), 3-methylcholanthrene (MC) (0.001, a prototypical PAH) and I3C (0.0001) as inhibitors of E2-induced proliferation of MCF-7 cells (Bjeldanes et al., 1991; Liu et al., 1994; Tiwari et al., 1994). Using these potency values and the estimated mass intake of I3C, ICZ, carcinogenic PAHs, and exodioxins in the human diet, the dietary intake of antiestrogen equivalents for these compounds can be estimated (see Table 2). The antiestrogen equivalency factors are based on *in vitro* studies, and undoubtedly the antiestrogen equivalency factors would be lower for compounds such as I3C, ICZ and the PAHs which are more readily metabolized *in vivo* . Previous studies indicate that both E2 and TCDD are approximately equipotent as estrogens and antiestrogens (Gierthy et al., 1987; Gierthy and Lincoln, 1988; Biegel and Safe, 1990; Zacharewski et al., 1991, 1994; Krishnan and Safe, 1993; Harper et al., 1994; Krishnan et al., 1995), respectively, and the current dietary intake of TCDD and related compounds is approximately 80 to 120 pg/day antiestrogen equivalents. The current estimated intake of estrogenic organochlorine compounds is 2.5 µg/day and their estrogenic potency relative to E2 is approximately 10^{-5} to 10^{-6}. Therefore, the estrogenic equivalents associated with organochlorine pesticides (2.5 to 25 pg/day) is comparable to the antiestrogen equivalents associated with dietary exposure to TCDD and related exodioxins, and is considerably lower than values observed for other natural TCDD-like compounds in food (Table 2).

Table 2: Dietary Intake of Ah Receptor Agonists and Their Estimated Antiestrogen Equivalents (Bjeldanes et al., 1991; Chaloupka et al., 1992; Liu et al., 1994; Tiwari et al., 1994).

Compounds	Mass Intake (pg/day)	Relative Potency	Antiestrogen Equivalents (pg/day)
PCDDs/PCDFs	1000 - 2000		80 - 120
PAHs	1,200,000 - 5,000,000	0.001	1200 - 5000
I3C	735,000,000	0.0001	73,500
ICZ	~ 73,500 ICZ	0.001	73.5

It should be noted that while there is no evidence that occupational exposure to high levels of PCBs or DDE is associated with increased breast cancer incidence, it was reported that for women accidentally exposed to TCDD in Seveso, Italy, "Breast cancer incidence among females was below expectations in the most contaminated zones, and a clear deficit for endometrial cancer was observed in Zones B and R" (Bertazzi et al., 1993). These observations suggest that exposure to TCDD resulted in antiestrogenic effects in females. Consequently, the overall hormone-dependent impacts of organochlorine compounds (estrogenic or antiestrogenic) must take into account the relative levels of exposure and potencies of the various pollutants as well as "natural" dietary chemicals which may exhibit both hormonal and antihormonal activities.

REFERENCES

Bergman Å, Klasson-Wehler E, Kuroki H (1994): Selective retention of hydroxylated PCB metabolites in blood. Environ Health Perspect 102:464-469.

Bertazzi PA, Pesatori AC, Consonni D, Tironi A, Landi MT, Zocchetti C (1993): Cancer incidence in a population accidentally exposed to 2,3,7,8-tetrachloro-dibenzo-p-dioxin. Epidemiology 4:398-406.

Biegel L, Safe S (1990): Effects of 2,3,7,8-tetrachlorodibenzo-p-dioxin (TCDD) on cell growth and the secretion of the estrogen-induced 34-, 52- and 160-kDa proteins in human breast cancer cells. J Steroid Biochem Mol Biol 37:725-732.

Bitman J, Cecil HC (1970): Estrogenic activity of DDT analogs and polychlorinated biphenyls. J Agric Food Chem 18:1108-1112.

Bitman J, Cecil HC, Harris SJ, Fries GF (1968): Estrogenic activity of o,p'-DDT in the mammalian uterus and avian oviduct. Science 162:371-372.

Bjeldanes LF, Kim JY, Grose KR, Bartholomew JC, Bradfield CA (1991): Aromatic hydrocarbon responsiveness-receptor agonists generated from indole-3-carbinol *in vitro* and *in vivo* - comparisons with 2,3,7,8-tetrachlorodibenzo-*p*-dioxin. Proc Natl Acad Sci USA 88:9543-9547.

Brown DP (1987): Mortality of workers exposed to polychlorinated biphenyls - an update. Arch Environ Health 42:333-339.

Brown NM, Lamartiniere CA (1995): Xenoestrogens alter mammary gland differentiation and cell proliferation in the rat. Environ Health Perspect 103:708-713.

Chaloupka K, Krishnan V, Safe S (1992): Polynuclear aromatic hydrocarbon carcinogens as antiestrogens in MCF-7 human breast cancer cells. Role of the Ah receptor. Carcinogenesis 13:2223-2239.

Colborn T, Vom Saal FS, Soto AM (1993): Developmental effects of endocrine-disrupting chemicals in wildlife and humans. Environ Health Perspect 101:378-384.

Davis DL, Bradlow HL, Wolff M, Woodruff T, Hoel DG, Anton-Culver H (1993): Medical hypothesis: xenoestrogens as preventable causes of breast cancer. Environ Health Perspect 101:372-377.

Dewailly E, Dodin S, Verreault R, Ayotte P, Sauvé L, Morin J, Brisson J (1994): High organochlorine body burden in women with estrogen receptor-positive breast cancer. J Natl Cancer Inst 86:232-234.

Ecobichon DJ, MacKenzie DO (1974): The uterotropic activity of commercial and isomerically-pure chlorobiphenyls in the rat. Res Comm Chem Pathol Pharmacol 9:85-95.

Falck F, Ricci A, Wolff MS, Godbold J, Deckers P (1992): Pesticides and polychlorinated biphenyl residues in human breast lipids and their relation to breast cancer. Arch Environ Health 47:143-146.

Gallo MA, Hesse EJ, MacDonald GJ, Umbreit TH (1986): Interactive effects of estradiol and 2,3,7,8-tetrachlorodibenzo-*p*-dioxin on hepatic cytochrome P-450 and mouse uterus. Toxicol Lett 32:123-132.

Gierthy JF, Lincoln DW (1988): Inhibition of postconfluent focus production in cultures of MCF-7 breast cancer cells by 2,3,7,8-tetrachlorodibenzo-*p*-dioxin. Breast Cancer Res 12:227-233.

Gierthy JF, Bennett JA, Bradley LM, Cutler DS (1993): Correlation of *in vitro* and *in vivo* growth suppression of MCF-7 human breast cancer by 2,3,7,8-tetrachlorodibenzo-*p*-dioxin. Cancer Res 53:3149-3153.

Gierthy JF, Lincoln DW, Gillespie MB, Seeger JI, Martinez HL, Dickerman HW, Kumar SA (1987): Suppression of estrogen-regulated extracellular plasminogen activator activity of MCF-7 cells by 2,3,7,8-tetrachlorodibenzo-*p*-dioxin. Cancer Res 47:6198-6203.

Giesy JP, Ludwig JP, Tillitt DE (1994): Deformities of birds in the Great Lakes region: assigning causality. Environ Sci Technol 28:128A-135A.

Goldstein JA, Safe S (1989): Mechanism of action and structure-activity relationships for the chlorinated dibenzo-*p*-dioxins and related compounds. Kimbrough RD, Jensen AA (eds): "Halogenated Biphenyls, Naphthalenes, Dibenzodioxins and Related Compounds." Amsterdam: Elsevier-North Holland, pp 239-293.

Hammond B, Katzenellenbogen BS, Krauthammer N, McConnell J (1979): Estrogenic activity of the insecticide chlordecone (Kepone) and interaction with uterine estrogen receptor. Proc Natl Acad Sci USA 76:6641-6645.

Harper N, Wang X, Liu H, Safe S (1994): Inhibition of estrogen-induced progesterone receptor in MCF-7 human breast cancer cells by aryl hydrocarbon (Ah) receptor agonists. Mol Cell Endocrinol 104:47-55.

Henderson AK, Rosen D, Miller GL, Figgs LW, Zahm SH, Sieber SM, Humphrey HEB, Sinks T (1995): Breast cancer among women exposed to polybrominated biphenyls. Epidemiology 6:544-546.

Higginson J (1985): DDT epidemiologic evidence. IARC Sci Publ 65:107-117.

Holcomb M, Safe S (1994): Inhibition of 7,12-dimethylbenzanthracene-induced rat mammary tumor growth by 2,3,7,8-tetrachlorodibenzo-*p*-dioxin. Cancer Letters 82:43-47.

Hulka BS, Liu ET, Lininger RA (1994): Steroid hormones and risk of breast cancer. Cancer 74:1111-1124.

Hunter DJ, Kelsey KT (1993): Pesticide residues and breast cancer: the harvest of a Silent Spring. J Natl Cancer Inst 85:598-599.

Kociba RJ, Keyes DG, Beger JE, Carreon RM, Wade CE, Dittenber DA, Kalnins RP, Frauson LE, Park CL, Barnard SD, Hummel RA, Humiston CG (1978): Results of a 2-year chronic toxicity and oncogenicity study of 2,3,7,8-tetrachlorodibenzo-*p*-dioxin (TCDD) in rats. Toxicol Appl Pharmacol 46:279-303.

Korach KS, Sarver P, Chae K, McLachlin JA, McKinney JD (1988): Estrogen receptor-binding activity of polychlorinated hydroxybiphenyls: conformationally restricted structural probes. Mol Pharmacol 33:120-126.

Krieger N, Wolff MS, Hiatt RA, Rivera M, Vogelman J, Orentreich N (1994): Breast cancer and serum organochlorines: a prospective study among white, black, and Asian women. J Natl Cancer Inst 86:589-599.

Krishnan V, Porter W, Santostefano M, Wang X, Safe S (1995): Inhibition of estrogen-induced cathepsin D gene expression by 2,3,7,8-tetrachlorodibenzo-*p*-dioxin (TCDD) in MCF-7 cells: molecular mechanism. Mol Cell Biol 15:6710-6719.

Krishnan V, Safe S (1993): Polychlorinated biphenyls (PCBs), dibenzo-*p*-dioxins (PCDDs) and dibenzofurans (PCDFs) as antiestrogens in MCF-7 human breast cancer cells: quantitative structure-activity relationships. Toxicol Appl Pharmacol 120:55-61.

Kuhnau J (1976): The flavonoids. A class of semi-essential food components: their role in human nutrition. Wld Rev Nutr Diet 24:117-191.

Lake CA, Lake JL, Haebler R, McKinney R, Boothman WS, Sadove SS (1995): Contaminant levels in Harbor seals from the northeastern United States. Arch Environ Contam Toxicol 29:128-134.

Liu H, Wormke M, Safe S, Bjeldanes LF (1994): Indolo[3,2-b]carbazole: a dietary factor which exhibits both antiestrogenic and estrogenic activity. J Natl Cancer Inst 86:1758-1765.

Markaverich BM, Roberts RR, Alejandro MA, Johnson GA, Middleditch BS, Clark JH (1988): Bioflavonoid interaction with rat uterine type II binding sites and cell growth inhibition. J Steroid Biochem 30:71-78.

Markaverich BM, Webb B, Densmore CL, Gregory RR (1995): Effects of coumestrol on estrogen receptor function and uterine growth in ovariectomized rats. Environ Health Perspect 103:574-581.

Mäkelä SI, Davis VL, Tally WC, Korkman J, Salo L, Vihko R, Santti R, Korach KS (1994): Dietary estrogens act through estrogen receptor-mediated processes and show no antiestrogenicity in cultured breast cancer cells. Environ Health Perspect 102:572-578.

Mäkelä SI, Pylkkanen LH, Santti RS, Adlercreutz H (1995): Dietary soybean may be antiestrogenic in male mice. J Nutr 125:437-445.

Mussalo-Rauhamaa H, Häsänen E, Pyysalo H, Antervo K, Kauppila R, Pantzar P (1990): Occurrence of â-hexachlorocyclohexane in breast cancer patients. Cancer 66:2124-2128.

Robinson AK, Mukku VT, Spalding DM, Stancel GM (1984): The estrogenic activity of DDT: the *in vitro* induction of an estrogen-inducible protein by *o,p*-DDT. Toxicol Appl Pharmacol 76:537-543.

Robinson PE, Mack GA, Remmers J, Levy R, Mohadjer L (1990): Trends of PCB, hexachlorobenzene, and β-benzene hexachloride levels in the adipose tissue of the U.S. population. Environ Res 53:175-192.

Ruh MF, Zacharewski T, Connor K, Howell J, Chen I, Safe S (1995): Naringenin: a weakly estrogenic bioflavonoid which exhibits antiestrogenic activity. Biochem Pharmacol 50:1485-1493.

Safe S (1994): Polychlorinated biphenyls (PCBs): environmental impact, biochemical and toxic responses, and implications for risk assessment. C R C Crit Rev Toxicol 24:87-149.

Safe S (1995a): Do environmental estrogens play a role in development of breast cancer in women and male reproductive problems. Human Ecol Risk Assess 1:17-23.

Safe S (1995b): Environmental and dietary estrogens and human health - is there a problem? Environ Health Persp 103:346-351.

Safe S (1995c): Modulation of gene expression and endocrine response pathways by 2,3,7,8-tetrachlorodibenzo-*p*-dioxin and related compounds. Pharmacol Therap 67:247-281.

Safe S, Washburn K, Zacharewski T, Phillips TD (1995): Synthesis and characterization of hydroxylated polychlorinated biphenyls (PCBs) identified in human serum. Chemosphere 31:3017-3023.

Schmitt CJ, Zajicek JL, Peterman PH (1990): National contaminant biomonitoring program: residues of organochlorine chemicals in U.S. freshwater fish, 1976-1984. Arch Environ Contam Toxicol 19:748-781.

Sharpe RM, Skakkebaek NF (1993): Are oestrogens involved in falling sperm counts and disorders of the male reproductive tract. Lancet 341:1392-1395.

Soto AM, Chung KL, Sonnenschein C (1994): The pesticides endosulfan, toxaphene, and dieldrin have estrogenic effects on human estrogen-sensitive cells. Environ Health Perspect 102;380-383. Swanson HI, Bradfield CA (1993): The Ah-receptor: genetics, structure and function. Pharmacogenetics 3:213-223.

Tanabe S, Iwata H, Tatsukawa R (1994): Global contamination by persistent organochlorines and their ecotoxicological impact on marine mammals. Sci Total Environ 154:163-177.

Thomas KB, Colborn T (1992): Organochlorine endocrine disruptors in human tissue. Colborn T, Clement C (eds): "Chemically Induced Alterations in Sexual Development: the Wildlife/Human Connection." Princeton, NJ: Princeton Scientific Publishing, pp 365-394.

Tiwari RK, Guo L, Bradlow HL, Telang NT, Osborne MP (1994): Selective responsiveness of breast cancer cells to indole-3-carbinol, a chemopreventative agent. J Natl Cancer Inst 86:126-131.

Turle R, Norstrom RJ, Collins B (1991): Comparison of PCB quantitation methods: re-analysis of archived specimens of herring gull eggs from the Great Lakes. Chemosphere 22:201-213.

Unger M, Kiaer H, Blichert-Toft M, Olsen J, Clausen J (1984): Organochlorine compounds in human breast fat from deceased with and without breast cancer and in biopsy material from newly diagnosed patients undergoing breast surgery. Environ Res 34:24-28.

Verdeal K, Ryan DS (1979): Naturally-occurring estrogens in plant foodstuffs - a review. J Food Protection 42:577-583.

Welch RM, Levin W, Conney AH (1969): Estrogenic action of DDT and its analogs. Toxicol Appl Pharmacol 14:358-367.

Whitlock JP, Jr. (1993): Mechanistic aspects of dioxin action. Chem Res Toxicol 6:754-763.

Winter CK (1992): Dietary pesticide risk assessment. Rev Environ Contam Toxicol 127:23-67.

Wolff MS, Toniolo PG, Leel EW, Rivera M, Dubin N (1993): Blood levels of organochlorine residues and risk of breast cancer. J Natl Cancer Inst 85:648-652.

Zacharewski T, Bondy K, McDonell P, Wu ZF (1994): Antiestrogenic effects of 2,3,7,8-tetrachlorodibenzo-p-dioxin on 17β-estradiol-induced pS2 expression. Cancer Res 54:2707-2713.

Zacharewski T, Harris M, Safe S (1991): Evidence for a possible mechanism of action of the 2,3,7,8-tetrachlorodibenzo-p-dioxin-mediated decrease of nuclear estrogen receptor levels in wild-type and mutant Hepa 1c1c7 cells. Biochem Pharmacol 41:1931-1939.

Etiology of Breast and
Gynecological Cancers, pages 147–158
© 1997 Wiley-Liss, Inc.

DIET AND BREAST CANCER: OPPORTUNITIES FOR PREVENTION AND INTERVENTION

David P. Rose, Jeanne M. Connolly, and Xin-Hua Liu

Division of Nutrition and Endocrinology, American Health Foundation, Valhalla, New York 10595

INTRODUCTION

It is more than 50 years since Tannenbaum (1942) reported an association between fat consumption and experimental mammary carcinogenesis, yet the relevance of this repeatedly confirmed observation to human breast cancer remains in doubt (Willett, et al., 1992; Whittemore and Henderson, 1993; Freedman, et al., 1993; Rose, 1994). It seems unlikely that the tools of descriptive epidemiology are capable of resolving the issue; any significant progress is likely to emerge from mechanistic studies directed at providing biological plausibility, from focusing on identified biomarkers of breast cancer risk (Slattery, et al., 1995) and their interaction with specific components of dietary fat and their biologically active metabolic products, and from the results of appropriately designed dietary intervention trials.

In this discussion, the focus will be on the need to make two major distinctions. The first is that any discussion of the influence which dietary fat may have on the initial steps in the carcinogenic process, with the implication that epidemiological investigation and any intervention should be initiated relatively early in life, must be separated from effects on the progression of dysplastic breast lesions and carcinoma *in situ* to invasive breast cancer. The second is that the increasingly recognized interactions between diet and hormonal status and their biological significance in the context of breast cancer, are quite separate from the effects which specific fatty acids, and the autocoids derived from them, have on breast cancer cell biology.

DIETARY FAT, SERUM ESTROGENS, AND BREAST CANCER

It is generally recognized that estrogenic hormones are involved in breast cancer development (Key and Pike, 1988; Rose, 1993; Toniolo, et al., 1995) and progression (Jordan, 1991). But, although some case-control studies demonstrated higher levels of circulating estrogens (Adami, et al., 1979; Moore, et al., 1982), and increases in their biological availability (Moore, et al., 1982; Jones, et al., 1987; Takatani, et al., 1987), it is only recently that the association has been supported by a substantial study of prospective design (Toniolo, et al., 1995).

A relationship between blood estrogen levels and breast cancer was also suggested by two epidemiological studies which compared the serum estradiol and estrone concentrations in women from populations with markedly different risks for the disease. Shimizu, et al. (1990) assayed these two principal biologically active estrogens in serum samples from rural-dwelling healthy postmenopausal Japanese women (low risk), and postmenopausal white American women (high risk), and found significantly lower levels in the Japanese group. A similar study by Key, et al. (1990) compared estradiol levels of both premenopausal and postmenopausal rural Chinese with British women of corresponding menopausal status. Again, the Chinese women had significantly lower levels of the circulating estrogen.

While these observed variations in serum estrogens between Asian and western European and American women may be ascribable to several cultural characteristics, one prominent difference is the level of dietary fat intake. Thus, while the average fat consumption in Japan has increased from 9% of total calories in 1955 to 25% in 1987 (Wynder et al., 1991), little change has occurred in the rural areas. Clearly, this implies that the shift towards a western style dietary pattern in the urban centers includes a considerably higher fat intake than the 25% of total calories average figure. In this context, it is noteworthy that the overall breast cancer mortality rate in Japan has shown a sizable increase since 1960 (Wynder et al., 1991), and that a comparison of serum estradiol concentrations between British women and Japanese women resident in the Tokyo area did not show any significant difference (Bulbrook et al., 1976). Similar dietary differences apply to the British-Chinese study (Key et al., 1990). Here, a nutritional survey showed that the rural Chinese women were obtaining an average of 15% of their calories from dietary fat, but in the United Kingdom it continues to be as high as 40%.

Goldin et al. (1986) compared the plasma estrogen levels of white American women resident in Hawaii (high breast cancer risk; high-fat diet), and recent immigrants from Southeast Asia (low breast cancer risk; low fat diet). On average, the estradiol concentration for the group of premenopausal Asian women was only 56% that of the Caucasians, and individual values were positively correlated with the estimated dietary fat intake.

While these, and similar comparisons provide indirect support for the hypothesis that dietary fat affects estrogen status, and so may influence breast cancer risk, it should be recognized that the observed associations are not necessarily causal. However, several experimental studies have provided direct evidence of a fat-estrogen interaction. Rose, et al. (1987) performed a dietary intervention in which the fat consumption of 16 American white premenopausal women was decreased from an average of 37% to approximately 20% of total calories. After 3 months, the estradiol and estrone concentrations were significantly reduced in serum samples obtained in the midluteal stage of the menstrual cycle. Since this initial report, several groups of investigators have confirmed the suppressive effect of low-fat diets on the circulating estrogens in both pre-menopausal (Taylor, et al., 1992; Goldin, et al., 1994) and postmenopausal (Prentice, et al., 1990) women.

Although the reductions in serum estradiol and estrone obtained in these experimental studies are statistically significant, they amount to changes in the order of 15-20%. While it may be questioned whether these somewhat modest reductions are also of significance in the context of breast cancer risk, the data obtained from the prospective study performed by Toniolo, et al. (1995) are reassuring; here the difference between the cases (women who subsequently developed breast cancer) and controls (those healthy at the time of the data analysis) amounted to 18-20%. Prentice et al. (1990), using data from published case-control studies, calculated that a reduction of 17% in the serum estradiol concentrations of postmenopausal women would have a significant effect on breast cancer risk. Also, Bernstein et al. (1990), on the basis of a similar analysis performed on serum assay results from their own Chinese-American comparisons, concluded that differences in the range of 11 to 20% are likely to be important in the extent of their influence on mammary tissue, and may explain the differing levels of breast cancer risk.

If we accept the arguments presented above, the timing of a low-fat dietary intervention becomes important; is it really necessary to initiate this early in life? Experience from the adjuvant therapy tamoxifen trials suggests otherwise (Early Breast Cancer Trialists' Collaborative Group, 1992). Here, it was found that not only did the antiestrogen favorably impact on the outcome of the pre-existing breast cancer, but it also produced a significant reduction in the risk of the patients, notably those beyond the menopause, developing a new primary cancer in the opposite breast. If such a benefit accrues from blocking estrogen action, it seems reasonable to argue that this should also result from reducing the levels of biologically active estrogens by dietary means.

FATTY ACIDS, EICOSANOIDS, AND BREAST CANCER PROGRESSION

While total fat consumption may affect breast cancer risk and progression by hormonal mechanisms, specific fatty acids may do the same by more direct effects on tumor cell biology.

Several epidemiological studies have associated a high fat consumption with a poor prognosis in postsurgically resected breast cancer (Gregorio, et al., 1985; Nomura, et al., 1991; Holm, et al., 1993; Rohan, et al., 1993; Zhang, et al., 1995), and in two of these relatively high intakes of polyunsaturated omega-6 fatty acids were related to more advanced disease at the time of diagnosis (Nomura, et al., 1991), and reduced survival (Rohan, et al., 1993).

In a series of studies, we showed that linoleic acid, an omega-6 fatty acid, stimulates the growth and metastasis of estrogen-independent breast cancer cell lines in athymic nude mice (Rose, et al., 1991; Rose, et al., 1993; Rose, et al., 1994). In contrast, the long-chain omega-3 fatty acids, which are present at high concentrations in some fish oils, inhibit breast cancer progression in the nude mouse model (Rose, et al., 1995).

Linoleic acid, the principal omega-6 fatty acid in some vegetable oils, is metabolized to arachidonic acid, which is incorporated into cell membrane phospholipids, but is available for mobilization by way of phospholipase A_2 activity and subsequent conversion to bioactive eicosanoids. Among the families of eicosanoids, cyclooxygenase is responsible for the biosynthesis of prostaglandins and thromboxanes, and lipoxygenases for the formation of 5-, 12-, and 15-hydroxyeicosatetraenoic acids (HETEs), and a series of leukotrienes (Fig. 1)

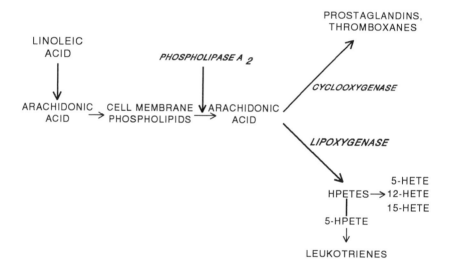

Fig. 1. The biosynthesis of eicosanoids from dietary linoleic acid via arachidonic acid. HPETE, hydroperoxyeicosatetraenoic acid; HETE, hydroxyeicosatetraenoic acid.

We, and others, have shown that the growth of some human breast cancer cell lines *in vitro* is also stimulated by linoleic acid, and that this effect is mediated via the production of one or more lipoxygenase products (Rose and

Connolly, 1989; Rose and Connolly, 1990; Buckman, et al., 1991; Earashi, et al., 1996). Earashi, et al. (1996) related this growth stimulation to expression of c-*myc* mRNA.

Regional and systemic metastases are the principal causes of treatment failure in patients with breast cancer. As well as their stimulating effects on tumor cell growth, eicosanoids derived from linoleic acid have been associated with metastasis. The formation of systemic metastases involves a series of critical steps, the first of which is the invasive process by which tumor cells penetrate the epithelial basement membrane and enter the underlying interstitial stroma. Invasion itself requires the successful completion of three steps: tumor cell adhesion to the membrane surface, secretion and activation of proteolytic enzymes, and cell migration into the digested zone and attachment to the exposed area of matrix (Stracke and Liotta, 1982).

In addition to its stimulatory effects on breast cancer cell growth, we found that linoleic acid stimulates the capacity of the MDA-MB-435 human breast cancer cell line for invasion in an *in vitro* assay (Connolly and Rose, 1993). This effect is associated with induction of the 92 kDa isoform of type IV collagenase (matrix metalloproteinase-9; MMP-9), a key proteinase in breast cancer metastasis, is mediated by way of 12-HETE biosynthesis from the omega-6 fatty acid, and is blocked by a pharmacological inhibitor of 12-lipoxygenase activity (Liu and Rose, 1994; Liu, et al., 1996).

While 12-HETE, and perhaps other lipoxygenase products, is involved in breast cancer invasion, products of cyclooxygenase activity appear to be involved in other steps in the metastatic process. Elevated prostaglandin E_2 production by the primary tumor has been related to a high risk of developing metastasis in breast cancer patients (Rolland, et al., 1980), and also shown to be correlated with metastatic capacity in a series of mouse mammary carcinoma cell lines (Fulton and Heppner, 1985). In the MDA-MB-435 breast cancer cell model, the non-steroidal anti-inflammatory drug indomethacin inhibited dietary linoleic acid-stimulated growth and metastasis in nude mice at doses which reduced tumor levels of several cyclooxygenase products, including prostaglandin E_2, but did not affect the concentrations of 5-, 12-, or 15-HETE (Connolly, et al., 1996).

Feeding diets supplemented with eicosapentaenoic acid (EPA) or docosahexaenoic acid (DHA), long-chain omega-3 fatty acids, partially suppresses MDA-MB-435 breast cancer cell growth in the mammary fat pads of nude mice, and also inhibits the development of metastatic lung nodules (Rose and Connolly, 1993; Rose, et al., 1995). These inhibitory effects on lung metastasis are associated with reduced levels of MMP-9 in the primary tumors, and in experiments *in vitro* EPA was also found to suppress MMP-9 mRNA expression in the cultured cell line (Liu and Rose, 1995). While several mechanisms may be postulated to explain the effects of omega-3 fatty acids on breast cancer cell metastases, their inhibitory effects on eicosanoid biosynthesis may be important; the concentrations of both prostaglandin E_2 and lipoxygenase products, notably 12-HETE, were reduced in mammary fat pad tumors from mice fed EPA or DHA (Rose, et al., 1995).

APPLICATIONS FOR PREVENTION AND THERAPY: CLINICAL TRIALS

Several approaches to breast cancer prevention and intervention in the established disease emerge from the epidemiological, clinical, and experimental data which are now available. The most straightforward in concept, but most difficult in implementation, is the prescription of a low-fat diet in which total intake is reduced to 15-20% of total calories. The feasibility of conducting a clinical trial in which women are randomly assigned to a control or low-fat intervention group has been demonstrated by several groups of independent investigators (Prentice, et al., 1988; Boyd, et al., 1992; Chlebowski, et al., 1992).

Two of the low-fat intervention trials have breast cancer prevention as their end-point. One, the "Women's Health Initiative", is a National Institutes of Health-funded trial in which the planned recruitment is approximately 48,000 healthy women aged 50-79 years. The experimental design of this trial, which incorporates two other intervention arms -- hormone replacement, and calcium and vitamin D supplementation -- for the prevention of cardiovascular disease and osteoparotic fractures, respectively, has been aggressively criticized (Whittemore and Henderson, 1993; Willett and Hunter, 1994) and defended (Freedman, et al., 1993). The other prevention trial focuses on women who are identified as being at an increased risk of breast cancer because they have densities on mammographic examination which are indicative of breast cancer dysplasia (Boyd, et al., 1992; Byrne, et al., 1995; Boyd, et al., 1995). The advantages of this Canadian trial are that the populations to be studied have a defined, and quantifiable, breast cancer risk, and that a readily available intermediate endpoint exists; regression of the mammographic and associated histologically identified dysplasia.

The Women's Intervention Nutrition Study (WINS) has as its purpose the prevention of recurrent disease in postmenopausal, surgically-treated, breast cancer patients. This is a multi-center, randomized, trial which is funded by the National Cancer Institute. As in the case of the two prevention trials, the primary dietary intervention is a reduction in total fat intake to 15-20% of total calories, which is achieved by substituting a dietary pattern high in fiber-rich fruits and vegetables. Consequently, an interaction between a low-fat and a high-fiber intake cannot be excluded, which may itself be favorable to the desired outcome (Rose, 1992) .

Although one of the principal mechanistic arguments which has been presented in support of the three low-fat dietary interventions is a reduction in the circulating estrogens, a decrease in fat intake to 15-20% of total calories will also have a pronounced effect on linoleic acid intake. This is the most common polyunsaturated fatty acid in the western diet, with a mean intake in the United States of 6-7% of calories (National Research Council, 1989). However, on the basis of our experience with the nude mouse model for breast cancer progression described earlier, we advocate a clinical trial, perhaps with mammographic dysplasia or the presence of carcinoma *in situ* as entry criteria, of a dietary intervention comprising a less aggressive reduction in total fat intake and a partial substitution of omega-6 fatty acid sources with omega-3 fatty acids.

REFERENCES

Adami H-O, Johansson EDB, Vegelius J, Victor A (1979): Serum concentrations of estrone, androstenedione, testosterone and sex-hormone-binding globulin in postmenopausal women with breast cancer and in age-matched controls. Ups J Med Sci 84:259-261.

Bernstein L, Yuan J-M, Ross RK, Pike MC, Hanisch R, Lobo R, Stanczyk F, Gao Y-T, Henderson BE (1990): Serum hormone levels in pre-menopausal Chinese women in Shanghai and white women in Los Angeles: results from two breast cancer case-control studies. Cancer Causes Control 1:51-58.

Boyd NF, Connelly P, Byng J, Yaffe M, Draper H, Little L, Jones D, Martin LJ, Lockwood G, Tritchler D (1995): Plasma lipids, lipoproteins, and mammographic densities. Cancer Epidemiol Biomarkers & Prev 4:727-733.

Boyd NF, Cousins M, Lockwood G, Tritchler D (1992): Dietary fat and breast cancer risk: the feasibility of a clinical trial of breast cancer prevention. Lipids 27:821-826.

Buckman DK, Hubbard NE, Erickson KL (1991): Eicosanoids and linoleate-enhanced growth of mouse mammary tumor cells. Prostaglandins Leukotrienes Essential Fatty Acids 44:177-184.

Bulbrook RD, Swain MC, Wang DY, Hayward JL, Kumaoka S, Takatani O, Abe O, Utsunomiya J (1976): Breast cancer in Britain and Japan: plasma oestradiol-17ß, oestrone and progesterone, and their urinary metabolites in normal British and Japanese women. Eur J Cancer 12:725-735.

Byrne C, Schairer C, Wolfe J, Parekh N, Salane M, Brinton LA, Hoover R, Haile R (1995): Mammographic features and breast cancer risk: effects with time, age, and menopause status. J Natl Cancer Inst 87:1622-1629.

Chlebowski RT, Rose DP, Buzzard IM, Blackburn GL, Insull W Jr, Grosvenor M, Elashoff R, Wynder EL (1992): Adjuvant dietary fat intake reduction in postmenopausal breast cancer patient management. Breast Cancer Res Treat 20:73-84.

Connolly JM, Liu X-H, Rose DP (1996) Dietary linoleic acid-stimulated human breast cancer cell growth and metastasis in nude mice and their suppression by indomethacin, a cyclooxygenase inhibitor. Nutr Cancer in press.

Connolly JM, Rose DP (1993): Effects of fatty acids on invasion through reconstituted basement membrane ("Matrigel") by a human breast cancer cell line. Cancer Lett 75:137-142.

Early breast cancer trialists' collaborative group (1992): Systemic treatment of early breast cancer by hormonal, cytotoxic or immune therapy. Lancet 339:1-15.

Earashi M, Endo Y, ObataT, Minami M, Noguchi M, Miyazaki I, Sasaki T (1996): Effects of linoleic acid and eicosanoid synthesis inhibitors on the growth and c-*myc* oncogene expression of human breast cancer cells. Int J Oncol 8:145-151.

Freedman LS, Prentice RL, Clifford C, Harlan W, Henderson M, Rossouw J (1993): Dietary fat and breast cancer: where we are. J Natl Cancer Inst 85:764-765.

Fulton AM, Heppner GH (1985): Relationships of prostaglandin E and natural killer sensitivity to metastatic potential in murine mammary adenocarcinomas. Cancer Res 45:4779-4784.

Goldin BR, Adlercreutz H, Gorbach SL, Woods MN, Dwyer JT, Conlon T, Bohn E, Gershoff SN (1986): The relationship between estrogen levels and diets of Caucasian American and Oriental immigrant women. Am J Clin Nutr 44:945-953.

Goldin BR, Woods MN, Spiegelman DL, Longcope C, Morrill-LaBrode A, Dwyer JT, Gualtieri LJ, Hertzmark E, Gorbach SL (1994): The effect of dietary fat and fiber on serum estrogen concentrations in premenopausal women under controlled dietary conditions. Cancer 74:1125-1131.

Gregorio DI, Emrich LJ, Graham S, Marshall JR, Nemato T (1985): Dietary fat consumption and survival among women with breast cancer. J Natl Cancer Inst 75:37-41.

Holm L-E, Nordevang E, Hjalmar M-L, Lidbrink E, Callmer E, Nilsson B (1993): Treatment failure and dietary habits in women with breast cancer. J Natl Cancer Inst 85:32-36.

Jones LA, Ota DM, Jackson GA, Jackson PM, Kemp K, Anderson DE, McCamant SK, Bauman DH (1987): Bioavailability of estradiol as a marker for breast cancer risk assessment. Cancer Res 47:5224-5229.

Jordan VC (1991): Chemosuppression of breast cancer with long-term tamoxifen therapy. Prev Med 20:3-14.

Key TJA, Chen J, Wang DY, Pike MC, Boreham J (1990): Sex hormones in women in rural China and in Britain. Br J Cancer 62:631-636.

Key TJA, Pike MC (1988). The role of oestrogens and progestogens in the epidemiology and prevention of breast cancer. Eur J Cancer Clin Oncol 24:29-43.

Liu X-H, Connolly JM, Rose DP (1996): Eicosanoids as mediators of linoleic acid-stimulated invasion and type IV collagenase production by a metastatic human breast cancer cell line. Clin Exp Metastasis 14: in press.

Liu X-H, Rose DP (1994): Stimulation of type IV collagenase expression by linoleic acid in a metastatic human breast cancer cell line. Cancer Lett 76:71-77.

Liu X-H, Rose DP (1995): Suppression of type IV collagenase in MDA-MB-435 human breast cancer cells by eicosapentaenoic acid *in vitro* and *in vivo*. Cancer Lett 92:21-26.

Moore JW, Clark GMG, Bulbrook RD, Hayward JL, Murai JT, Hammond GL, Siiteri PK (1982): Serum concentrations of total and non-protein-bound oestradiol in patients with breast cancer and in normal controls. Int J Cancer 29:17-21.

National Research Council (1989): Diet and Health: Implications for Reducing Chronic Disease Risk. Washington DC: National Academy Press, pp 159-258.

Nomura AMY, Le Marchand L, Kolonel LN, Hankin JH (1991): The effect of dietary fat on breast cancer survival among Caucasian and Japanese women in Hawaii. Breast Cancer Res Treat 18:S135-141.

Prentice R, Thompson D, Clifford C, Gorbach S, Goldin B, Byar D (1990): Dietary fat reduction and plasma estradiol concentration in healthy post-menopausal women. J Natl Cancer Inst 82:129-134.

Prentice RL, Kakar F, Hursting S, Sheppard L, Klein R, Kushi LH (1988): Aspects of the rationale for the Women's Health Trial. J Natl Cancer Inst 80:802-814.

Rohan TE, Hiller JE, McMichael AJ (1993): Dietary factors and survival from breast cancer. Nutr Cancer 20:167-177.

Rolland PH, Martin PM, Jacquemier J, Rolland AM, Toga M (1980): Prostaglandin in human breast cancer: evidence suggesting that an elevated prostaglandin production is a marker of high metastatic potential for neoplastic cells. J Natl Cancer Inst 64:1061-1070.

Rose DP (1992): Dietary fiber, phytoestrogens and breast cancer. Nutrition 8:47-51.

Rose DP (1993): Diet, hormones, and cancer. Annu Rev Publ Health 14:1-17.

Rose DP (1994): Dietary fat and breast cancer: controversy and biological plausibility (ed. EK Weisburger) Diet and Breast Cancer. New York: Marcel Dekker, pp 1-13.

Rose DP, Boyar AP, Cohen C, Strong LE (1987): Effect of a low-fat diet on hormone levels in women with cystic breast disease. I. Serum steroids and gonadotropins. J Natl Cancer Inst 78:623-626.

Rose DP, Connolly JM (1989): Stimulation of growth of human breast cancer cell lines in culture by linoleic acid. Biochem Biophys Res Commun 164:277-283.

Rose DP, Connolly JM (1990): Effects of fatty acids and inhibitors of eicosanoid synthesis on the growth of a human breast cancer cell line in culture. Cancer Res 50:7139-7144.

Rose DP, Connolly JM (1993): Effects of omega-3 fatty acids on human breast cancer growth and metastasis in nude mice. J Natl Cancer Inst 85:1743-1747.

Rose DP, Connolly JM, Liu X-H (1994): Effects of linoleic acid on the growth and metastasis of two human breast cancer cell lines in nude mice, and the invasive capacity of these cell lines in vitro. Cancer Res 54:6557-6562.

Rose DP, Connolly JM, Meschter CL (1991): Effect of dietary fat on human breast cancer growth and lung metastasis in nude mice. J Natl Cancer Inst 83:1491-1495.

Rose DP, Connolly JM, Rayburn J, Coleman M. (1995): Influence of diets containing different levels of eicosapentaenoic or docosahexaenoic acid on the growth and metastasis of human breast cancer cells in nude mice. J Natl Cancer Inst 87:587-592.

Rose DP, Hatala MA, Connolly JM, Rayburn J (1993): Effect of diets containing different levels of linoleic acid on human breast cancer growth and lung metastasis in nude mice. Cancer Res 53:4686-4690.

Shimizu H, Ross RK, Bernstein L, Pike MC, Henderson BE (1990): Serum oestrogen levels in postmenopausal women: comparison of American whites and Japanese in Japan. Br J Cancer 62:451-453.

Slattery ML, O'Brien E, Mori M (1995) Disease heterogeneity: does it impact our ability to detect dietary associations with breast cancer? Nutr Cancer 24:213-220.

Stracke ML, Liotta LA (1992): Multi-step cascade of tumor cell metastasis. In Vivo 6:309-316.

Takatani O, Kosano H, Okumoto T, Akamatsu K, Tamakuma S, Hiraide H (1987): Distribution of estradiol and percentage of free testosterone in sera of Japanese women: preoperative breast cancer patients and normal controls. J Natl Cancer Inst 79:1199-1204.

Tannenbaum A (1942): The genesis and growth of tumors. III. Effects of a high-fat diet. Cancer Res 2:468-475.

Taylor PR, Judd JT, Jones DY, Nair PP, Campbell WS (1992): Influence of type and amount of dietary fat on plasma estradiol (E) in premenopausal women. Am J Clin Nutr (Suppl) Am Soc Clin Nutr Annu Meet abstr 130.

Toniolo PG, Levitz M, Zeleniuch-Jacquotte A, Banerjee S, Koenig KL, Shore RE, Strax P, Pasternack BS (1995): A prospective study of endogenous estrogens and breast cancer in postmenopausal women. J Natl Cancer Inst 87:190-197.

Whittemore AS, Henderson BE (1993): Dietary fat and breast cancer: where are we? J Natl Cancer Inst 85:762-763.

Willett WC, Hunter DJ (1994): Prospective studies of diet and breast cancer. Cancer 74:1085-1089.

Willett WC, Hunter DJ, Stampfer MJ, Colditz G, Manson JE, Spiegelman D, Rosner B, Hennekens CH, Speizer FE (1992): Dietary fat and fiber in relation to risk of breast cancer. An 8-year follow-up. JAMA 268:2037-2044.

Wynder EL, Fujita Y, Harris RE, Hirayama T, Hiyama T (1991): Comparative epidemiology of cancer between the United States and Japan. Cancer 67:746-763.

Zang S, Folsom AR, Sellers TA, Kushi LH, Potter JD (1995): Better breast cancer survival for postmenopausal women who are less overweight and eat less fat. Cancer 76:275-283.

Etiology of Breast and
Gynecological Cancers, pages 159–183
© 1997 Wiley-Liss, Inc.

PERSPECTIVES AND PROGRESS IN DEVELOPMENT OF BREAST CANCER CHEMOPREVENTIVE DRUGS

Gary J. Kelloff, Charles W. Boone, James A. Crowell, Susan G. Nayfield, Ernest T. Hawk, Vernon E. Steele, Ronald A. Lubet, and Caroline C. Sigman

Chemoprevention Branch, Division of Cancer Prevention and Control (DCPC), National Cancer Institute (NCI), National Institutes of Health, Bethesda, MD 20892 (GJK, CWB, JAC, SGN, ETH, VES, RAL)

CCS Associates, Mountain View, CA 94043 (CCS)

INTRODUCTION

Cancer chemoprevention is defined as the use of specific chemical compounds to prevent, inhibit, or reverse carcinogenesis (Sporn and Newton, 1979; Kelloff et al., 1994a,b). Chemoprevention can be applied throughout or at any phase of the 20–40 year process of carcinogenesis. Its scope includes both healthy subjects at normal risk and populations at intermediate risk from environmental and lifestyle factors, genetic predisposition, and precancerous lesions. Also included are previous cancer patients at high risk for second primaries. A multidisciplinary approach to the development of chemopreventive drugs has been described previously (Kelloff et al., 1994a,c,d, 1995a). This strategy considers experimental and epidemiological evidence that defines cancer risk at major target sites, as well as the underlying molecular, cellular, and tissue level mechanisms that contribute to the development and progression of human cancers. As previously described (e.g., Kelloff et al., 1994e), there are three critical components to the successful development of chemopreventive drugs: well-characterized agents with potential for inhibiting the target cancer, biomarkers correlating to cancer incidence for measuring chemopreventive effect, and suitable cohorts for clinical efficacy studies. The objective of this review is to describe the approach to and progress in developing chemopreventive drugs for breast cancer. The important considerations in this approach are summarized in Table 1, and some have been reviewed previously (Kelloff et al., 1993, 1995b).

An important aspect of chemoprevention is understanding the associated risk factors and mechanisms of carcinogenesis that contribute to these risks. It is well-known that breast cancer accounts for the highest proportion of new cancer cases (32%) and is the second highest cause of cancer mortality ($\approx$18%) estimated for US women in 1995 (Wingo et al., 1995). The Gail model (Gail et al., 1989) summarizes and interrelates most of the factors which confer increased risk for breast cancer. These factors can be categorized as age, estrogen exposure (including parity), genetic susceptibility, lifestyle and histological/previous lesions. Age is the most important single factor (Henderson, 1993). A primary contributor to this factor is probably duration of estrogen exposure, and other important factors in breast cancer risk are also associated with estrogen—e.g., early age

Table 1. Considerations in Chemoprevention of Breast Cancer[a]

The Problem

In US most common cancer in females

32% (182,000) of total new cases in females (estimated 1995)

18% (46,000) of cancer deaths in females (estimated 1995)

Etiology/Risk Factors/Risk Biomarkers Defining Cohorts for Chemoprevention

Age ≥50 years

Familial history of breast cancer or genetic syndrome (*e.g.*, Li-Fraumeni, BRCA1)

Past history of breast, endometrial, or ovarian cancer

Atypical hyperplasia, DCIS, LCIS

Estrogen exposure (*e.g.*, early menarche, late menopause, late age at first full-term pregnancy)

Lifestyle (*e.g.*, high-fat diet)

Proposed Chemopreventive Mechanisms (Promising Agents)

Antiestrogens (*e.g.*, tamoxifen, toremifene, raloxifene)

Antiproliferatives (*e.g.*, DFMO, DHEA, Fluasterone, 4-HPR, 9-*cis*-RA, selenium compounds)

Antioxidants (*e.g.*, perillyl alcohol, selenium compounds, vitamin E)

Apoptosis inducers (*e.g.*, DHEA, 4-HPR, 9-*cis*-RA, *p*-XSC)

Aromatase inhibitors (*e.g.*, 4-OHA, exemestane, anastrazole, (+)-vorozole)

Carcinogen detoxicants (*e.g.*, indole-3-carbinol, oltipraz)

Differentiating agents (*e.g.*, retinoids)

Estrogen detoxicants (*e.g.*, indole-3-carbinol)

Signal transduction inhibitors (*e.g.*, *ras* inhibitors such as DHEA and perillyl alcohol, retinoids)

Combinations: 4-HPR (or other retinoid) + tamoxifen (or other antiestrogen), selenium + vitamin E

Table 1. (continued)

Preclinical Models

Rats treated with DMBA or MNU

Intermediate Biomarkers of Breast Cancer, Potential Clinical Trial Endpoints

Histological: DCIS, LCIS, atypical hyperplasia (measure nuclear morphometry, ploidy)

Proliferation: Nucleolar organizer regions, S-phase, PCNA, Ki-67

Differentiation: Myoepithelial cell markers (*e.g.*, S-100, keratin 17, vimentin), altered cytoplasmic glycoprotein expression (*e.g.*, human milk fat globule protein), altered cell surface antigen expression (*e.g.*, antibodies GB3, DF3, A-80)

Genetic/Regulatory: Altered oncogene expression (*e.g.*, c-*erb*B-2, c-*myc*, c-*fos*, c-*ras*), altered tumor suppressors (*e.g.*, p53), altered growth factor expression (*e.g.*, TGFβ), loss of heterozygosity (*e.g.*, chromosomes 17p, 1p, 18q)

Biochemical: Estradiol metabolism

Clinical Cohorts for Phase II Chemoprevention Trials

Patients with mammographic lesions requiring biopsy (DCIS)

High-risk subjects with atypical hyperplasia and multiple early biomarker abnormalities

Clinical Cohorts for Longer Phase II and III Chemoprevention Trials

Patients with previous breast cancer

Patients with LCIS

High-risk subjects without evidence of disease: Women ≥60 or 35–59 years old with risk = 60 year old, women carrying germline mutation (*e.g.*, BRCA1)

---

* This table summarizes material discussed and referenced in text. Abbreviations are as follows: 9-*cis*-RA=9-*cis*-retinoic acid, DCIS=ductal carcinoma *in situ*, DFMO=2-difluoromethylornithine, DHEA=dehydroepiandrosterone, DMBA=7,12-dimethylbenz(*a*)anthracene, 4-HPR=all-*trans*-N-(4-hydroxyphenyl)retinamide, LCIS=lobular carcinoma *in situ*, MNU=N-methyl-N-nitrosourea, PCNA=proliferating cell nuclear antigen, *p*-XSC=*para*-xylylselenocyanate

at menarche, late menopause, nulliparity, age at first full-term pregnancy, and years of oral contraceptive use (MacMahon *et al.*, 1970; Henderson *et al.*, 1981; Russo *et al.*, 1992; Henderson, 1993). As will be discussed below, these observations, supported by experimental and clinical data, have led to the development of chemopreventve agents that specifically inhibit the proliferative effects of excess estrogen.

Several genetic lesions have been identified which confer susceptibility to breast cancer. One is the Li-Fraumeni syndrome, which is characterized by a germline mutation in the p53 gene. Affected germlines have high incidences of six cancers; the relative risk for premenopausal breast cancer has been estimated to be 17.9 (Garber *et al.*, 1991; Li *et al.*, 1991). Most inherited breast cancer has been attributed to modifications in the tumor suppressor BRCA1 gene located on chromosome 17q21 (King, 1992; Smith *et al.*, 1992). Easton and colleagues (Easton *et al.*, 1993, 1995; Goldgar *et al.*, 1994) have estimated that 60% of families with three or more breast cancer patients and virtually all families with multiple cases of both breast and ovarian cancer carry alterations in BRCA1. More than 100 different BRCA1 mutations have been detected, and some have been seen frequently (Collins, 1996). Perhaps the best known is the frameshift mutation in exon2 called 185delAG that has been identified in Jewish families with familial breast or ovarian cancer and is found in approximately 1% of Ashkenazi Jews (Struewing *et al.*, 1995; Collins, 1996). It has been suggested that changes in BRCA1 may be linked to breast cancer in the general population as well as to inherited susceptibility (Smith *et al.*, 1992; Langston *et al.*, 1996). The observation that tumor suppressor function may be depressed in these populations implies that agents which enhance cell cycle control function, such as apoptosis inducers, may have potential as breast cancer chemopreventives.

Including all cases where a specific inherited lesion has not been identified, the overall risk from familial predisposition is much less, but still significant (reviewed in Mettlin, 1992; Henderson, 1993). The relative risk for a woman with first-degree (mother, sister, both) family history of breast cancer ranges from 1.8–5.6 (Bain *et al.*, 1980).

The presence of certain histological lesions the risk for breast cancer. For example, a diagnosis of atypical hyperplasia increases the relative risk to 3.7–4.5. Both types of atypical hyperplasia (ductal, lobular) predict carcinoma of the ipsilateral and contralateral breast with equal frequency (Dupont *et al.*, 1993; Connolly and Schnitt, 1993); this is also true for lobular carcinoma *in situ* (LCIS, RR=7–10) (Ponten *et al.*, 1990; Harris *et al.*, 1992; Posner and Wolmark, 1992). These lesions appear to be risk markers, but not direct precursors of breast cancer. In contrast, ductal carcinoma *in situ* (DCIS) is recognized as a precursor lesion in the breast (Posner and Wolmark, 1992). The rate of invasive cancer after the initial diagnosis of DCIS has been reported as 20–50%, usually within the ipsilateral breast (Schnitt *et al.*, 1988; Ponten *et al.*, 1990). Previous breast cancer also increases risk. The rate of recurrence of Stage I/II breast cancer after lumpectomy alone is 39% within 8 years, which decreases to 10% with radiation treatment (Harris *et al.*, 1992).

It should be noted that 60–70% of women diagnosed with breast cancer have none of the risk factor(s) discussed above (Seidman *et al.*, 1982; Marshall, 1993). Lifestyle, such as diet, and environment may also influence the development of breast cancer, as suggested by international differences in breast cancer rates. For example, the age-adjusted rate in Japan (19/100,000) is one-fifth that in the US (77–86/100,000) (Henderson, 1993). When Japanese migrate to the US, breast cancer incidence among their offspring approaches the US incidence.

High fat intake has been suggested as a risk factor based on preclinical studies showing a higher incidence of carcinogen-induced mammary carcinomas in rats given high fat (20% corn oil, w/w, *i.e.*, ≈36% of calories) compared with low fat diets (5% corn oil, *i.e.*,

≈10% of calories) (*e.g.*, Ip and Ip, 1981; Ip, 1987). Two large prospective cohort studies in the US (Nurse's Study, National Health and Nutrition Examination Survey), did not find an association between calorie-adjusted fat intake and breast cancer risk (Jones *et al.*, 1987; Willett *et al.*, 1987, 1992; Carroll, 1992). However, these studies compared fat intake levels of >30% of calories, exceeding the highest level in the rat studies. International comparisons show a linear relationship between mortality from breast cancer and dietary fat as percent of calories within the 10–30% range of the rat studies (reviewed in Carroll, 1992). Since estrogen synthesis takes place in adipocytes, the association of high fat to breast cancer may result from excess estrogen exposure. It has been shown, for example, that estrogen synthesis is higher in adipose tissue near malignant breast tumors than that near benign breast lesions (O'Neill and Miller, 1987; Manni, 1993).

In the sections following, approaches to breast cancer chemoprevention that take these risks into account are discussed, along with progress to date in the development of promising breast cancer chemopreventive drugs.

IDENTIFICATION AND EVALUATION OF BREAST CANCER CHEMOPREVENTIVES

The primary criterion for selecting agents for clinical development is evidence of chemopreventive efficacy, with high likelihood that the agent will be active in preventing cancer at the target site. Because chemopreventive agents may be given to relatively healthy subjects for long periods of time, a high margin of safety is also necessary to warrant considering an agent for clinical evaluation. This second criterion implies that sufficient prior clinical use or preclinical efficacy, toxicity, and pharmacodynamics data are available to allow estimation of an efficacy/safety ratio. Often, dose-titration studies to determine the optimal dose and dosing regimen will be performed as part of Phase II trials (Kelloff *et al.*, 1994e, 1995a).

The third criterion is that there is a logical, presumed mechanism of chemopreventive activity of the agent. Such mechanisms guide the selection of both cohorts and endpoints for clinical trials. For example, an antiproliferative agent like 2-difluoromethylornithine (DFMO) is expected to be effective against cancers with a pronounced proliferative component, such as those in breast. An antimutagenic agent like oltipraz may be more effectively evaluated in a cohort such as smokers, who are constantly exposed to the DNA-damaging effects of carcinogens. Likewise, indicators of proliferation such as S-phase fraction and proliferating cell nuclear antigen (PCNA) may prove to be more reliable and easily quantified measures of the effects of antiproliferative agents than would be the identification of specific mutations. In other words, the intermediate endpoint and ultimately the cancer should be modulatable by the chemopreventive agent.

PROMISING CHEMOPREVENTIVE AGENTS IN BREAST

Five drugs—DFMO, dehydroepiandrostenedione (DHEA), exemestane, all-*trans*-*N*-(4-hydroxyphenyl)retinamide (4-HPR), and tamoxifen citrate—are currently being evaluated in Phase II and Phase III clinical studies as potential breast cancer chemopreventive drugs. Of these, the retinoid, 4-HPR, and the antiestrogen, tamoxifen, are furthest in development.

4-HPR

As a retinoid, 4-HPR, a synthetic amide of all-*trans*-retinoic acid, is an antiprolifera-tive and differentiation-inducing agent (reviewed in Kelloff *et al.*, 1994c) with less toxicity than its parent and other efficacious retinoids. An important mechanism contributing to its antiproliferative activity is induction of apoptosis (reviewed in Kelloff *et al.*, 1994c, Oridate *et al.*, 1995). Another activity that may be associated with its antiproliferative effects is inhibition of the induction of ornithine decarboxy-lase (ODC), a critical enzyme in polyamine biosynthesis; polyamine biosynthesis has been implicated in cell proliferation (Luk and Casero, 1987, McCann *et al.*, 1987). Other relevant activities are inhibition of prostaglandin synthesis (ElAttar and Lin, 1991) and tyrosine kinase activity, as well as enhancement of immunoglobulin secretion (Dillehay *et al.*, 1991). 4-HPR may also have a very specific antiproliferative effect on terminal end buds in mammary glands (Radcliffe and Moon, 1983). It has been shown to be an effective inhibitor of mammary gland carcinomas *in vivo* in rat models (*e.g.*, Moon *et al.*, 1979, McCormick *et al.*, 1982) and in mouse mammary tumor virus (MMTV)-positive C_3H mice (*e.g.*, Osborne *et al.*, 1990).

The National Cancer Institute (NCI) is sponsoring a Phase III trial of 4-HPR in patients surgically treated for Stage I/II breast cancer. This study is assessing prevention of a second primary in the contralateral breast after five years treatment with 4-HPR and two years follow-up (Costa *et al.*, 1992, 1994; De Palo *et al.*, 1995). Interim results suggest a protective effective on incidence of contralateral breast cancer in premenopausal patients and in patients ≤45 years of age. A protective effect against local relapse of breast cancer is also seen in premenopausal patients (44 cases in 4-HPR treatment group *vs.* 71 cases in control group). There is also some indication of a protective or delaying effect against ovarian cancer. No ovarian cancers were seen in evaluable patients in the 4-HPR group during the five-year treatment period, while six were seen in the control group. Three ovarian cancers have developed in the 4-HPR treatment group–all during the follow-up period after 4-HPR treatment had ended.

Tamoxifen

Tamoxifen citrate (Nolvadex®) is being evaluated in a large NCI-sponsored Phase III clinical chemoprevention trial (*e.g.*, Fisher, 1992). Its pharmacology and potential as a chemopreventive drug have been reviewed (*e.g.*, Nayfield *et al.*, 1991). This triphenylethylene-based antiestrogen that competitively blocks binding of estrogen to its receptor is used in the treatment of advanced breast cancer. The agent has additional effects that may be related to chemoprevention and to its antiestrogenic activity, such as inhibition of protein kinase C activity, induction of transforming growth factor β (TGFβ), regulation of calcium-dependent events, and modulation of hormone secretion. Depending on species, age and the endpoint measured, however, tamoxifen may also have estrogenic effects.

4-HPR + Tamoxifen

Additional clinical development work is in progress for both 4-HPR and tamoxifen citrate. For example, Phase II trials have been initiated to evaluate the effects of these agents on intermediate biomarkers of cancer in neoplastic breast tissue (Kelloff *et al.*,

1994e; Dhingra, 1995). The agents are being tested individually and in combination. Combination treatment with the two agents showed synergistic inhibitory activity in carcinogen-induced rat mammary gland carcinogenesis (Moon *et al.*, 1992). The combination was also more effective in reducing the induction of subsequent rat mammary carcinomas after removal of the first cancer than either agent alone (Ratko *et al.*, 1989). A further advantage of the combination is that is may allow lower doses of each agent, thereby reducing the potential for toxicity.

DFMO

DFMO is an irreversible inhibitor of ODC and, as stated above, a potent antiproliferative. In animal studies, DFMO is effective against many cancers, including both MNU- and DMBA-induced rat mammary gland cancers (reviewed in Kelloff *et al.*, 1994f; Steele *et al.*, 1994). A Phase II chemoprevention trial to evaluate the effects of DFMO on intermediate biomarkers in neoplastic breast tissue has been initiated, and a Phase II trial in subjects at high risk for breast cancer is planned (Kelloff *et al.*, 1994f).

DHEA

Free DHEA and its sulfate conjugate, DHEA-S, are major steroid precursors secreted by the adrenal cortex. In peripheral tissues, they are metabolized to androstenedione, which can be converted to testosterone and estrogen; in fact, this is the source of much of the estrogen in postmenopausal women. Epidemiological data suggest that serum DHEA or its urinary metabolites inversely correlate to human cancer risk. Positive associations of low levels of DHEA and cancer incidence have been reported for breast (*e.g.*, Cameron *et al.*, 1970; Bulbrook *et al.*, 1971; Brownsey *et al.*, 1972; Wang *et al.*, 1974, 1975; Thomas *et al.*, 1976; Rose *et al.*, 1977), gastric (Gordon *et al.*, 1993), ovarian (Cuzick *et al.*, 1983), and bladder cancer (Gordon *et al.*, 1991). DHEA is a potent inhibitor of glucose-6-phosphate dehydrogenase (G6DPH), which catalyzes formation of extramitochondrial NAD(P)H and ribose-6-phosphate. The chemopreventive activity of DHEA may be due to a lack of these substances for DNA synthesis and cell proliferation (*e.g*, Pashko *et al.*, 1981). Depressed levels of NAD(P)H may also lead to decreased carcinogen metabolism, due to reduced activity of mixed function oxidases, which also require NAD(P)H (reviewed in Schwartz and Pashko, 1986, 1993). It has been noted that individuals with G6PDH deficiency have lower rates of cancer, and their lymphocytes are less efficient in metabolizing B(a)P (Mbensa *et al.*, 1978; Feo *et al.*, 1987). Also, DHEA has been shown *in vitro* to block cell transformation by aflatoxin B_1 or DMBA (Schwartz and Peratoni, 1975). Another activity, inhibition of protein isoprenylation, has been shown for both DHEA and DHEA-S (Schulz and Nyce, 1991, 1994; Schulz *et al.*, 1992). G proteins, including the *ras* oncogene, require posttranslational isoprenylation to appropriately associate with the cell plasma membrane. Thus, this activity of DHEA and DHEA-S could help to slow cell growth by damping aberrant signal transduction through the *ras* and other G protein-mediated pathways. Other metabolic effects of DHEA include anti-glucocorticoid activity (reviewed in Kalimi *et al.*, 1994), anti-obesity, and anti-diabetic effects (reviewed in Regelson and Kalimi, 1994), as well as inhibition of superoxide formation (Whitcomb and Schwartz, 1985).

DHEA has been effective in rat mammary gland (*e.g.*, Ratko *et al.*, 1991) and prostate (cited in Kelloff *et al.*, 1994g) as well as several other animal cancer models (reviewed in Schwartz and Pashko, 1995). Like DFMO, it is currently being evaluated in a Phase II trial for its effective on intermediate biomarkers in breast and a Phase II trial in a cohort at high risk for breast cancer is planned.

Exemestane

Another method of inhibiting estrogen influence on breast carcinogenesis is by specifically damping or preventing estrogen synthesis. Steroid aromatase, a cytochrome P450 enzyme, catalyzes the first step in estrogen biosynthesis from androgens in humans: namely, C-19 hydroxylation and subsequent oxidative cleavage in the androgens androstenedione and testosterone to give estrone and estradiol, respectively (reviewed in Kelloff *et al.*, 1994c). Several compounds that inhibit aromatase also inhibit chemical carcinogenesis in estrogen-sensitive tissues. For example, the androstenedione derivative, 4-hydroxyandrost-4-ene-3,17-dione (4-OHA), a suicide inhibitor of aromatase, inhibits MNU-induced tumors in rat mammary glands (Lubet *et al.*, 1994). 4-OHA has been used clinically to inhibit estrogen synthesis in postmenopausal metastatic breast cancer (*e.g.*, Coombes *et al.*, 1992; Bajetta *et al.*, 1993). Exemestane is an androstenedione derivative and aromatase inhibitor with better oral activity than 4-OHA. It has been shown to induce mammary gland tumor regression in rat models and reduces estrogen levels in postmenopausal advanced breast cancer patients (reviewed in Zilembo *et al.*, 1995). A Phase II clinical chemoprevention trial to evaluate its effects on breast cancer intermediate biomarkers is in progress.

Additional agents are under consideration for Phase II clinical trials in breast including oltipraz, DHEA analog 8354 (fluasterone), indole-3-carbinol, perillyl alcohol, 9-*cis*-retinoic acid, antiestrogens as alternatives to tamoxifen (*e.g.*, raloxifene and toremifene), nonsteroidal aromatase inhibitors (*e.g.*, vorozole), *para*-xylylselenocyanate (*p*-XSC), and the combination of vitamin E with selenium.

Oltipraz

Oltipraz is a synthetic dithiolthione that is structurally related to naturally occurring dithiolthiones found in cruciferous vegetables. This highly lipophilic drug was originally developed by Rhône-Poulenc for the treatment of schistosomiasis. It was also found to increase glutathione (GSH) levels in rodents in several target organs and to enhance several phase II metabolic enzyme activities in animals, particularly the GSH-*S*-transferases (GST), which are involved in carcinogen detoxification (reviewed in Kensler *et al.*, 1992; Kelloff *et al.*, 1994h). Oltipraz is now regarded as a prototypic phase II enzyme inducer. In animal cancer models, oltipraz is one of the most widely effective agents tested, showing chemopreventive activity in lung, colon, skin, mammary glands, and bladder (reviewed in Steele *et al.*, 1994). In rat mammary glands, the agent inhibited cancers in both MNU- and DMBA-induced rat models.

DHEA Analog 8354 (Fluasterone)

The 16α-fluoroderivative of DHEA, DHEA analog 8354 or fluasterone, has also been shown to be an effective chemopreventive agent in rat mammary gland and colon (reviewed in Kelloff *et al.*, 1994g), and it has less androgenic and liver toxicity than the parent compound (reviewed in Schwartz and Pashko, 1995).

Indole-3-carbinol

Indole-3-carbinol is a non-nutritive component of cruciferous vegetables (Bradfield and Bjeldanes, 1987, Yound and Wolf, 1988); consumption of these vegetables has been associated with decreased human cancer risk (Sparnins *et al.*, 1982; Young and Wolf, 1988). Indole-3-carbinol is effective against a wide variety of carcinogens. Much of its chemopreventive activity stems from its capacity to induce both phase I and II enzymes involved in carcinogen metabolism (*e.g.*, Fong *et al.*, 1990). Although many agents, including indole-3-carbinol, induce several different phase II enzymes, the indole's capacity to induce multiple families of cytochrome P450-dependent isozymes is relatively unique. Indole-3-carbinol induces TCDD-type (CYP 1A family), phenobarbital-type (CYP 2B family) and dexamethasone-type (CYP 3A family) isozymes (*e.g.*, Stresser *et al.*, 1994). These enzyme-inducing effects are due to indole-3-carbinol condensation products formed under the acid conditions in the stomach (*e.g.*, De Kruif *et al.*, 1991); some of the products formed also have chemopreventive activity (*e.g.*, Dashwood *et al.*, 1994). The potentially different enzyme-inducing activities of the acid condensation products may partially explain the pleiotropic effects on cytochrome P450 enzymes (De Kruif *et al.*, 1991).

Indole-3-carbinol also inhibits spontaneous tumorigenesis and tumor induction by direct-acting carcinogens in estrogen-responsive tissues (Bradlow *et al.*, 1991; Kojima *et al.*, 1994,). Increased estrogen conjugation and excretion via induction of phase II enzymes may contribute to these effects. Additionally, the suppressive effects have been attributed to modulation of cytochrome P450-dependent estradiol hydroxylation. Essentially, estradiol is metabolized via two mutually exclusive pathways. Hydroxylation at C-2 yields 2-hydroxyestrone; hydroxylation at C-16α yields 16α-hydroxyestrone which is reduced to form estriol. Increased estradiol-16α-hydroxylation has been associated with increased risk for breast cancer in women (Schneider *et al.*, 1982) and mice (Bradlow *et al.*, 1985), and 16α-hydroxyestrone has been reported to be genotoxic to mammary cells (Swaneck and Fishman, 1991). Indole-3-carbinol may lessen 16α-hydroxylation indirectly by enhancing C-2 hydroxylation (Bradlow *et al.*, 1994). In rodents, indole-3-carbinol increases estradiol 2-hydroxylation under the same experimental conditions in which it reduces mammary and endometrial tumor development, and it also enhances estradiol 2-hydroxylation in humans (reviewed in Bradlow *et al.*, 1994).

Perillyl Alcohol

Perillyl alcohol is a hydroxylated derivative of *d*-limonene; both compounds inhibit isoprenylation of G proteins, including the *ras* oncogene product (Crowell *et al.*, 1992; Khosravi-Far *et al.*, 1992; Ren and Gould, 1995). As stated above, chemopreventive activity associated with isoprenylation inhibition may arise from interfering with aberrant signal transduction via the *ras* and other G protein-mediated pathways. The monoterpenes also interfere with synthesis of ubiquinone (CoQ), at least partially accounting for their ability to inhibit proliferation of tumor cells (Bronfen *et al.*, 1994; Cerda *et al.*, 1994), which often rely on glycolysis for ATP production (Ren and Gould, 1994). Perillyl alcohol has also been reported to induce apoptosis (Mills *et al.*, 1995) and differentiation (Ren and Gould, 1993). *d*-Limonene (Jirtle *et al.*, 1993) and perillyl alcohol (Mills *et al.*, 1995) increase cellular levels of the IGF-II receptor, TGFβ type I receptor, and TGFβ. Finally, *d*-limonene and its hydroxylated analogs such as perillyl alcohol induce cytochrome P450, GST, and glucuronyl transferase activities (Gould, 1993a).

There is only limited preclinical data supporting perillyl alcohol's chemopreventive activity. It inhibits promotion of DEN-induced rat liver tumors (Mills *et al.*, 1995) and causes regression of established mammary gland tumors and prevents secondary tumors in DMBA-induced rats (Haag and Gould, 1994). However, there are several preclinical studies demonstrating the chemopreventive activity of *d*-limonene. It both inhibits lung (*e.g.*, van Duuren and Goldschmidt, 1976), skin (Elson *et al.*, 1988), mammary gland (Maltzman *et al.*, 1989; Gould, 1991, 1993b) and liver (Wattenberg *et al.*, 1989) tumorigenesis, and causes regression of established mammary tumors (Elegbede *et al.*, 1986; Haag *et al.*, 1992).

9-*cis*-Retinoic Acid (9-*cis*-RA)

As evidenced by the activity of the 4-HPR, retinoids appear to have high potential as breast cancer chemopreventive agents. The retinoid, 9-*cis*-RA, is a stereo- and photoisomer of all-*trans*-retinoic acid which may have more potent chemopreventive activity in breast than 4-HPR. The retinoid is a highly effective inhibitor of MNU-induced rat mammary gland tumorigenesis; furthermore, it significantly enhances the efficacy of suboptimal doses of tamoxifen (Anzano *et al.*, 1994)

Antiestrogens

As indicated above, tamoxifen, alone and in combination with 4-HPR has demonstrated significant chemopreventive potential in breast; however, it has estrogenic effects that may contribute to carcinogenicity in other tissues, particularly liver in animals (Greaves *et al.*, 1993; Hard *et al.*, 1993; Hirsamaki *et al.*, 1993) and endometrium in humans (*e.g.*, Fisher *et al.*, 1994; van Leeuwen *et al.*, 1994). As discussed previously, combination with 4-HPR is one strategy to allow possible lower efficacious doses that are less toxic. Another alternative is to develop similar compounds with purer antiestrogenic activity. Toremifene (Moon *et al.*, 1994) and raloxifene (Jordan and Assikis, 1995) are two examples of such compounds that have demonstrated chemopreventive activity in rat mammary gland. Toremifene has also demonstrated efficacy similar to that of tamoxifen as adjuvant therapy for advanced breast cancer (reviewed in Hayes *et al.*, 1995; Jordan, 1995). Like tamoxifen, the chemopreventive effect of raloxifene in MNU-induced rat mammary gland carcinogenesis is synergistic with 9-*cis*-RA (Anzano *et al.*, 1996).

Nonsteroidal Aromatase Inhibitors

Besides the androstenedione analogs described above, nonsteroidal aromatase inhibitors have been developed which have the advantages of high specificity (hence, high potency) and relatively low toxicity. Several of these appear to have potential as chemopreventive agents. For example, the triazole derivative anastrazole (Arimidex®) is being evaluated for estrogen repression in postmenopausal advanced breast cancer patients (Plourde *et al.*, 1994, 1995). Also, another triazole-derived aromatase inhibitor, (+)-vorozole, has shown potent chemopreventive activity in the MNU-induced rat mammary gland model (Lubet *et al.*, 1994).

Selenium Compounds

p-XSC. El-Bayoumy (El-Bayoumy, 1994, El-Bayoumy *et al.*, 1995) has recently reviewed the chemopreventive efficacy of selenium compounds against rodent mammary cancer. A significant problem with selenium compounds is toxicity. The search for effective, less toxic organoselenium agents has led to the synthesis of *p*-XSC, the most promising of a series of organoselenium compounds (Ip *et al.*, 1994). *p*-XSC was shown to have chemopreventive activity in the rat DMBA-induced mammary gland model as well as in the AOM-induced colon carcinogenesis model and the mouse NNK lung model. In the rat mammary gland, *p*-XSC was effective in both initiation and post initiation phases at higher doses but at lower doses, it showed an effect only in the initiation phase (El Bayoumy *et al.*, 1992; Ip *et al.*, 1994). *p*-XSC also suppressed DMBA-DNA adduct formation in the mammary gland (El-Bayoumy *et al.*, 1992). Several other mechanisms have been investigated to explain the antiinitiation effects. *p*-XSC shares antioxidant activity of other selenium compounds in the ability to replete GSH peroxidase in selenium-deficient animals, inhibits prostaglandin E_2 synthesis in the colon, and enhances UDP-glucuronyl transferase activity in the liver (Ip *et al.*, 1994; El-Bayoumy *et al.*, 1995). The ability of *p*-XSC to stimulate apoptosis (Tillotson *et al.*, 1994) may contribute to its post-initiation effect.

l-Selenomethionine + vitamin E. Another approach is to administer selenium in combination with other chemopreventive agents—allowing lower doses to obtain efficacy while lessening toxicity. In an unpublished study sponsored by the NCI Chemoprevention Branch, the combination of sodium selenite (2 ppm in diet) with vitamin E acetate (1 g/kg diet) was effective against DMBA-induced rat mammary gland cancers. No significant toxicity (*i.e.*, primarily, weight loss) was seen in the treated animals compared with controls. Neither compound was active alone. This result along with the previous demonstration of the activity of selenium compounds against DMBA-induced rat mammary cancer (reviewed in El-Bayoumy, 1994) suggests the possibility of clinical testing a selenium compound in combination with vitamin E against breast cancer. A Phase II trial of the combination is planned (the agents will also be tested individually). *l*-Selenomethionine is the probable source of selenium because of previous clinical experience with high-selenium yeast (containing *l*-selenomethionine) at doses up to 400 mg *l*-selenomethionine/ day and its activity against DMBA-induced carcinogenesis alone (Ip, 1986; Ip and White, 1987) and in combination with vitamin E (Ip and White, 1987).

INTERMEDIATE BIOMARKERS WITH POTENTIAL AS SURROGATE ENDPOINTS FOR BREAST CANCER

A primary focus of chemoprevention drug development in general and, specifically, in breast is to review the current status of early markers in the target tissue and to develop research strategies for identifying and validating these intermediate biomarkers for cancer, particularly those that are useful in clinical trials as surrogate endpoints for cancer incidence. As discussed previously (Boone *et al.*, 1992, 1993; Boone and Kelloff, 1993; Kelloff *et al.*, 1994b,e, 1995a), the most reliable of these markers are those directly on a causal pathway to cancer, are closely and specifically associated with cancer, and are quantifiable. Two types of biomarkers are most likely to meet these criteria—precancerous histological lesions and proliferation indices within these lesions. An appropriate strategy is to identify a well-established histological lesion with significant malignant potential (*i.e.*, dysplasia) in both preclinical models and the human cancer. Computer-assisted image analysis (CAIA) of nuclear and nucleolar morphometry is used to quantify changes in the lesions. Cytometric CAIA is used to quantify proliferation indices. Other types of biomarkers are then investigated within the histological lesion and surrounding tissue. As described above, the best-recognized premalignant lesion in human breast is DCIS, which essentially differs from cancer only in the lack of basement membrane invasion. Thus, this lesion is late in the malignant process for very effective chemoprevention; however, other types of biomarkers identified in this lesion may be explored in earlier stages of carcinogenesis. Also, as described above, there is evidence suggesting that atypical hyperplasia is an earlier lesion which may progress (reviewed in Kelloff *et al.*, 1993); chemopreventive intervention at this stage would be more effective. However, atypia is detected in only 7% of women with proliferative breast disease, and it is also difficult to follow or sample serially. There are studies indicating that cytomorphometric and cytophotometric measurements will be useful surrogate endpoints. For example, cytomorphometric analysis has demonstrated aneuploidy in 50–71% of DCIS (Crissman *et al.*, 1990; Pallis *et al.*, 1992). Similar evaluation of atypical hyperplasia found a smaller incidence of aneuploidy (35%); thus, this biomarker appeared to be differentially expressed in early and late precancerous lesions (Crissman *et al.*, 1990).

Additional potential intermediate biomarkers are listed in Table 1. Although some such as p53 overexpression (Smith *et al.*, 1993), c-*erb*B-2 overexpression (*e.g.*, Smith *et al.*, 1993), and loss of myoepithelial cytokeratin 17 and other myoepithelial markers (Wetzels *et al.*, 1991; Bocker *et al.*, 1992) have been demonstrated in DCIS, they still will need to be investigated in atypical hyperplasia or normal-appearing tissue in a cancerous breast. An important aspect of early Phase II chemoprevention trials in breast is to demonstrate modulation of these promising biomarkers by chemopreventive agents.

COHORTS FOR CLINICAL TRIALS OF BREAST CANCER CHEMOPREVENTIVE AGENTS

The critical role of Phase II trials for evaluating surrogate endpoints and providing early evidence of efficacy in chemoprevention drug development has been described previously (*e.g.*, Kelloff *et al.*, 1994b,e) and recounted above. In Phase II trials, the most important criterion for a cohort is that it be matched to the chemopreventive agent being evaluated. A chemopreventive agent is likely to be most effective in subjects whose disease or risk of disease can be modulated by the presumed mechanism of the agent within the relatively short duration of Phase II trials (one month to three years). An example is patients with a premalignant lesion. There are cohorts at high risk for cancer who are not good candidates for these Phase II chemoprevention trials. An example is subjects at risk because of germline mutations who do not also have premalignant lesions. Such cohorts may only be practical for large Phase III trials. Often, good cohorts for both Phase II and Phase III chemoprevention trials are cancer patients who have undergone previous treatment. These patients are continually monitored for possible recurrences.

For all cohorts, It is important that chemoprevention trials work within the constraints of standard treatment so that patients are not at unusual risk. In early Phase II trials where the goal is identification and standardization of biomarkers as endpoints, standard treatment may also lead to very short-term trials prior to surgery in patients who are scheduled for excision of cancers or high-risk tissue. With these considerations in mind, several cohorts have been identified for Phase II and Phase III chemoprevention trials in breast.

For Phase II trials, an obvious potential cohort from the above discussion is patients with DCIS, which accounts for approximately 70% of breast CIS. The histological subtypes have been grouped as comedo and non-comedo (papillary/ micropapillary, cribriform, solid) (Swain, 1992). Comedo-type, which consists of a thickened layer of duct cells surrounding a central area of necrosis and microcalcifications, progresses to invasive carcinoma at a much higher rate than non-comedo. After local excision of DCIS, the recurrence rate ranges up to 50%; recurrence of non-comedo DCIS is approximately 25–30% within 15 years. A study group for chemoprevention clinical trials is patients biopsied for mammographic lesions suspected as being DCIS. These patients are treated with chemopreventive agents from the time of the diagnostic biopsy to surgical removal of the lesion (1–2 months). Effects of chemopreventive agents on DCIS and associated intermediate biomarkers are then evaluated in the excised breast tissue. Currently, four chemoprevention trials are underway in such cohorts. The agents in these trials are DFMO, DHEA, exemestane, and the combination of 4-HPR with tamoxifen.

A second promising cohort for Phase II chemoprevention trials, first described by Fabian (Fabian *et al.*, 1993) is women with breast atypical hyperplasia associated with biomarker abnormalities (*e.g.*, in ploidy, estrogen receptor, EGFR, p53, and c-*erb*B-2). These subjects could be given chemopreventive agents and monitored by fine needle aspiration over several months (≥6) to evaluate effects of the agents on the hyperplasia and, particularly, the other associated biomarkers.

As noted above, LCIS is a risk marker, rather than a precursor lesion (Gump, 1993). The lifetime risk of invasive breast cancer for LCIS patients has been estimated to be approximately 20% (Ponten *et al.*, 1990). LCIS patients may be most useful as cohorts for longer Phase II and Phase III trials, since the risk is not related to the original biopsy site. Both breasts are at similar risk for cancer, and biopsy is not usually performed (Page and Dupont, 1990; Ponten *et al.*, 1990; Harris *et al.*, 1992; Posner and Wolmark, 1992). Instead, the patients are monitored by physical examination and mammography. During this monitoring period, chemopreventive intervention would be possible. One problem, however, may be the difficulty in detecting this lesion by noninvasive methods (*i.e.*, mammography).

Another cohort for Phase III trials is previous breast cancer patients. Chemopreventive agents may be administered to such patients after treatment for the cancer. Such patients are typically followed closely for recurrence and second primary tumors, and so monitoring for effects of chemopreventive agents would not exceed the limits of standard treatment. One such promising chemoprevention trial, of 4-HPR, was described above and is currently in progress (*e.g.*, De Palo *et al.*, 1995).

Because of the high incidence of breast cancer, ultimately it is desirable to identify chemopreventive strategies for all high-risk populations, including those with germline mutations. Currently, such trials are encumbered by the requirements for large cohorts and long duration to evaluate effects on breast cancer incidence, even with potent drugs such as tamoxifen (Fisher, 1992). During Phase II, and even Phase III, clinical development it may not be possible to test chemopreventive agents in subjects with germline mutations or other high-risk factors and no early lesions. For many of these high-risk subjects, other treatment options may now appear to be more immediate and clear cut (*e.g.*, prophylactic mastectomy). Hopefully, successes in early Phase II trials in identifying surrogate endpoints for cancer will lead to Phase III trials appropriate for evaluating and confirming chemopreventive efficacy in these cohorts.

CURRENT AND FUTURE PROSPECTS FOR BREAST CANCER CHEMOPREVENTION

Because of its increasing incidence, breast cancer is an important target for chemoprevention. Addressing this challenge through chemoprevention is now at the stage of discovery and early development. The current intensive effort is in Phase II intervention trials that evaluate endpoints that are potential surrogates for cancer incidence reduction. Similarly, chemopreventive mechanisms appropriate to breast and agents with these mechanisms are being identified and pursued. This approach allows many agents and leads to be followed until the best strategies can be selected. Once strategies are selected in Phase II trials, they may be confirmed in Phase III trials.

REFERENCES

Anzano MA, Byers SW, Smith JM, Peer CW, Mullen LT, Brown CC, Roberts AB, Sporn MB (1994): Prevention of breast cancer in the rat with 9-*cis*-retinoic acid as a single agent and in combination with tamoxifen. Cancer Res 54:4614–4617.

Anzano MA, Peer CW, Smith JM, Mullen LT, Shrader MW, Logsdon DL, Driver CL, Brown CC, Roberts AB, Sporn MB (1996): Chemoprevention of mammary carcinogenesis in the rat: combined use of raloxifene and 9-*cis*-retinoic acid. J Natl Cancer Inst 88:123–125.

Bain C, Speizer FE, Rosner B, Belanger C, Hennekens CH (1980): Family history of breast cancer as a risk indicator for the disease. Am J Epidemiol 111:301–308.

Bajetta E, Zilembo N, Buzzoni R, Noberasco C, Celio L, Bichisao E (1993): Efficacy and tolerability of 4-hydroxyandrostenedione (4-OHA) as first-line treatment in postmenopausal patients with breast cancer after adjuvant therapy. Cancer Treat Rev 19:31–36.

Bocker W, Bier B, Freytag G, Brommelkamp B, Jarasch E-D, Edel G, Dockhorn-Dworniczak B, Schmid KW (1992): An immunohistochemical study of the breast using antibodies to basal and luminal keratins, α-smooth muscle actin, vimentin, collagen IV and laminin. Part II. Epitheliosis and ductal carcinoma *in situ*. Virchows Arch [A] Pathol Anat Histopathol 421:323–330.

Boone CW, Kelloff GJ, Steele VE (1992): Natural history of intraepithelial neoplasia in humans with implications for cancer chemoprevention strategy. Cancer Res 52:1651– 1659.

Boone CW, Kelloff GJ (1993): Intraepithelial neoplasia, surrogate endpoint biomarkers, and cancer chemoprevention. J Cell Biochem 17F:37–48.

Boone CW, Kelloff GJ, Freedman LS (1993): Intraepithelial and postinvasive neoplasia as a stochastic continuum of clonal evolution, and its relationship to mechanisms of chemopreventive drug action. J Cell Biochem 17G:14–25.

Bradfield CA, Bjeldanes LF (1987): High-performance liquid chromatographic analysis of anticarcinogenic indoles in *Brassica oleracea*. J Agric Food Chem 35:46–49.

Bradlow HL, Hershcopf RJ, Martucci CP, Fishman J (1985): Estradiol 16α-hydroxylation in the mouse correlates with mammary tumor incidence and presence of murine mammary tumor virus: a possible model for the hormonal etiology of breast cancer in humans. Proc Natl Acad Sci USA 82:6295–6299.

Bradlow HL, Michnovicz JJ, Halper M, Miller DG, Wong GYC, Osborne MP (1994): Long-term responses of women to indole-3-carbinol or a high fiber diet. Cancer Epidemiol Biomarkers Prev 3:591–595.

Bradlow HL, Michnovicz JJ, Telang NT, Osborne MP (1991): Effects of dietary indole-3-carbinol on estradiol metabolism and spontaneous mammary tumors in mice. Carcinogenesis 12:1571–1574.

Bronfen JH, Stark MJ, Crowell PL (1994): Inhibition of human pancreatic carcinoma cell proliferation by perillyl alcohol. Proc Am Assoc Cancer Res 35:431, abst. no. 2572.

Brownsey B, Cameron EHD, Griffiths K, Gleave EN, Forrest APM, Campbell H (1972): Plasma dehydroepiandrosterone sulphate levels in patients with benign and malignant breast disease. Eur J Cancer Clin Oncol 8:131–137.

Bulbrook RD, Hayward JL, Spicer CC (1971): Relation between urinary androgen and corticoid excretion and subsequent breast cancer. Lancet 2:395–398.

Cameron EHD, Griffiths K, Gleave EN, Stewart HJ, Forrest APM, Campbell H (1970): Benign and malignant breast disease in South Wales: a study of urinary steroids. Br Med J 4:768–771.

Carroll KK (1992): Dietary fat and breast cancer. Lipids 27:793–797.

Cerda S, Wilkinson J IV, Broitman SA (1994): Enhanced antitumor activity of lovastatin and perillyl alcohol combinations in the colonic adenocarcinoma cells line SW480. Proc Am Assoc Cancer Res 35:335, abst. no. 1996.

Collins FS (1996): BRCA—-Lots of mutations, lots of dilemmas. N Engl J Med 334:186– 188.

Connolly JL, Schnitt SJ (1993): Clinical and histologic aspects of proliferative and non-proliferative benign breast disease. J Cell Biochem 17G:45–48.

Coombes RC, Hughes SWM, Dowsett M (1992): 4-Hydroxyandrostenedione: a new treatment for postmenopausal patients with breast cancer. Eur J Cancer 28A:1941–1945.

Costa A, Formelli F, Chiesa F, Decensi A, De Palo G, Veronesi U (1994): Prospects of chemoprevention of human cancers with the synthetic retinoid fenretinide. Cancer Res 54:2032S–2037S.

Costa A, Veronesi U, De Palo G, Chiesa F, Formelli F, Marubini E, Del Vecchio M, Nava M (1992): Chemoprevention of cancer with the synthetic retinoid fenretinide: clinical trials in progress at the Milan Cancer Institute. In Wattenberg L, Lipkin M, Boone CW, Kelloff GJ (eds): "Cancer Chemoprevention." Boca Raton: CRC Press, pp 95–112.

Crissman JD, Visscher DW, Kubus J (1990): Image cytophotometric DNA analysis of atypical hyperplasias and intraductal carcinomas of the breast. Arch Pathol Lab Med 114:1249–1253.

Crowell PL, Elegbede JA, Elson CE, Lin S, Vedejs E, Cunningham D, Bailey HH, Gould MN (1992): Human metabolism of orally administered d-limonene. Proc Am Assoc Cancer Res 33:524, abst. no. 3134.

Cuzick J, Bulstrode JC, Stratton I, Thomas BS, Bulbrook RD, Hayward JL (1983): A prospective study of urinary androgen levels and ovarian cancer. Int J Cancer 32:723– 726.

Dashwood RH, Fong AT, Arbogast DN, Bjeldanes LF, Hendricks JD, Bailey GS (1994): Anticarcinogenic activity of indole-3-carbinol acid products: ultrasensitive bioassay by trout embryo microinjection. Cancer Res 54:3617–3619.

De Kruif CA, Marsman JW, Venekamp JC, Falke HE, Noordhoek J, Blaauboer BJ, Wortelboer HM (1991): Structure elucidation of acid reaction products of indole-3-carbinol: detection in vivo and enzyme induction in vitro. Chem Biol Interact 80:303– 315.

De Palo G, Veronesi U, Marubini E, Camerini T, Chiesa F, Nava M, Formelli F, Del Vecchio M, Costa A, Boracchi P, Mariani L (1995): Controlled clinical trials with fenretinide in breast cancer, basal cell carcinoma and oral leukoplakia. J Cell Biochem 22:11–17.

Dhingra K (1995): A phase II chemoprevention trial design to identify surrogate endpoint biomarkers in breast cancer. J Cell Biochem 23:19–24.

Dillehay DL, Jiang XL, Lamon EW (1991): Differential effects of retinoids on pokeweed mitogen induced B-cell proliferation vs immunoglobulin synthesis. Int J Immunopharmacol 13:1043–1048.

Dupont WD, Parl FF, Hartmann WH, Brinton LA, Winfield AC, Worrell JA, Schuyler PA, Plummer WD (1993): Breast cancer risk associated with proliferative breast disease and atypical hyperplasia. Cancer 71:1258–1265.

Easton DF, Bishop DT, Ford D, Crockford GP (1993): Genetic linkage analysis in familial breast and ovarian cancer: results from 214 families. The Breast Cancer Linkage Consortium. Am J Hum Genet 52:678–701.

Easton DF, Ford D, Bishop DT (1995): Breast and ovarian cancer incidence in BRCA1-mutation carriers. Am J Hum Genet 56:265–271.

El-Bayoumy K (1994): Evaluation of chemopreventive agents against breast cancer and proposed strategies for future clinical intervention trials. Carcinogenesis 15:2395–2420.

El-Bayoumy K, Chae Y-H, Upadhyaya P, Meschter C, Cohen LA, Reddy BS (1992): Inhibition of 7,12-dimethylbenz(a)anthracene-induced tumors and DNA adduct formation in the mammary glands of female Sprague-Dawley rats by the synthetic organoselenium compound, 1,4-phenylenebis(methylene)selenocyanate. Cancer Res 52:2402– 2407.

El-Bayoumy K, Upadhyaya P, Chae Y-H, Sohn O-S, Rao CV, Fiala E, Reddy BS (1995): Chemoprevention of cancer by organoselenium compounds. J Cell Biochem 22:92–100.

ElAttar TM, Lin HS (1991): Effect of retinoids and carotenoids on prostaglandin formation by oral squamous carcinoma cells. Prostaglandins Leukot Essent Fatty Acids 43:175–178.

Elegbede JA, Elson CE, Tanner MA, Qureshi A, Gould MN (1986): Regression of rat primary mammary tumors following dietary d-limonene. J Natl Cancer Inst 76:323– 325.

Elson CE, Maltzman TH, Boston JL, Tanner MA, Gould MN (1988): Anti-carcinogenic activity of d-limonene during the initiation and promotion/progression stages of DMBA-induced rat mammary carcinogenesis. Carcinogenesis 9:331–332.

Fabian CJ, Zalles C, Kamel S, McKittrick R, Moore WP, Zeiger S, Simon C, Kimler B, Cramer A, Garcia F, Jewell W (1993): Biomarkers and cytologic abnormalities in women at high and low risk for breast cancer. J Cell Biochem 17G:153–160.

Feo F, Ruggiu ME, Lenzerini L, Garcea R, Daino L, Frassetto S, Addis V, Gaspa L, Pascale R (1987): Benzo(a)pyrene metabolism by lymphocytes from normal individuals and individuals carrying the Mediterranean variant of glucose-6-phosphate dehydrogenase. Int J Cancer 39:560–564.

Fisher B (1992): Experimental and clinical justification for the use of tamoxifen in a breast cancer prevention trial: a description of the NSABP effort. Proc Am Assoc Cancer Res 33:567–568.

Fisher B, Costantino JP, Redmond CK, Fisher ER, Wickerham DL, Cronin WM (1994): Endometrial cancer in tamoxifen-treated breast cancer patients: findings from the National Surgical Adjuvant Breast and Bowel Project (NSABP) B-14. J Natl Cancer Inst 86:527–537.

Fong AT, Swanson HI, Dashwood RH, Williams DE, Hendricks JD, Bailey GS (1990): Mechanisms of anti-carcinogenesis by indole-3-carbinol. Studies of enzyme induction, electrophile-scavenging, and inhibition of aflatoxin B_1 activation. Biochem Pharmacol 39:19–26.

Gail MH, Brinton LA, Byar DP, Corle DK, Green SB, Schairer C, Mulvihill JJ (1989): Projecting individualized probabilities of developing breast cancer for white females who are being examined annually. J Natl Cancer Inst 81:1879–1886.

Garber JE, Goldstein AM, Kantor AF, Dreyfus MG, Fraumeni JF Jr, Li FP (1991): Follow-up study of twenty-four families with Li-Fraumeni syndrome. Cancer Res 51:6094–6097.

Goldgar DE, Fields P, Lewis CM, Tran TD, Cannon-Albright LA, Ward JH, Swensen J, Skolnick MH (1994): A large kindred with 17q-linked breast and ovarian cancer: genetic, phenotypic, and genealogical analysis. J Natl Cancer Inst 86:200–209.

Gordon GB, Helzlsouer KJ, Comstock, GW (1991): Serum levels of dehydroepiandrosterone and its sulfate and the risk of developing bladder cancer. Cancer Res 51:1366– 1369.

Gordon GB, Helzlsouer KJ, Alberg AJ, Comstock GW (1993): Serum levels of dehydroepiandrosterone and dehydroepiandrosterone sulfate and the risk of developing gastric cancer. Cancer Epidemiol Biomarkers Prev 2:33–35.

Gould MN (1991): Chemoprevention and treatment of experimental mammary cancers by limonene. Proc Am Assoc Cancer Res 32:474–475.

Gould MN (1993a): Chemoprevention of mammary cancer by monoterpenes. Proc Am Assoc Cancer Res 34:572–573.

Gould MN (1993b): The introduction of activated oncogenes to mammary cells *in vivo* using retroviral vectors: a new model for the chemoprevention of premalignant lesions of the breast. J Cell Biochem 17G:66–72.

Greaves P, Goonetilleke R, Nunn G, Topham J, Orton T (1993): Two-year carcinogenicity study of tamoxifen in Alderly Park Wistar-derived rats. Cancer Res 53:3919–3924.

Gump FE (1993): Lobular carcinoma *in situ* (LCIS): pathology and treatment. J Cell Biochem 17G:53–58.

Haag JD, Gould MN (1994): Mammary carcinoma regression induced by perillyl alcohol, a hydroxylated analog of limonene. Cancer Chemother Pharmacol 34:477–483.

Haag JD, Lindstrom MJ, Gould MN (1992): Limonene-induced regression of mammary carcinomas. Cancer Res 52:4021–4026.

Hard GC, Iatropoulos MJ, Jordan K, Radi L, Kaltenberg OP, Imondi AR, Williams GM (1993): Major difference in the hepatocarcinogenicity and DNA adduct forming ability between toremifene and tamoxifen in female Crl:CD(BR) rats. Cancer Res 53:4534– 4541.

Harris JR, Lippman ME, Veronesi U, Willett W (1992): Breast cancer (Second of three parts). N Engl J Med 327:390–398.

Hayes DF, Van Zyl JA, Hacking A, Goedhals L, Bezwoda WR, Mailliard JA, Jones SE, Vogel CL, Berris RF, Shemano I, Schoenfelder J (1995): Randomized comparison of tamoxifen and two separate doses of toremifene in postmenopausal patients with metastatic breast cancer. J Clin Oncol 13:2556–2566.

Henderson BE, Pike MC, Casagrande JT (1981): Breast cancer and the oestrogen window hypothesis. Lancet 2:363–364.

Henderson IC (1993): Risk factors for breast cancer development. Cancer 71:2127–2140.

Hirsimaki P, Hirsimaki Y, Nieminen L, Payne BJ (1993): Tamoxifen induces hepatocellular carcinoma in rat liver: a 1-year study with 2 antiestrogens. Arch Toxicol 67:49–54.

Ip C (1986): Interaction of vitamin C and selenium supplementation in the modification of mammary carcinogenesis in rats. J Natl Cancer Inst 77:299–234.

Ip C (1987): Fat and essential fatty acid in mammary carcinogenesis. Am J Clin Nutr 45:218–224.

Ip C, White G (1987): Mammary cancer chemoprevention by inorganic and organic selenium: single agent treatment or in combination with vitamin E and their effects on *in vitro* immune functions. Carcinogenesis 8:1763–1766.

Ip C, El-Bayoumy K, Upadhyaya P, Ganther H, Vadhanavikit S, Thompson H (1994): Comparative effect of inorganic and organic selenocyanate derivatives in mammary cancer chemoprevention. Carcinogenesis 15:187–192.

Jirtle RL, Haag JD, Ariazi EA, Gould MN (1993): Increased mannose 6-phosphate/ insulin-like growth factor II receptor and transforming growth factor β1 levels during monoterpene-induced regression of mammary tumors. Cancer Res 53:3849–3852.

Jones DY, Schatzkin A, Green SB, Block G, Brinton LA, Ziegler RG, Hoover R, Taylor PR (1987): Dietary fat and breast cancer in the National Health and Nutrition Examination Survey I Epidemiologic Follow-up Study. J Natl Cancer Inst 79:465–471.

Jordan VC (1995): Alternate antiestrogens and approaches to the prevention of breast cancer. J Cell Biochem 22:51–58.

Jordan VC, Assikis VJ (1995): Endometrial carcinoma and tamoxifen: clearing up a controversy. Clin Cancer Res 1:467–472.

Kalimi M, Shafagoj Y, Loria R, Padgett D, Regelson W (1994): Anti-glucocorticoid effects of dehydroepiandrosterone (DHEA). Mol Cell Biochem 131:99–104.

Kelloff GJ, Boone CW, Steele VE, Crowell JA, Lubet R, Doody LA, Greenwald P (1993): Development of breast cancer chemopreventive drugs. J Cell Biochem 17G:2– 13.

Kelloff GJ, Boone CW, Crowell JA, Steele VE, Lubet R, Sigman CC (1994a): Chemopreventive drug development: perspectives and progress. Cancer Epidemiol Biomarkers Prev 3:85–98.

Kelloff GJ, Boone CW, Steele VE, Crowell JA, Lubet R, Sigman CC (1994b): Progress in cancer chemoprevention: perspectives on agent selection and short-term clinical intervention trials. Cancer Res 54:2015S–1024S.

Kelloff GJ, Boone CW, Steele VE, Fay JR, Lubet RA, Crowell JA, Sigman CC (1994c): Mechanistic considerations in chemopreventive drug development. J Cell Biochem 20:1–24.

Kelloff GJ, Crowell JA, Boone CW, Steele VE, Lubet RA, Greenwald P, Alberts DS, Covey JM, Doody LA, Knapp GG, Nayfield S, Parkinson DR, Prasad VK, Prorok PC, Sausville EA, Sigman, CC (1994d): Strategy and planning for chemopreventive drug development: Clinical Development Plans. J Cell Biochem 20:55–62.

Kelloff GJ, Boone CW, Crowell JA, Steele VE, Lubet R, Doody LA (1994e): Surrogate endpoint biomarkers for phase II cancer chemoprevention trials. J Cell Biochem 19:1–9.

Kelloff GJ, Crowell JA, Boone CW, Steele VE, Lubet RA, Greenwald P, Alberts DS, Covey JM, Doody LA, Knapp GG, Nayfield S, Parkinson DR, Prasad VK, Prorok

PC, Sausville EA, Sigman CC (1994f): Clinical Development Plan: 2-difluoromethylornithine (DFMO). J Cell Biochem 20:147–165.

Kelloff GJ, Crowell JA, Boone CW, Steele VE, Lubet RA, Greenwald P, Alberts DS, Covey JM, Doody LA, Knapp GG, Nayfield S, Parkinson DR, Prasad VK, Prorok PC, Sausville EA, Sigman CC (1994g): Clinical Development Plan: DHEA analog 8354. J Cell Biochem 20:141–146.

Kelloff GJ, Crowell JA, Boone CW, Steele VE, Lubet RA, Greenwald P, Alberts DS, Covey JM, Doody LA, Knapp GG, Nayfield S, Parkinson DR, Prasad VK, Prorok PC, Sausville EA, Sigman CC (1994h): Clinical Development Plan: oltipraz. J Cell Biochem 20:205–218.

Kelloff GJ, Johnson JR, Crowell JA, Boone CW, DeGeorge JJ, Steele VE, Mehta MU, Temeck JW, Schmidt WJ, Burke G, Greenwald P, Temple RJ (1995a): Approaches to the development and marketing approval of drugs that prevent cancer. Cancer Epidemiol Biomarkers Prev 4:1–10.

Kelloff GJ, Boone CW, Crowell JA, Nayfield SG, Hawk E, Steele VE, Lubet RA, Sigman CC (1995b): Development of breast cancer chemopreventive drugs. The Breast J 1:271–283.

Kensler TW, Groopman JD, Roebuck BD (1992): Chemoprotection by oltipraz and other dithiolethiones. In Wattenberg L, Lipkin M, Boone CW, Kelloff GJ (eds): "Cancer Chemoprevention." Boca Raton: CRC Press, pp 205–226.

Khosravi-Far R, Cox AD, Kato K, Der CJ (1992): Protein prenylation: key to *ras* function and cancer intervention? Cell Growth Differ 3:461–469.

King M-C (1992): Breast cancer genes: how many, where and who are they? Nat Genet 2:89–90.

Kojima T, Tanaka T, Mori H (1994): Chemoprevention of spontaneous endometrial cancer in female Donryu rats by dietary indole-3-carbinol. Cancer Res 54:1446–1449.

Langston AA, Malone KE, Thompson JD, Daling JR, Ostrander EA (1996): *BRCA1* mutations in a population-based sample of young women with breast cancer. N Engl J Med 334:137–142.

Li FP, Correa P, Fraumeni JF Jr (1991): Testing for germline p53 mutations in cancer families. Cancer Epidemiol Biomarkers Prev 1:91–94.

Lubet RA, Steele VE, Casebolt TL, Eto I, Kelloff GJ, Grubbs CJ (1994): Chemopreventive effects of the aromatase inhibitors vorozole (R-83842) and 4-hydroxyandrostenedione in the methylnitrosourea (MNU)-induced mammary tumor model in Sprague-Dawley rats. Carcinogenesis 15:2775–2780.

Luk GD, Casero RA Jr (1987): Polyamines in normal and cancer cells. Adv. Enzyme Regul. 26:91–105.

MacMahon B, Cole P, Lin TM, Lowe CR, Mirra AP, Ravnihar B, Salber EJ, Valaoras VG, Yuasa S (1970): Age at first birth and breast cancer risk. Bull WHO 43:209–221.

Maltzman TH, Hurt LM, Elson CE, Tanner MA, Gould MN (1989): The prevention of nitrosomethylurea-induced mammary tumors by *d*-limonene and orange oil. Carcinogenesis 10:781–783.

Manni A (1993): Clinical use of aromatase inhibitors in the treatment of breast cancers. J Cell Biochem 17G:242–246.

Marshall E (1993): The politics of breast cancer. Science 259:616–617.

Mbensa M, Rwakunda C, Verwilghen RL (1978): Glucose-6-phosphate dehydrogenase deficiency and malignant hepatoma in a Bantu population. East Afr Med J 55:17–19.

McCann PP, Pegg AE, Sjoerdsma A (1987): "Inhibition of Polyamine Metabolism: Biological Significance and Basis for New Therapies." New York: Academic Press.

McCormick DL, Mehta RG, Thompson CA, Dinger N, Caldwell JA, Moon RC (1982): Enhanced inhibition of mammary carcinogenesis by combined treatment with N-(4-hydroxyphenyl)retinamide and ovariectomy. Cancer Res 42:508–512.

Mettlin C (1992): Breast cancer risk factors. Contributions to planning breast cancer control. Cancer 69:1904–1910.

Mills JJ, Chari RS, Boyer IJ, Gould MN, Jirtle RL (1995): Induction of apoptosis in liver tumors by the monoterpene perillyl alcohol. Cancer Res 55:979–983.

Moon RC, Thompson HJ, Becci PJ, Grubbs CJ, Gander RJ, Newton DL, Smith JM, Phillips SL, Henderson WR, Mullen LT, Brown CC, Sporn MB (1979): N-(4-hydroxyphenyl)retinamide, a new retinoid for prevention of breast cancer in the rat. Cancer Res 39:1339–1346.

Moon RC, Kelloff GJ, Detrisac CJ, Steele VE, Thomas CF, Sigman CC (1992): Chemoprevention of MNU-induced mammary tumors in the mature rat by 4-HPR and tamoxifen. Anticancer Res 12:1147–1154.

Moon RC, Steele VE, Kelloff GJ, Thomas CF, Detrisac CJ, Mehta RG, Lubet RA (1994): Chemoprevention of MNU-induced mammary tumorigenesis by hormone response modifiers: toremifene, RU 16117, tamoxifen, aminoglutethimide and progesterone. Anticancer Res 14:889–893.

Nayfield SG, Karp JE, Ford LG, Dorr FA, Kramer BS (1991): Potential role of tamoxifen in prevention of breast cancer. J Natl Cancer Inst 83:1450–1459.

O'Neill JS, Miller WR (1987): Aromatase activity in breast adipose tissue from women with benign and malignant breast diseases. Br J Cancer 56:601–604.

Oridate N, Lotan D, Mitchell MF, Hong WK, Lotan R (1995): Inhibition of proliferation and induction of apoptosis in cervical carcinoma cells by retinoids: implications for chemoprevention. J Cell Biochem 23:80–86.

Osborne MP, Telang NT, Kaur S, Bradlow HL (1990): Influence of chemopreventive agents on estradiol metabolism and mammary preneoplasia in the C3H mouse. Steroids 55:114–119.

Page DL, Dupont WD (1990): Anatomic markers of human premalignancy and risk of breast cancer. Cancer 66:1326–1335.

Pallis L, Skoog L, Falkmer U, Wilking N, Rutquist LE, Auer G, Cedermark B (1992): The DNA profile of breast cancer *in situ*. Eur J Surg Oncol 18:108–111.

Pashko LL, Schwartz AG, Abou-Gharbia M, Swern D (1981): Inhibition of DNA synthesis in mouse epidermis and breast epithelium by dehydroepiandrosterone and related steroids. Carcinogenesis 2:717–721.

Plourde PV, Dyroff M, Dukes M (1994): Arimidex: a potent and selective fourth-generation aromatase inhibitor. Breast Cancer Res Treat 30:103–111.

Plourde PV, Dyroff M, Dowsett M, Demers L, Yates R, Webster A (1995): Arimidex™: a new oral, once-a-day aromatase inhibitor. J Steroid Biochem Mol Biol 53:175–179.

Ponten J, Holmberg L, Trichopoulos D, Kallioniemi O-P, Kvale G, Wallgren A, Taylor-Papadimitriou J (1990): Biology and natural history of breast cancer. Int J Cancer Suppl 5:5–21.

Posner MC, Wolmark N (1992): Non-invasive breast carcinoma. Breast Cancer Res Treat 21:155–164.

Radcliffe JD, Moon RC (1983): Effect of N-(4-hydroxyphenyl)retinamide on food intake, growth, and mammary gland development in rats (41736). Proc Soc Exp Biol Med 174:270–275.

Ratko TA, Detrisac CJ, Dinger NM, Thomas CF, Kelloff GJ, Moon RC (1989): Chemopreventive efficacy of combined retinoid and tamoxifen treatment following surgical excision of a primary mammary cancer in female rats. Cancer Res 49:4472–4476.

Ratko TA, Detrisac CJ, Mehta RG, Kelloff GJ, Moon RC (1991): Inhibition of rat mammary gland chemical carcinogenesis by dietary dehydroepiandrosterone or a fluorinated analogue of dehydroepiandrosterone. Cancer Res 51:481–486.

Regelson W, Kalimi M (1994): Dehydroepiandrosterone (DHEA)—The multifunctional steroid II. Effects on the CNS, cell proliferation, metabolic and vascular, clinical and other effects. Mechanism of action? Ann NY Acad Sci 719:564–575.

Ren Z, Gould MN (1993): Inhibition of ubiquinone biosynthesis by the monoterpene perillyl alcohol. Proc Am Assoc Cancer Res 34:548, abst. no. 3265.

Ren Z, Gould MN (1994): Inhibition of ubiquinone and cholesterol synthesis by the monoterpene perillyl alcohol. Cancer Lett 76:185–190.

Ren Z, Gould MN (1995): Inhibition of protein isoprenylation by the monoterpene perillyl alcohol in intact cells and in cell lysates. Proc Am Assoc Cancer Res 36:585, abst. no. 3484.

Rose DP, Stauber P, Thiel A, Crowley JJ, Milbrath JR (1977): Plasma dehydroepiandrosterone sulfate, androstenedione and cortisol, and urinary free cortisol excretion in breast cancer. Eur J Cancer Clin Oncol 13:43–47.

Russo J, Rivera R, Russo IH (1992): Influence of age and parity on the development of the human breast. Breast Cancer Res Treat 23:211–218.

Schneider J, Kinne D, Fracchia A, Pierce V, Anderson KE, Bradlow HL, Fishman J (1982): Abnormal oxidative metabolism of estradiol in women with breast cancer. Proc Natl Acad Sci USA 79:3047–3051.

Schnitt SJ, Silen W, Sadowsky NL, Connolly JL, Harris JR (1988): Ductal carcinoma in situ (intraductal carcinoma of the breast). N Engl J Med 318:898–903.

Schulz S, Nyce JW (1991): Inhibition of protein isoprenylation and p21 *ras* membrane association by dehydroepiandrosterone in human colonic adenocarcinoma cells *in vitro*. Cancer Res 51:6563–6567.

Schulz S, Nyce JW (1994): Inhibition of protein farnesyltransferase: a possible mechanism of tumor prevention by dehydroepiandrosterone sulfate. Carcinogenesis 15:2649–2652.

Schulz S, Klann RC, Schonfeld S, Nyce JW (1992): Mechanisms of cell growth inhibition and cell cycle arrest in human colonic adenocarcinoma cells by dehydroepiandrosterone: role of isoprenoid biosynthesis. Cancer Res 52:1372–1376.

Schwartz AG, Pashko LL (1986): Food restriction inhibits [3H] 7,12-dimethylbenz(*a*) anthracene binding to mouse skin DNA and tetradecanoylphorbol-13-acetate stimulation of epidermal [3H] thymidine incorporation. Anticancer Res 6:1279–1282.

Schwartz AG, Pashko LL (1993): Cancer chemoprevention with the adrenocortical steroid dehydroepiandrosterone and structural analogs. J Cell Biochem 17G:73–79.

Schwartz AG, Pashko LL (1995): Cancer prevention with dehydroepiandrosterone and non-androgenic structural analogs. J Cell Biochem 22:210–217.

Schwartz AG, Perantoni A (1975): Protective effect of dehydroepiandrosterone against aflatoxin B$_1$- and 7,12-dimethylbenz(*a*)anthracene-induced cytotoxicity and transformation in cultured cells. Cancer Res 35:2482–2487.

Seidman H, Stellman SD, Mushinski MH (1982): A different perspective on breast cancer risk factors: some implications of the nonattributable risk. CA Cancer J Clin 32:301–313.

Smith HS, Lu Y, Deng G, Martinez O, Krams S, Ljung B-M, Thor A, Lagios M (1993): Molecular aspects of early stages of breast cancer progression. J Cell Biochem 17G:144–152.

Smith SA, Easton DF, Evans DGR, Ponder BAJ (1992): Allele losses in the region 17q12-21 in familial breast and ovarian cancer involve the wild-type chromosome. Nat Genet 2:128–131.

Sparnins VL, Venegas PL, Wattenberg LW (1982): Glutathione S-transferase activity: enhancement by compounds inhibiting chemical carcinogenesis and by dietary constituents. J Natl Cancer Inst 68:493–496.

Sporn MB, Newton DL (1979): Chemoprevention of cancer with retinoids. Fed Proc 38:2528–2534.

Steele VE, Moon RC, Lubet RA, Grubbs CJ, Reddy BS, Wargovich M, McCormick DL, Pereira MA, Crowell JA, Bagheri D, Sigman CC, Boone CW, Kelloff GJ (1994): Preclinical efficacy evaluation of potential chemopreventive agents in animal carcinogenesis models: methods and results from the NCI Chemoprevention Drug Development Program. J Cell Biochem 20:32–54.

Stresser DM, Bailey GS, Williams DE (1994): Indole-3-carbinol and β-naphthoflavone induction of aflatoxin B$_1$ metabolism and cytochromes P-450 associated with bioactivation and detoxication of aflatoxin B_1 in the rat. Drug Metab Dispos 22:383–391.

Struewing JP, Abeliovich D, Peretz T, Avishai N, Kaback MM, Collins FS, Brody LC (1995): The carrier frequency of the *BRCA1* 185delAG mutation is approximately 1 percent in Ashkenazi Jewish individuals. Nat Genet 11:198–200.

Swain SM (1992): Ductal carcinoma *in situ*. Cancer Invest 10:443–454.

Swaneck GE, Fishman J (1991): Estrogen actions on target cells: evidence for different effects by products of two alternative pathways of estradiol metabolism. In Hochberg RB, Naftolin F (eds): "The New Biology of Steroid Hormones." New York: Raven Press, pp 45–70.

Thomas BS, Kirby P, Symes EK, Wang DY (1976): Plasma dehydroepiandrosterone concentration in normal women and in patients with benign and malignant breast disease. Eur J Cancer Clin Oncol 12:405–409.

Tillotson JK, Upadhyaya P, Ronai Z (1994): Inhibition of thymidine kinase in cultured mammary tumor cells by the chemopreventive organoselenium compound, 1,4-phenylenebis(methylene)selenocyanate. Carcinogenesis 15:607–610.

van Duuren BL, Goldschmidt BM (1976): Cocarcinogenic and tumor-promoting agents in tobacco carcinogenesis. J Natl Cancer Inst 56:1237–1242.

van Leeuwen FE, Benraadt J, Coebergh JWW, Kiemeney LALM, Gimbrere CHF, Otter R, Schouten LJ, Damhuis RAM, Bontenbal M, Diepenhorst FW, van den Belt-Dusebout AW, van Tinteren H (1994): Risk of endometrial cancer after tamoxifen treatment of breast cancer. Lancet 343:448–452.

Wang DY, Bulbrook RD, Hayward JL (1975): Urinary and plasma androgens and their relation to familial risk of breast cancer. Eur J Cancer Clin Oncol 11:873–877.

Wang DY, Bulbrook RD Herian M, Hayward JL (1974): Studies on the sulphate esters of dehydroepiandrosterone and androsterone in the blood of women with breast cancer. Eur J Cancer Clin Oncol 10:477–482.

Wattenberg LW, Sparnins VL, Barany G (1989): Inhibition of *N*-nitrosodiethylamine carcinogenesis in mice by naturally occurring organosulfur compounds and monoterpenes. Cancer Res 49:2689–2692.

Wetzels RHW, Kuijpers HJH, Lane EB, Leigh IM, Troyanovsky SM, Holland R, van Haelst UJGM, Ramaekers FCS (1991): Basal cell-specific and hyperproliferation-related keratins in human breast cancer. Am J Pathol 138:751–763.

Whitcomb JM, Schwartz AG (1985): Dehydroepiandrosterone and 16α-Br-epiandrosterone inhibit 12-*O*-tetradecanoylphorbol-13-acetate stimulation of superoxide radical production by human polymorphonuclear leukocytes. Carcinogenesis 6:333–335.

Willett WC, Stampfer MJ, Colditz GA, Rosner BA, Hennekens CH, Speizer FE (1987): Dietary fat and the risk of breast cancer. N Engl J Med 316:22–28.

Willett WC, Hunter DJ, Stampfer MJ, Colditz G, Manson JE, Spiegelman D, Rosner B, Hennekens CH, Speizer FE (1992): Dietary fat and fiber in relation to risk of breast cancer: an 8-year follow-up. JAMA 268:2037–2044.

Wingo PA, Tong T, Bolder S (1995): Cancer statistics, 1995. CA Cancer J Clin 45:8–30.

Young TB, Wolf DA (1988): Case-control study of proximal and distal colon cancer and diet in Wisconsin. Int J Cancer 42:167–175.

Zilembo N, Noberasco C, Bajetta E, Martinetti A, Mariani L, Orefice S, Buzzoni R, Di Bartolomeo M, Di Leo A, Laffranchi A, di Salle E (1995): Endocrinological and clinical evaluation of exemestane, a new steroidal aromatase inhibitor. Br J Cancer 72:1007–1012.

Etiology of Breast and
Gynecological Cancers, pages 185–203
© 1997 Wiley-Liss, Inc.

THE MOLECULAR GENETICS OF ENDOMETRIAL CARCINOMA

Christina A. Bandera and Jeff Boyd
Division of Gynecologic Oncology
Department of Obstetrics and Gynecology
University of Pennsylvania Medical Center
Philadelphia, PA 19104

INTRODUCTION

The endometrial lining of the uterine cavity is a dynamic glandular tissue which proliferates and regresses continually throughout a woman's reproductive years. Occasionally, the control of endometrial growth is aberrant. Overgrowth of the endometrium may lead to benign hyperplasia, hyperplasia with malignant potential, or endometrial carcinoma.

In 1996 approximately 34 thousand new cases of uterine cancer will be diagnosed in the United States (Cancer Facts-96, 1996). Fortunately, the cure rate for endometrial carcinoma is 80% by surgery (Zaino, 1995), and some inoperable patients respond to radiation therapy or hormonal therapy. Nonetheless, in 1996, an estimated 6000 American women will die secondary to advanced disease (Cancer Facts-96, 1996). Studying the molecular basis of endometrial carcinoma necessitates an appreciation of the clinical categorization of the disease.

Classically, risk factors for endometrial cancer are conditions which are associated with increased endogenous estrogen levels. Estrogen stimulation leads to complex atypical hyperplasia. It has been observed that 29% of women with untreated complex atypical hyperplasia will develop endometrial carcinoma (Kurman et al., 1984). Pro-estrogenic factors include obesity, nulliparity, late menopause, early menarche, and the use of estrogen replacement. In addition, tamoxifen acts as an estrogen analog in uterine tissue, and is also associated with the progression to hyperplasia and carcinoma (Ross and Whitehead, 1995). Estrogen-related endometrial carcinoma is categorized as type I disease. Histopathology typically reveals a well-differentiated glandular pattern with frequent foam cells and an increased number of progesterone receptors indicating estrogenic effect. Patients tend to be premenopausal, or in early menopause. Symptoms of abnormal vaginal bleeding occur in early stage disease, and prognosis is excellent

(Delgidisch and Holinka, 1987). Interestingly, women who have a family history of cancer in other hormonally-responsive organs such as breast and ovary do not appear to have an increased risk of endometrial carcinoma (Schildkraut et al., 1989; Parazzini et al., 1994).

The type II category of endometrial carcinoma occurs in patients without identifiable hyperestrogenism. Typically, these patients present many years after menopause with more advanced disease. No precursor lesion such as hyperplasia has been associated with this category of endometrial carcinoma which arises from atrophic endometrium (Kurman et al., 1984). Most commonly, type II disease is associated with adenocarcinoma, papillary serous, and clear cell histologic subtypes. Prognosis is poorer than in patients with type I estrogen-related disease (Delgidisch and Holinka, 1987).

Finally, we propose that a type III endometrial carcinoma be defined. These are the patients who have an inherited predisposition for endometrial neoplasia. They tend to develop the disease 15 years earlier than the general population and prognosis is favorable (Watson et al., 1994; Vasen et al., 1994). Usually the pedigrees of these patients reveal a hereditary nonpolyposis colorectal carcinoma (HNPCC) syndrome where colon cancer predominates as the most common cancer in the family, and endometrial carcinoma is the second most common malignancy occurring in 20 to 40% of women in the family (Watson and Lynch, 1993; Hakala et al., 1991). In a minority of families, endometrial carcinoma is the primary malignancy, suggesting a heritable site-specific uterine cancer syndrome (Boltenberg et al., 1990; Lynch et al., 1994; Sandles et al., 1992).

It is important to note that the three types of endometrial carcinoma are rarely considered separately in molecular studies of the disease, and important patterns may be obscured by the heterogeneity of a study population. For example, some tertiary referral centers may have an abnormally large number of patients with a familial cancer syndrome who would be expected to have a very unique genetic profile. Furthermore, not all random populations have the same ratio of type I and type II endometrial carcinoma. Many studies cited in this review are from Japan where the incidence of endometrial cancer is lower than in the US, probably because of the relative infrequency of pro-estrogenic factors such as hormone replacement therapy and obesity (Enomoto et al., 1994b).

This chapter will survey the current lines of investigation in the field of the molecular genetics of endometrial carcinoma. Expanded discussion will be devoted to DNA content, genomic alterations, and receptor status. Correlations between the molecular genetic profile of endometrial carcinoma and the clinical understanding of the disease process will be explored.

ENDOMETRIAL CARCINOMA
and the MULTISTEP MODEL of CARCINOGENESIS

Cancer is now thought of as a disease caused by a series of genetic events occurring within a cell. In 1971 Alfred Knudson suggested that retinoblastoma is the result of an inherited mutation and an additional acquired mutation in the other allele of the same gene leading to the development of cancer (Knudson, 1971). This two-step model has been expanded into a broadly applicable multistep model of carcinogenesis in which inherited mutations and additional genetic events resulting from carcinogenic exposures (for hereditary cancers), or a series of somatic mutations only (for sporadic cancers) contribute to the progression towards a neoplastic phenotype (Vogelstein and

Kinzler, 1993). In colon cancer, the genetic events leading from normal epithelium to hyperproliferation, adenoma, and carcinoma have been well-characterized and include allelic deletions, mutations in tumor suppressor genes and activation of oncogenes (Fearon and Jones, 1992).

In type I endometrial carcinoma, the progression from complex atypical endometrial hyperplasia to adenocarcinoma has been described on a histopathologic level (Kurman et al., 1984); however, the genetic basis for this progression is poorly understood. Studies based on X chromosome inactivation and heterozygous markers have confirmed the clonal nature of endometrial carcinoma, which proves that the cancer arises from the genetic transformation and proliferation of a single cell (Enomoto et al., 1994a; Mutter et al., 1995). One model suggests that estrogen stimulates endometrial hyperplasia which is associated with poor oxygenation of cells leading to enzyme-alterations within cells (Coroncleanu, 1993). In the altered intracellular environment, destabilization of the genome could result in the progression to cancer. This model helps explain the high frequency of endometrial carcinoma in women with hypertension (associated with hypoxia due to vasoconstriction) and diabetes mellitus (associated with hypoxia due to vasculitis).

In type II endometrial carcinoma, a precursor lesion has not been identified, making the study of tumor progression more difficult. Type III endometrial carcinoma is associated with inherited genetic mutations which predispose the patient to developing cancer when additional genetic events occur.

Understanding the molecular basis of the development and progression of endometrial carcinoma may lead to improved screening protocols, aggressive therapy for high risk patients, and genetically-based treatments. For example, women who are identified as members of families with the HNPCC syndrome are aggressively monitored for signs of endometrial malignancy, and prophylactic hysterectomy may be recommended (Hakala et al., 1991; Slattery and Kerher, 1994; Suomi et al., 1995; Vasen et al., 1994; Watson et al., 1994). Although most cases of endometrial carcinoma are curable, 20-30% of stage I and II cancers will recur in two to five years despite standard therapy (Britton et al., 1989; Lindahl et al., 1987; Turnos et al., 1992), and 10% of patients will eventually die of disease (Moore et al., 1991). Characterization of the molecular genetic basis of the disease may enable us to identify and aggressively treat patients with a high risk of developing recurrent disease. Furthermore, gene therapy (e.g., the replacement of defective genes via viral vectors) has already been applied with some success in several diseases including cystic fibrosis, and may be applicable to cancer prevention and cure (Hanania et al., 1995).

DNA CONTENT as a PROGNOSTIC INDICATOR

Flow cytometry provides a rapid method of quantifying the DNA content of cells by measuring the fluorescence of nuclear DNA tagged with propidium iodide. In cancers of the breast, bladder, and colon, determining the DNA content of tumor cells has been shown to be a useful predictor of survival (Coon et al., 1987; Williams and Daly, 1990). This type of analysis has been applied to endometrial carcinoma; however, its utility is still unclear. Generally, in endometrial carcinoma, aneuploidy correlates with factors which are associated with a poor prognosis such as high grade of tumor, advanced stage, and advanced age of the patient (Friedlander et al., 1984).

Several studies suggest that aneuploidy may be an independent risk factor for recurrence of early stage disease (Ambros and Kurman, 1992; Britton et al., 1989; Coleman et al., 1991; Friberg et al., 1994; Ikeda et al., 1993; Lukes et al., 1994; Melchiorri et al., 1993; Rosenberg et al., 1989; Susini et al., 1994; Van der Putten et al., 1989). One study surveying tissue from stage I and II endometrial carcinomas concludes that aneuploidy associated with more than 50% myometrial invasion is predictive of poor outcome (Lindahl et al., 1994); this study recommends that these cases be treated more aggressively than they would be on the basis of myometrial invasion alone. However, additional investigations of aneuploidy in early stage endometrial carcinoma fail to identify DNA content as an independent prognostic indicator (Pfisterer et al., 1995; Tornos et al., 1992). Inconsistencies between studies may be the result of multiple factors such as flow cytometry technique, use of paraffin-embedded tissue as opposed to fresh tissue, and heterogeneity of study populations.

S-phase fraction (SPF) reflecting the proportion of cells involved in DNA synthesis is another characteristic which can be assessed by flow cytometry. In normal endometrium the SPF is 1-3%, and increases to 4-5% in the peri-ovulatory period when estrogen levels peak. In hyperplasia the SPF is 4-5%. An SPF greater than 7 to 10% has been associated with endometrial carcinoma with a poor prognosis (Pfisterer et al., 1995; Rosenberg et al., 1989). However, the validity of SPF as an independent predictor of outcome is also controversial (Coleman et al., 1991; Goodman et al., 1993; Lindahl et al., 1987). Despite a large amount of literature addressing the issue, neither DNA ploidy nor SPF determinations are considered standard in the diagnostic evaluation of endometrial carcinoma at the present time.

A more precise reflection of DNA content in cancer cells is cytogenic evaluation to identify structural chromosomal aberrations. Traditionally, cytogenic evaluation involves karyotype analysis. More recently, fluorescent in situ hybridization (FISH) techniques have enabled researchers to perform rapid screening of specific chromosomes. In endometrial carcinoma both techniques have been employed to identify frequent chromosomal anomalies. Duplication of chromosome 1 is the most common abnormality found, although genes implicated in endometrial carcinoma have yet to be identified in this area (Bardi et al., 1995; Deger et al., 1994; Ketter et al., 1995). Additional studies have found numerical abnormalities and structural rearrangements in chromosomes 1, 2, 3, 6, 7, 10, 12, 22 and X (Bardi et al., 1995; Couturier et al., 1986; Deger et al., 1994; Dutrillaux et al., 1986; Fujita et al., 1985; Gibas and Rubin, 1987; Jenkyn et al., 1986; Milatovich et al., 1990; Shah et al., 1994; Simon et al., 1990; Yoshida et al., 1986). These chromosomes may contain genes involved in tumor progression.

ONCOGENES

An oncogene is a dominantly acting gene whose expression converts a normal cell into a cell with an enhanced malignant potential. A protooncogene is the normal form of the gene that does not confer malignant potential. Generally, protooncogenes are involved in the control of cellular division or differentiation. Protooncogene activation may involve a point mutation, deletion, chromosomal rearrangement, or abnormal amplification (Sasano et al, 1992). Mutations of protooncogenes, with rare exception, occur somatically.

The three oncogenes which have been most thoroughly studied in endometrial carcinoma are the *RAS* family of genes, *ERBB-2* (also called *HER-2* or *neu*), and *C-MYC*. The *RAS* family of oncogenes encode p21 proteins which appear to be involved in signal transduction across the plasma membrane (Barbacid, 1987), and may also regulate a mitogen-activated protein kinase via interaction with the raf oncogene product (Stokoe et al., 1994). Mutations in this gene are common in a variety of cancers. For example, in pancreatic cancer the *K-RAS* mutation rate is 75-95%; in colon cancer and pulmonary adenocarcinoma the rate of mutation is greater than 30% (Bos et al., 1989, Vogelstein et al., 1988). In endometrial carcinoma, immunohistochemical studies show that expression of ras^{p21} is consistently elevated compared with normal endometrial tissue (Scambia et al., 1992). *K-RAS* activating mutations have been identified in 6-16% of hyperplasia specimens (Enomoto et al., 1990; Enomoto et al., 1993; Sasaki et al., 1993), and in 10-37% of endometrial carcinoma specimens (Boyd and Risinger, 1991; Caduff et al., 1995; Enomoto et al., 1990; Enomoto et al., 1991; Enomoto et al., 1993; Ignar-Trowbridge et al., 1992; Lester and Cauchi, 1990; Mizuuchi et al., 1992; Pisani et al., 1995; Sasaki et al., 1993; Sato et al., 1991; Yaginuma and Ishikawa, 1993). The significance of *K-RAS* mutations is controversial. In one study, no association was found between *K-RAS* mutations and stage, grade, depth of invasion or clinical outcome (Caduff et al., 1995). Another study suggests that the presence of a *K-RAS* mutation improves prognosis; in this study, all 15 patients with mutations were alive and well at the completion of the study, while 22 of 69 patients without *K-RAS* mutations were dead of disease (Sasaki et al., 1993). This data contrasts with a Japanese study reporting a series 49 endometrial carcinoma cases revealing an association between *K-RAS* mutation and poor outcome (Imamura et al., 1992).

K-RAS mutations appear to be more common in endometrial carcinoma cases in Japan than in the United States, as illustrated by a study reporting *K-RAS* mutations two times more frequently in Japanese cases (23%) than in American cases (12%) (Sasaki et al., 1993). However, the type of mutation occurring is similar in both populations, involving primarily point mutations in codon 12. Furthermore, in both American and Japanese series, *K-RAS* mutations are found most frequently in endometrioid carcinomas, and rarely in papillary serous and clear cell carcinomas (Caduff et al., 1995; Sasaki et al., 1993). Despite the difference in *K-RAS* mutation rate in Japan and the US, the cumulative data suggest that *K-RAS* mutations occur early in the development of endometrial carcinoma, but are not necessary for malignant transformation.

ERBB-2 is a protooncogene which encodes a transmembrane tyrosine kinase receptor. *ERBB-2* amplification and overexpression have been identified in a variety of cancers, and are noted to be associated with metastases in breast and gastric cancer. Additional *in vitro* models associate the *ERBB-2* oncogene with metastatic potential (Hung et al., 1995). In endometrial carcinoma, erbB-2 overexpression occurs in approximately 9-15% of cases (Berchuck et al., 1991; Borst et al., 1990; Hetzel et al., 1992; Lukes et al., 1994; Pisani et al., 1995), and has been associated with the presence of intraperitoneal metastases (Berchuck et al., 1991; Hetzel et al., 1992). In general, ERBB-2 overexpression in endometrial carcinoma appears to be associated with poor prognosis; however, multivariate analysis of two series of cases has failed to reveal a statistically significant association (Lukes et al., 1994; Pisani et al., 1995).

C-MYC encodes a nuclear protein involved with gene regulation, and its activation has been demonstrated in colon, lung, breast and ovarian cancer (Sato et al., 1993). C-MYC mRNA and protein expression were also identified in all 10 endometrial carcinoma cases screened in a recent study (Sato et al., 1993). Another series of 15 endometrial carcinomas revealed *C-MYC* amplification in 67% of cases (Borst et al., 1990). However, a similar analysis using an appropriate loading control found *C-MYC* amplification in only 1 of 51 cases (Boyd, 1994). Furthermore, screening of 11 endometrial carcinoma cell lines revealed only one cancer (an aggressive papillary serous carcinoma of the endometrium) with *C-MYC* amplification (Boyd and Risinger, 1991).

In summary, *K-RAS* activation appears to be associated with 10-37% of endometrial carcinomas, whereas *ERBB-2* and *C-MYC* activation are associated with less than 15%. The low rates of involvement of these oncogenes suggest that on a molecular level endometrial carcinoma is heterogeneous, and that additional oncogenes involved in the disease process have yet to be identified.

TUMOR SUPPRESSOR GENES

Loss of tumor suppressor gene function predisposes a cell towards progression to cancer. Typically, loss of function of a recessive tumor suppressor gene requires a mutation in one allele and a deletion of the remaining allele. The *P53* gene controls cell proliferation, and is the most commonly mutated gene known in human cancers. In lung cancer the *P53* mutation rate is greater than 50%, and it is thought to be an event occurring early in carcinogenesis. In colon cancer and breast cancer *P53* mutation is probably a late event. A minority of cancers fail to display *P53* mutations (Greenblatt et al., 1994). In endometrial carcinoma, *P53* overexpression and mutation have also been extensively studied.

The rate of *P53* mutation in endometrial carcinoma is approximately 22% (Greenblatt et al., 1994). Mutations are most common in late stage disease (Honda et al., 1994; Kohler et al., 1992). In endometrial hyperplasia, *P53* mutations or overexpression have not been identified (Jiko et al., 1993; Kohler et al., 1993). Multiple studies suggest that *P53* mutation and overexpression in endometrial carcinoma are associated with advanced stage, high grade, serous phenotype, and lymph node metastases (Enomoto et al., 1993; Inoue et al., 1994; Kohler et al., 1992; Pisani et al., 1995; Tsuda and Hirohashi, 1992). As is the case with the *K-RAS* protooncogene, *P53* mutations may occur more commonly in endometrial carcinoma in Japan than in the US. One study reports a rate of 23% in 40 Japanese cases, and 13% in 38 US cases. The type of mutation occurring most commonly in Japan (G:C to A:T) was not identified in the comparison group from Colorado (Enomoto et al., 1994b). This information suggests that *P53* mutation occurs more commonly in Japan, and is a late event in the progression to endometrial carcinoma.

Expression of the *DCC* tumor suppressor gene on chromosome 18q is found to be absent or decreased in at least 50% of colorectal, pancreatic, breast and prostatic carcinomas, and gliomas. High rates of LOH on 18q are also observed in these malignancies. The *DCC* gene encodes a transmembrane protein whose structure is similar to neural cell adhesion molecules, and it may be important in regulating cell proliferation, differentiation, and aggregation (Cho and Fearon, 1995; Fearon and Pierceall, 1995). In endometrial carcinoma, LOH on 18q has also been reported; however, the screening of 29 known DCC exons in 60 cases failed to identify mutations (Fujino et al., 1994). On the other hand, a series of 38 endometrial carcinoma cases from Japan revealed abnormal DCC mRNA expression in 50% of cases (Gima et al., 1994). A second series of 8 endometrial carcinoma cases from Japan revealed 37% with decreased DCC mRNA expression, but only 14% of informative cases displayed LOH (Enomoto et al., 1995). These studies suggest that abnormal DCC expression may be a result of transcriptional variation due to mutations outside the gene.

The E-cadherin gene is a tumor suppressor which resides on 16q22 and encodes a calcium-dependent protein which contributes to the maintenance of epithelial integrity (Takeichi, 1991). This protein appears to behave as a cell adhesion molecule (Birchemeier et al., 1995). It is hypothesized that loss of E-cadherin function results in a breakdown of intercellular junctions leading to invasive behavior. E-cadherin mutations and down-regulation have been identified in gastric, ovarian, breast, colon, head and neck, and bladder malignancies (Birchmeier et al., 1995; Mareel et al., 1995). In endometrial carcinoma, one study found only 3 mutations in 72 cases, suggesting it plays a role in a minority of endometrial malignancies (Risinger et al., 1994).

The search for additional tumor suppressor genes is largely focused on screening chromosomal regions with high rates of allelic loss. In endometrial carcinoma, allelic deletions have been identified on all chromosomes except chromosome X (Fujino et al., 1994; Imamura et al.,1992; Jones et al., 1994; Okamoto et al., 1991; Peiffer et al., 1995). One region of particular interest is chromosome 14q, where loss of heterozygosity appears to correlate with poor prognosis (Fujino et al., 1994). Other areas warranting further investigation include 3p where the h*MLH1* DNA mismatch repair gene resides, and 8p where the *VHL* tumor suppressor gene resides (Fujino et al., 1994; Jones et al., 1994). The 18q21 locus has been identified to be a region of minimal deletion in endometrial carcinoma (Fujino et al., 1994). This locus harbors two known tumor suppressor genes, *DCC* and *DPC-4* (Hahn et al., 1996). However, the screening of both of these genes in endometrial carcinoma has yielded no evidence of mutations, suggesting that this region may contain at least one more tumor suppressor gene (Bandera et al., unpublished observations; Fujino et al., 1994).

Microcell-mediated chromosomal transfer also provides clues to the location of tumor suppressor genes. When transfer of an entire chromosome or part of a chromosome into a cancer cell line suppresses tumorgenicity then it is concluded that a wild-type allele of a tumor suppressor is present in that DNA fragment. Transfer of chromosome 1, 6, 9, 11, or 18 into endometrial carcinoma cell lines results in complete or partial suppression of tumorgenicity (Sasaki et al.,1994; Yamada et al., 1995). As noted earlier in the chapter, chromosome 1 is frequently duplicated in endometrial carcinoma karyotype evaluations, it displays a high rate of LOH, and it has the ability to suppress the growth of endometrial carcinoma cells in chromosome transfer studies. These observations suggest the role of chromosome 1 in endometrial tumorigenesis deserves further investigation.

MICROSATELLITE INSTABILITY

A DNA microsatellite is a simple sequence repeat, consisting of one to six nucleotides repeated 10 to 50 times. Microsatellites are located throughout the genome; however, their function is unknown. Microsatellite instability (MI) is characterized by changes in the lengths of microsatellites. MI is detected by a shift in the electorphoretic mobility of the microsatellite DNA sequence in tumor tissue compared to the normal tissue DNA sequence.

This type of genetic instability was first identified in colorectal carcinoma in 1993 (Aaltusen et al., 1993; Ionov et al., 1993; Thibodeau et al., 1993). In cases of HNPCC, 75-89% of tumors demonstrate MI. In endometrial carcinoma associated with the HNPCC syndrome, 75% of the tumors are reported to display MI (Risinger et al., 1993). Furthermore, MI has been identified in 17-23% of sporadic endometrial carcinoma cases (Risinger et al., 1993; Peltomaki et al., 1993; Burks et al., 1994; Duggan et al., 1994). Type I endometrial carcinomas with MI appear to have a good prognosis (Risinger et al., 1993); it has been suggested that, in general, neoplasms associated with microsatellite instability tend to display indolent behavior (Honchel et al., 1995).

Genetic mutations in four genes involved in mismatch repair have been identified in HNPCC: hMSH2 on 2p, hMLH1 on 3p, hPMS1 on 2q and hPMS2 on 7p. These genes are thought to be responsible for the high rate of MI in HNPCC. The hMSH2 gene has also been found to be mutated in endometrial carcinoma cell lines (Risinger et al., 1995; Umar et al., 1994). Evaluation of the DNA mismatch repair genes in nine cases of sporadic endometrial carcinoma with MI revealed two cases with somatic mutations in the hMSH2 gene (Katabuchi et al., 1995). These data suggest that additional genes may be responsible for MI in the majority of endometrial carcinomas.

HORMONES and GROWTH FACTORS

Production of the ovarian steroid hormones estrogen and progesterone is stimulated by the anterior pituitary, and cause the endometrium to undergo cyclic growth and regression. The growth of the endometrium involves glandular proliferation, neovascularization and glycogen storage. Endometrial regression requires necrosis, shedding of the endometrial lining, platelet aggregation, and thrombosis. When pregnancy occurs, the endometrium facilitates the creation of the fetoplacental unit. The importance of steroid hormones in these processes is well established. It is now becoming clear that the actions of these hormones are coordinated by a variety of polypeptide growth factors and cytokines (Tabibzadeh, 1991; McLachlan et al., 1992). The persistence or overexpression of these growth factors and their receptors in endometrial carcinoma cells leads to speculation about their role in the malignant transformation of the endometrium (Murphy, 1994). The growth factors of interest in endometrial carcinoma will be reviewed in this section.

Epidermal growth factor (EGF) and transforming growth factor-α (TGF-α) are single-chain polypeptides which exert their effects through the EGF receptor. Both of these growth factors and their receptor are expressed in normal endometrial tissue (Murphy et al., 1991), and both growth factors are found to stimulate growth of multiple endometrial cancer cell lines in vitro (Anzai et al., 1992; Gretz et al., 1994; Korc et al., 1980). The EGF receptor does not appear to be overexpressed in endometrial carcinoma (Berchuck et al., 1989). Several studies have examined the characteristics of EGF and TGF-α expression in endometrial carcinoma cell lines, and interesting observations have been made. First, EGF mRNA expression by northern blotting was low, whereas TGF-α mRNA expression was moderate in these cell lines (Anzai et al., 1992). In a non-aggressive estrogen-responsive cell line (Ishikawa), TGF-α mRNA expression was two times higher than in a more aggressive estrogen-unresponsive cell line (HEC-50) (Gong et al., 1992). Additional data revealed that TGF-α may promote the growth of estrogen-responsive endometrial carcinoma. It was shown that TGF-α was a more effective growth stimulator in the estrogen-responsive Ishikawa cell line, and the growth-stimulating effect was diminished by antibodies to the EGF receptor (Murphy et al., 1992). On the other hand, TGF-α has also been shown to be expressed at high levels in an endometrial carcinoma cell line which is highly tumorigenic in the absence of estrogen (HEC-1-A) (Gong et al., 1994). Of note, TGF-α mRNA expression was found in 66% of endometrial carcinoma tissue specimens studied, and did not correlate with histologic grade, or stage of disease (Xynos et al., 1992). Cumulatively, these studies suggest that the relationship between EGF, TGF-α, tumor aggressiveness, and steroid hormone responsiveness is not straightforward.

Transforming growth factor-ß (TGF-ß) is a growth inhibitor which has been implicated in the carcinogenic process. Mutations in a TGF-ß receptor gene are associated with colonic and gastric tumors with MI; however, they are reported in less than one fifth of endometrial carcinomas exhibiting MI (Myeroff et al., 1995). Both normal human endometrium and endometrial carcinoma cell lines have been shown to express TGF-ß mRNA (Kauma et al., 1990; Boyd and Kaufman, 1990). In some endometrial carcinoma cell lines TGF-ß appears to inhibit cell growth (Boyd and Kauffman, 1990). On the other hand, the 3 known isoforms of TGF-ß have been found to be overexpressed by immunohistochemical staining in the glandular epithelium of complex hyperplasia and endometrial carcinoma specimens compared with normal endometrium and simple hyperplasia (Gold et al., 1994). This overexpression might correlate with loss of the TGF-ß receptor, and a lack of negative feedback necessary to downregulate TGF-ß production. Studies relating TGF-ß overexpression and microsatellite instability in endometrial carcinoma have not been reported, but are an important area for future research.

The macrophage colony stimulating factor, CSF-1 and its receptor the c-fms protooncogene have also been studied in endometrial carcinoma. Studies employing immunohistochemical staining and northern blot analysis of mRNA expression confirm CSF-1 and c-fms overexpression in endometrial carcinoma when compared with normal endometrial tissue (Baiocchi et al., 1991; Kacinski et al., 1988; Leiserowitz et al., 1993; Suzuki et al., 1995). One study revealed that c-fms expression is low in normal secretory endometrium, elevated in proliferative and hyperplastic endometrium, and highest in endometrial carcinoma. Furthermore, the cancers with the highest levels of c-fms expression correlated with poor prognostic factors such as aneuploidy, high histologic grade, and possibly metastases (Leiserowitz et al., 1993). Serum CSF-1 levels are increased in all gynecologic malignancies; in endometrial carcinoma increased serum CSF-1 is notable in patients with advanced disease, and may be a useful marker for disease activity (Kacinski et al., 1990; Suzuki et al., 1995). The relationship between CSF-1 and steroid hormones is controversial. One study showed no change in CSF-1 or c-fms expression when endometrial carcinoma cell lines were exposed to estrogen and progesterone (Croxtall et al., 1992). This contrasts with data suggesting CSF-1 and c-fms are regulated by sex hormones in the uterus (Azuma et al., 1990). The role of the CSF-1 growth factor and the c-fms receptor in the horomonal stimulation of endometrial cancer is therefore still unclear.

Other growth factors which have been implicated in endometrial tumorigenesis include basic fibroblast growth factor (bFGF) and insulin-like growth factor I (IGF-I). bFGF is a heparin-binding growth factor which is overexpressed in complex hyperplasia and endometrial carcinoma (Rusnati et al., 1993; Gold et al., 1994). In an elegant study, an endometrial carcinoma cell line which produces low levels of bFGF (HEC-1-B) was transfected with a vector containing bFGF cDNA. The resulting cell population displayed accelerated growth when injected into mice, and showed an angiogenic response in the rabbit cornea assay (Coltrini et al., 1995). These data suggest that bFGF activity may be implicated in aggressive endometrial carcinoma.

The IGF-I growth factor receptor is overexpressed in endometrial neoplasms (Talavera et al., 1990). Furthermore, the endometrial expression of the IGF-I growth factor and its receptor is responsive to estrogen stimulation (Murphy and Ghary, 1990; Kleinman et al., 1995). In vitro study of the Ishikawa endometrial carcinoma cell line reveals enhanced IGF-I expression when the cell culture is exposed to estradiol and tamoxifen (Hana and Murphy, 1994). IGF-I is also regulated by insulin, and women with endometrial carcinoma have been found to have alterations in the circulating IGF regulating system when compared with controls (Rutanenn et al., 1993). These data link IGF-I and its receptor to a role as an autocrine modulator of steroid hormone effects. However, further studies are necessary to assess the significance of IGF-I and the IGF-I receptor in endometrial carcinoma.

In summary, multiple growth factors which are probably regulated by steroid hormones appear to be implicated in the paracrine and autocrine regulation of endometrial function. These growth factors are likely to be important in type I estrogen-related endometrial carcinoma. In type II, non-estrogen related endometrial carcinoma, growth factors may also play a role in upregulating the stimulatory effects of low-levels of steroid hormones circulating in the post-menopausal female.

CONCLUSION

This chapter reviewed the molecular alterations which accompany the malignant transformation of the endometrium. These genetic events include structural chromosomal alterations, protooncogene mutations, tumor suppressor gene inactivation, and the deregulation of paracrine growth factors and their receptors. Microsatellite instability may also be implicated in the oncogenic process. Survey of the molecular data collected reveal that none of the genetic events which have been studied occur in more than a third of endometrial carcinoma cases. The heterogeneity of the molecular biology of endometrial carcinoma makes it difficult to propose a rational stepwise model of endometrial tumorigenesis.

Although the clinical classification of endometrial carcinoma may be oversimplified, further study of the molecular basis of endometrial cancer should be evaluated within this framework in order to identify patterns in the disease process. By matching the biology and physiology of the disease we can begin to create models of endometrial carcinogenesis. For example, type I estrogen-related disease may be associated with the overexpression of hormone sensitive growth factors and receptors. Type II estrogen-independent disease is more likely to be associated with factors such as aneuploidy, oncogene activation, and tumor suppressor deactivation associated with a poor prognosis. Type III inherited endometrial carcinoma probably reflects a variety of germline mutations including the HNPCC mutations associated with microsatellite instability.

As the molecular profile of endometrial carcinoma becomes more detailed, fastidious clinical correlation will enable us to better understand the mechanisms underlying the various types of endometrial carcinoma. Understanding these mechanisms will lead to innovative approaches to diagnosis, treatment, and prevention of endometrial carcinoma.

REFERENCES

Aaltonen LA, Peltomaki P, Leach FS, Sistonen P, Pylkkänen L, Mecklin J-P, Järvinen H, Powell SM, Jen J, Hamilton SR, Petersen GM, Kinzler KW, Vogelstein B, de la Chapelle A (1993): Clues to the pathogenesis of familial colorectal cancer. Science 260:812-816.

Ambros RA, Kurman RJ (1992): Identification of patients with stage I uterine endometrioid adenocarcinoma at high risk of recurrence by DNA ploidy, myometrial invasion and vascular invasion. Gynecol Oncol 45:235-239.

Anzai Y, Gong Y, Holinka CF, Murphy LJ, Murphy LC, Kuramoto H, Gurpide E (1992): Effects of transforming growth factors and regulation of their mRNA levels in two human endometrial adenocarcinoma cell lines. J Steroid Biochem Mol Biol 42: 449-455.

Azuma C, Saji F, Kimura T, Tokugawa Y, Takenura M, Samejimi Y, Tanizawa O (1990): Steroid hormones induce macrophage colony stimulating factor (MCSF) and MCSF receptor mRNAs in human endometrium. J Mol Endocrinol 5:103-108.

Baiocchi G, Kavanagh JJ, Talpaz M, Wharton JT, Culleman JU, Kurzrock R (1991): Expression of the macrophage colony stimulating factor and its receptor in gynecologic malignancies. Cancer 67:990-996.

Barbacid M (1987): ras genes. Annu Rev Biochem 56:1463-1467.

Bardi G, Pandis N, Schouboe K, Hollond B, Heim S (1995): Near diploid karyotype with recurrent chromosome abnormalities characterize early-stage endometrial cancer. Cancer Genet Cytogenet 80:110-114.

Berchuck A, Rodriguez G, Kinney RB, Soper JT, Dodge RK, Clarke-Pearson DL, Bast RC Jr (1991): Overexpression of HER-2/neu in endometrial cancer is associated with advanced stage disease. Am J Obstet Gynecol 164:15-21.

Berchuck A, Soisson AP, Olt GJ, Soper JT, Clarke-Pearson DL, Bast RC jr, McCarty KS jr, (1989): Epidermal growth factor receptor expression in normal and malignant endometrium. Am J Obstet Gynecol 161:1247-1252.

Birchmeier W., Hülsken J, Behrens J (1995). E-cadherin as an invasion suppressor. Ciba Foundation Symposia 189:124-136.

Boltenberg A, Fargyik S, Kullander S (1990): Familial cancer aggregation in cases of adenocarcinoma corporis uteri. Acta Obstet Gynecol Scand 69:249-258.

Borst MP, Baker V, Dixon D, Hatch KD, Shingleton H, Miller D (1990): Oncogene alterations in endometrial carcinoma. Gynecol Oncol 38:364-366.

Bos JL (1989): ras oncogenes in human cancer: a review. Cancer Res 49:4682-4689.

Boyd J, Kaufman DG (1990): Expression of transformating growth factor ß, by human endometrial carcinoma cell lines: inverse correlation with effects on growth rate and morphology. Cancer Res 50:3394-3399.

Boyd J, Risinger JJ (1991): Analysis of oncogene alterations in human endometrial carcinoma: prevalence of ras mutations. Mol Carcinog 4: 189-195.

Boyd J (1994): Molecular genetics of human endometrial carcinoma. In Khan SA, Stancel GM (eds): "Protooncogenes and Growth Factors in Steroid Hormone Induced Growth and Differentiation." Boca Raton: CRC Press Inc., pp 193-205.

Britton LC, Wilson TO, Gaffey TA, Cha SS, Wieand HS, Podratz KC (1990): DNA ploidy in endometrial carcinoma: major objective prognostic factor. Mayo Clin Proc 65:643-650.

Burks RT, Kessis TD, Cho KR, Hedrick L (1994): Microsatellite instability in endometrial carcinoma. Oncogene 9:1163-1166.

Britton LC, Wilson TO, Gaffey TA, Lieher MM, Wieand HS, Podratz KC (1989): Flow cytometric DNA analysis of stage I endometrial cancer. Gynecol Oncol 34:317-322.

Caduff RF, Johnston CM, Frank TS (1995): Mutation of the Ki-ras oncogene in carcinoma of the endometrium. Am J Pathol 146:182-188.

"Cancer facts and figures - 1996" New York: American Cancer Society, Inc, 1996.

Cho KR, Fearon ER (1995): DCC: linking tumour suppressor genes and altered cell surface interactions in cancer? Eu J Cancer 31:1055-1060.

Coleman RL, Schink JC, Miller DS, Bauer KD, August CZ, Rademaker AW, Lurain JR (1993): DNA flow cytometric analysis of clinical stage I endometrial carcinomas with lymph node metastases. Gyncol Oncol 50:20-24.

Coltrini D, Gaalandris A, Nelli EE, Parotini S, Molinari-Tossatti MP, Quarto N, Ziche M, Giavezzi R, Presta M (1995): Growth advantage and vascularization induced by basic fibroblast growth factor overexpression in endometrial HEC-1-B cells: an export dependent mechanism of action. Cancer Res 55:4729-4738.

Coon JS, Landay Al, Weinstein RS (1987): Biology of disease: Advances in flow cytometry for diagnostic pathology. Lab Invest 57: 453-479.

Corocleanu M (1993): Hypothesis for endometrial carcinoma carcinogenesis. Clin Exp Obstet Gynecol 20:254-258.

Couturier J, Vielh P, Salmon RJ, Lombard M, Dutrillaux B (1988): Chromosome imbalance in endometrial adenocarcinoma. Cancer Genet Cytogenet 33:67-76.

Croxtall JD, Pollard JW, Casey F, Forder A, White JO (1991): Colony stimulating factor-1 stimulates Ishikawa cell proliferation and lipocortin II synthesis. J Steroid Biochem Mol Biol 42:121-129.

Deger RB, Nuomoff JS, Faruqui SA (1994): A single clonal abnormality of chromosome 1 found in an adenocarcinoma of the uterus. Cancer Genet Cytogenet 78:105-107.

Deligdisch L, Holinka CF (1987): Endometrial carcinoma: two diseases. Cancer Detection Prev 10:237-246.

Duggan BD, Felix JC, Muderspach LI, Tourgeman D, Zheng J, Shibata D (1994): Microsatellite instability in sporadic endometrial carcinoma. J Natl Cancer Inst 86:1216-1221.

Dutrillaux B, Couturier J (1986): Chromossome imbalances in endometrial adenocarcinomas: a possible adaption to abnormal metabolic pathways. Ann Genet 29:76-81.

Enomoto T, Fujita M, Chang C, Nakashema R, Ozaki M, Inoue M, Nomura T (1995): Loss of expression and loss of heterozygosity in the DCC gene in neoplasms of the human female reproductive tract. Brit J Cancer 71:462-467.

Enomoto T, Fujita M, Inoue M, Rice JM, Nakajima R, Tanizawa O, Nomura T (1993): Alterations of the p53 tumor suppressor gene and its association with activation of the c-K-ras-2 protooncogene in premalignant and malignant lesions of the human endometrium. Cancer Res 53: 1883-1888.

Enomoto T, Fujita M, Inoue M, Tanizawa O, Nomura T, Shroyer KR (1994a): Analysis of clonality by amplification of short tandem repeats. Diagn Mol Pathol 3:292-297.

Enomoto T, Fujita M, Masake I, Nomura T, Shroyer K (1994b): Alteration of the p53 tumor suppressor gene and activation of c-K-ras-2 protooncogene in endometrial adenocarcinoma from Colorado. Am J Clin Pathol 103:224-230.

Enomoto T, Inoue M, Perantoni AO, Buzard GS, Tanizawa O, Rice JM (1991): K-ras activation in premalignant and malignant epithelial lesions of the human uterus. Cancer Res 51:5308-5314.

Fearon ER, Jones PA (1992): Progressing toward a molecular description of colorectal cancer development. FASEB J 6:2783-2790.

Fearon ER, Pierceall WE (1995): Deleted in colorectal cancer gene: a candidate tumour suppressor gene encoding a cell surface protein with similarity to neural cell adhesion molecules. Cancer Surveys 24:3-17.

Feichter GE, Höffken H, Heep J, Haag D, Heberling D, Brandt H, Rummel H, Goerttler K (1982): DNA-flow-cytometric measurements of the normal, atrophic, hyperplastic and neoplastic endometrium. Virchows Arch 398:53-65.

Friberg L-G, Norén H, Delle U (1994): Prognostic value of DNA ploidy and s-phase fraction in endometrial cancer stage I and II: a prospective 5-year survival study. Gynecol Oncol 53:357-372.

Friedlander ML, Hedley DW, Taylor IW (1984): Clinical and biological significance of aneuploidy in human tumors. J Clin Pathol 37:789-792.

Fujino T, Risinger JI, Collins NK, Liu F-S, Nishii H, Takahashi H, Westphal E-M, Barret JC, Sasaki H, Kohler MF, Berchuck A, Boyd J (1994): Allelotype of endometrial carcinoma. Cancer Res 54:4294-4298.

Fujita H, Wake N, Kutsuzawa T, Ichinoe K, Hreshchyshyn MM, Sandberg AA (1985): Marker chromosomes of the long arm of chromosome 1 in endometrial carcinoma. Cancer Genet Cytoget 18:283-293.

Gibas Z, Rubin SC (1987): Well-differentiated adnocarcinomas of endometrium with simple karyotypic changes: a case report. Cancer Genet Cytogenet 25:21-26.

Gima T, Kato H, Honda T, Imamura T, Sasazuk T, Wake N (1994): DCC gene alteration in human endometrial carcinoma. Int J Cancer 57:480-485.

Gold LI, Sazena B, Mittal KR, Goswami S, Nactigal L, Korc M, Demopoulos RI (1994): Increased expression of transforming growth factor ß isoforms and basic fibroblast growth factor in complex hyperplasia and adenocarcinoma of the endometrium: evidence for paracrine and autocrine function. Cancer Res 54:2347-2358.

Gong Y, Ballejo G, Bushy LC, Murphy LJ (1992): Differential effects of estrogen and antiestrogen on transforming growth factor gene expression in human endometrial adenocarcinoma cells. J Steroid Biochem Mol Biol 41:309-314.

Gong Y, Murphy LC, Murphy LJ (1994): Hormonal regulation of proliferation and transforming growth factors gene expression in a human endometrial adenocarcinoma xenograft. J Steroid Biochem Mol Biol 50:13-19.

Goodman AK, Bell DA, Rice LW (1993): DNA ploidy status: its impact on early-stage endometrial adenocarcinoma. Gynecol Oncol 51: 355-361.

Greenblatt MS, Bennett WP, Hollstein M, Harris CC (1994): Mutations in the p53 tumor suppressor gene: clues to cancer etiology and molecular pathogenesis. Cancer Res 54:4855-4878.

Gretz HF, Talavera F, Connor P, Pearl M, Lelle RJ, James AR, Menon KMJ (1994): Protein kinase c-dependent and independent pathways mediate epidermal growth factor (EGF) effects in human endometrial adenocarcinoma cell line KLE. Gynecol Oncol 53:228-233.

Hahn SA, Schutte M, Hoque ATMS, Moskaluk CA, daCosta LT, Rozenblum E, Weinstein CL, Fischer A., Yeo CJ, Hrugan RH, Kern SE (1996): DPC4, a candidate tumor suppressor gene at human chromosome 18q21.2. Science 271:350-353.

Hakala T, Mecklin JP, Forss M, Järvinen H, Lehtovirta P (1991): Endometrial carcinoma in cancer family syndrome. Cancer 68:1656-1659.

Hana V, Murphy LJ (1994): Expression of insulin-like growth factors and their binding proteins in the estrogen responsive Ishikawa human endometrial cancer cell line. Endocrinology 135:2511-2516.

Hanania EG, Kavanagh J, Hortobagyi G, Giles RE, Champlin R, Deisseroth AB (1995): Recent advances in the application of gene therapy to human disease. Am J Med 99:537-552.

Hetzel D, Wilson TO, Keeney GL, Roche PC, Cha SS, Podratz KC (1992): Her-2/neu expression: a major prognostic factor in endometrial cancer. Gynecol Oncol 47:179-185.

Honchel R, Halling KC, Thibodeau SN (1995): Genomic instability in neoplasia. Semin Cell Biol 6: 45-52.

Honda T, Kato H, Imamura T, Gima T, Nishida J, Sasaki M, Hoshi K, Sato a, Wake N (1993): Involvement of p53 gene mutations in human endometrial carcinomas. Int J Cancer 53:963-967.

Hung M-C, Matin A, Zhang Y, Xing X, Sorgi F, Huang L, Yu D (1995): HER-2/neu-targeting gene therapy - a review. Gene 159:65-71.

Ignar-Trowbridge D, Risinger JI, Dent GA, Kohler MF, Berchuck A, McLachlan JA, Boyd J (1992): Mutations of the Ki-ras oncogene in endometrial carcinoma. Am J Obstet Gynecol 167:227-232.

Ikeda M, Watanabe Y, Nanjoh T, Noda K (1993): Evaluation of DNA ploidy in endometrial cancer. Gynecol Oncol 50:25-29.

Imamura T, Arima T, Kato H, Miyamoto S, Sasazuk T, Wake N (1992): Chromosomal deletions and K-ras gene mutations in human endometrial carcinomas. Int J Cancer 51:47-52.

Inoue M, Okayama A, Fujita T, Sakata M, Tanizawa O, Ueshima H (1994): Clinicopathological characteristics of p53 overexpression in endometrial cancers. Int J Cancer 58:14-19.

Ionov Y, Peinado MA, Malkhosyan S, Shibata D, Perucho M (1993): Ubiquitous somatic mutations in simple repeated sequences reveal a new mechanism for colonic carcinogenesis. Nature 363:558-561.

Jenkyn DJ, McCartney AJ (1986): Primary cytogenetic abnormality detected in an endometrial adenocarcinoma. Cancer Genet Cytogenet 20:149-157.

Jiko K, Sasano H, Ito K, Ozawa N, Sato S, Yajima A (1993): Immunohistochemical and in situ hybridization analysis of p53 in human endometrial carcinoma of the uterus. Anticancer Res 13:305-310.

Jones MH, Koi S, Fujimoto I, Hasumi K, Kato K, Nakamura Y (1994): Allelotype of uterine cancer by analysis of RFLP and microsatellite polymorphisms: frequent loss of heterozygosity in chromosome arms 3p, 9q, 10q, 17p. Genes Chromosom Cancer 9:119-123.

Kacinski BM, Carter D, Mittal K, Kohorn EI, Bloodgood RS, Donahue J, Donofrio L, Edwards R, Schwartz PE, Chambers JT, Chambers SK (1988): High level expression of fms proto-oncogene mRNA is observed in clinically aggressive human endometrial adenocarcinomas. Int J Radiat Oncol Biol Phys 15:823-829.

Kacinski BM, Chambers SK, Stanley ER, Carter D, Tseng P, Scata KA, Chang DH-Y, Pirro MH, Nguyen JT, Ariza A, Rohrschneider LR, Rothwell VM (1990): Cytokine CSF-1 (M-CSF) expressed by endometrial carcinomas in vivo and in vitro, may also be a circulating tumor marker of neoplastic disease activity in endometrial carcinoma patients. Int J Radiat Oncol Biol Phys 19:619-626.

Katabuchi H, van Rees B, Lambers AR, Ronnett BM, Blazes MS, Leach FS, Cho KR, Hedrick L (1995): Mutations in DNA mismatch repair genes are not responsible for microsatellite instability in most sporadic endometrial carcinomas. Cancer Res 55:5556-5560.

Kauma S, Matt D, Strom S, Eiserman D, Tuner T, (1990): Interleukin-1ß (IL-1ß), HLA-DR-α , and transforming growth factor ß (TGF-ß) expression in endometrium, placenta and placental membranes. Am J Obstet Gynecol 163:1430--1437.

Ketter R, von Ballestrem C-L, Lampel S, Seitz G, Zang KD, Romanakis K, Wullich B (1995). Rearrangement of chromosome 1 is a frequent finding in endometrial carcinoma. Cancer Genet Cytogenet 81:109-114.

Kleinman D, Karas M, Roberts CT jr, LeRoith D, Phillip M, Segev Y, Levy J, Sharoni Y (1995): Modulation of insulin-like growth factor I (IGF-1) receptors and membrane associated IGF binding proteins in endometrial cancer by estradiol. Endocrinology 136: 2531-2537.

Kohler MF, Berchuck A, Davidoff AM, Humphrey PA, Dodge RK, Inglehart JD, Soper JT, Clarke-Pearson DL, Bast RC, Marks JR (1992): Overexpression and mutation of p53 in endometrial carcinoma. Cancer Res 52:1622-1627.

Kohler MF, Nishii H, Humphrey PA, Saski H, Marks J, Bast RC, Clarke-Pearson DL, Boyd J, Berchuck A (1993): Mutation of the p53 tumor-suppressor gene is not a feature of endometrial hyperplasias. Am J Obstet Gynecol 169:690-694.

Korc M, Padilla J, Gorso D (1980): Epidermal growth factor inhibits the proliferation of a human endometrial cancer cell line. J Clin Endocrinol Metab 62:874-880.

Knudson AG (1971): Mutation and cancer: statistical study of retinoblastoma. Proc Natl Acad Sci USA 68:820-823.

Kurman RJ, Kaminski PF, Norris HJ (1984): Behavior of endometrial hyperplasia. Cancer 56:403-412.

Leiserowitz GS, Harris SA, Subramaniam M, Keeney GL, Podratz KC, Spelsberg TC (1993). Proto-oncogene c-fms is overexpressed in endometrial cancer. Gynecol Oncol 49:190-196.

Lester DR, Cauchi MN (1990): Point mutations at codon 12 of C-K-ras in human endometrial carcinomas. Cancer Lett 51:7-10.

Lindahl B, Alm P, Ferno M, Killander D, Langstrom e, Norgen a, Trope C (1989): Prognostic value of steroid receptor concentration and flow cytometrical DNA measurements in stage I-II endometrial carcinoma. Acta Oncol 28:595-599.

Lindahl B, Ranstam J, Willén R (1994): Five year survival rate in endometrial carcinoma stages I-II: influence of degree of tumor differentiation, age, myometrial invasion and DNA content. Br J Obstet Gynaecol 101:621-625.

Lukes AS, Kohler MF, Pieper CF, Kerns BJ, Bentley R, Rodriguez GC, Soper JT, Clarke-Pearson DL, Bast RC, Berchuck A (1994): Multivariable analysis of DNA ploidy, p53 and HER--2/neu as prognostic factors in endometrial cancer. Cancer 73:2380-2385.

Lynch HT, Lynch J, Conway T, Watson P, Coleman RL (1994): Familial aggregation of carcinoma of the endometrium. Am J Obstet Gynecol 171:24-27.

Mareel M, Brache M, Van Roy F (1995): Cancer metastases: negative regulation by an invasion-suppressor complex. Cancer Detect Prev 19: 451-464.

Myeroff LL, Parsons R, Kim S-J, Hedrick L, Cho KR, Orth K, Mathis M, Kinzler KW, Lutterbaugh J, Park K, Bang Y-J, Lee HY, Park J-G, Lynch HT, Roberts AB, Vogelstein B, Markowitz SD (1995): Transforming growth factor ß receptor type II gene mutation common in colon and gastric but rare in endometrial cancers with microsatellite instability. Cancer Res 55:5545-5547.

McLachlan JA, Nelson KG, Takahashi T, Bossert NL, Newbold RR, Korach KS (1992): Do growth factors mediate estrogen action in the uterus? In Hochberg RB, Naftolin F (eds): "The New Biology of Steroid Hormones." New York: Raven Press, pp337-344.

Melchiorri C, Chieco P, Lisignoli G, Marahini A, Orlandi C (1993): Ploidy disturbances as an early indicator of intrinsic malignancy in endometrial carcinoma. Cancer 72:165-172.

Milatovich A, Heereman NA, Palmer CG (1990): Cytogenetic studies of endometrial malignancies. Cancer Genet Cytogenet 46:41-54.

Mizuuchi H, Nasim S, Kudo R, Silverberg SG, Greenhouse S, Garrett CT (1992): Clinical implications of K-ras mutations in malignant epithelial tumors of the endometrium. Cancer Res 52:2777-2781.

Moore TD, Phillips PH, Nerenstone SR, Chesom MD (1991): Systemic treatment and recurrent endometrial carcinoma: current status and future directions. J Clin Oncol 9:1071-1088.

Murphy LJ (1991): Estrogen induction of insulin-like growth factors and myc proto-oncogene expression in the uterus. J Steroid Biochem Mol Biol 40:223-230.

Murphy LJ (1994): Growth factors and steroid hormone action in endometrial cancer. J Steroid Biochem Mol Biol 48:419-423.

Murphy LJ, Ghahary A (1990): Uterine isulin-like growth factor-1: Regulation of expression and its role in estrogen-induced uterine proliferation. Endocr Rev 11:443-453.

Murphy LJ, Gong Y, Murphy LC (1992): Regulation of transforming growth factor gene expression in human endometrial adenocarcinoma cells. J Steroid Biochem Mol Biol 41:309-314.

Murphy LJ, Gong Y, Murphy LC, Bhavnani B (1991): Growth factors in normal and malignant uterine tissue. Ann NY Acad Sci 622:383-391.

Mutter GL, Chaponot ML, Fletcher JA (1995): Polymerase chain reaction assay for non-random X chromosome inactivation identifies monoclonal endometrial cancers and precancers. Am J Pathol 146:501-508.

Nyholm HCJ, Nielsen AL, Norup P (1993): Endometrial cancer in postmenopausal women with and without previous estrogen replacement treatment: comparison of clinical and histopathological characteristics. Gynecol Oncol 49:229-235.

Okamoto A, Sameshima Y, Yamada Y, Teshima S, Terashima Y, Terada M, Yokota J (1991): Allelic loss on chromosome 17p and p53 mutations in human endometrial carcinoma of the uterus. Cancer Res 51:5632-5635.

Parazzini F, LaVecchia, Moroni S, Chatenoud L, Ricci E (1994): Family history and the risk of endometrial cancer. Int J Cancer 59:460-462.

Peiffer SL, Herzog TJ, Tribune DJ, Mutch DG, Gersell DJ, Goodfellow PJ (1995): Allelic loss of sequences from the long arm of chromosome 10 and replication errors in endometrial cancer. Cancer Res 55:1922-1926.

Peltomäki P, Lothe RA, Aaltonen LA, Pylkkänen L, Nyström-Lahti M, Seruca R, David L, Holm R, Ryberg D, Haugen A, Brøgger A, Børresen A-L, laChapelle A (1993):

Microsatellite instability is associated with tumors that characterize the hereditary non-polyposis colorectal carcinoma syndrome. Cancer Res 53:5853-5855.

Pfisterer J, Kommoss F, Sauerbrei w, Rendl I, Kiechle M, Kleine W, Pfeiderer A (1995): Prognostic value of DNA ploidy and s-phase fraction in stage I endometrial carcinoma. Gynecol Oncol 58:149-156.

Pisani A, Barbuto DA, Chen D, Ramos L, Lagasse LD, Karlan BY (1995): Her2/neu, p53, and DNA analyses as prognosticators for survival in endometrial carcinoma. Int J Gynecol Obstet 42: 52-53.

Risinger JI, Berchuck A, Kohler M, Boyd J (1994): Mutations of the E-cadherin gene in human gynecologic cancers. Nat Genet 7:98-102.

Risinger JI, Berchuck A, Kohler MF, Watson P, Lynch HT, Boyd J (1993): Genetic instability of microsatellites in endometrial carcinoma. Cancer Res 53:5100-5103.

Risinger JI, Umar A, Barrett JC, Kunkel TA (1995): hPMS2 mutant cell line is defective in strand-specific mismatch repair. J Biol Chem 270:18,183-186.

Rosenberg P, Wingren S, Simonsen E, Stal O, Risberg B, Nordendkjold B (1989): Flow cytometric measurements of DNA index and s-phase in paraffin embedded early stage endometrial cancer: an important prognostic indiator. Gynecol Oncol 35:50-54.

Ross D, Whitehead M (1995): Hormonal manipulation and gynecological cancer: the tamoxifen dilemma. Curr Opin Obstet Gynecol 7:63-68.

Rusnati M, Casarotti G, Pecorelli S, Ragnotti G, Presta M (1993): Estro-progestinic replacement therapy modulates the levels of basic fibroblast growth factor (bFGF) in postmenopausal endometrium. Gynecol Oncol 48:88-93.

Rutanen EM, Stenman S, Blum W, Kurkkainen T, Lehtovirta P, Stenman UT (1993): Relationship between carbohydrate metabolism and serum insulin-like growth factor system in postmenopausal women: comparison of endometrial cancer patients with healthy controls. J Clin Endocrinol Metab 77: 199-204.

Sandles LG, Shulman LP, Elias S, Photopulus GJ, Smiley LM, Poster WM, Simpson JL (1992): Endometrial adenocarcinoma: genetic analysis suggesting heritable site-specific uterine cancer. Gynecol Oncol 47: 167-171.

Sasaki H, Nishii H, Takahashi H, Jada A, Furusato M, Terashima Y, Siegal GP, Parker SL Kohler MF, Berchuk A, Boyd J (1993): Mutation of the Ki-*ras* protooncogene in human endometrial hyperplasia and carcinoma. Cancer Res 53:1906-1910.

Sasaki M, Honda T, Yamada H, Wake N, Barrett JC, Oshimura M (1994): Evidence for multiple pathways to cellular senescence. Cancer Res 23:6090-6093.

Sasano H, Garret Ct (1992): Oncogenes in gynecological tumors. Current Top Pathol 85:357-372.

Sato S, Ito K, Ozawa N, Yajima a, Sasano H (1991): Analysis of point mutations at codon 12 of K-*ras* in human endometrial carcinoma and cervical adenocarcinoma by dot blot hybridization and polymerase chain reaction. Tokuhu J Exp Med 165:131-136.

Sato S, Jiko K, Ito K, Ozawa N, Yajima A, Miyazaki S, Sasano H (1993): Expression of *cmyc* mRNA and protein in human endometrial carcinoma; simultaneous study of in situ hybridization and immunohistochemistry. Tohuku J Exp Med 170:229-234.

Scambia G, Catozzi L, Benedetti-Panici P, Ferrandina g, Battaglia F, Giovannini G, Distefano M, Pellizzola D, Piffanelli A, Mancuso S (1993): Expression of ras p21 oncoprotein in normal and neoplastic human endometrium. Gynecol Oncol 50:339-346.

Schildkraut JM, Risch N, Thompson WD (1989): Evaluating genetic association among ovarian, breast and endometrial cancer: evidence for a breast/ovarian cancer relationship. Am J Hum Genet 45: 521-529.

Shah NK, Currie JL, Rosensheim N, Campbell J, Long P, Abbas F, Griffin CA (1994): Cytogenetic and FISH analysis of endometrial carcinoma. Cancer Genet Cytogenet 73:142-146.

Simon D, Heyner S, Satyaswaroop PG, Farber M, Noumoff JS (1990): Is chromosome 10 a primary chromosomal abnormality in endometrial adenocarcinomas? Cancer Genet Cytogenet 47:155-162.

Slattery ML, Kerher RA (1994): Family history of cancer and colon cancer risk: the Utah population data base. J Natl Cancer Inst 86:16189-1625.

Smythe WR, Kaiser LR, Hwang HC, Amen KM, Pilewski JM Eck SJ, Wilson JM, Albelda SM (1994): Successful adenovirus-mediated gene transfer in an in vivo model of human malignant mesothelioma. Ann Thorac Surg 57:1395-1401.

Stokoe D, Macdonald SG, Cadwallader K, Symons M, Hancock JF (1994): Activation of Raf as a result of recruitment to the plasma membrane. Science 564:1463-1467.

Susini T, Rapi S, Savino L, Boddi V, Berti P, Massi G (1994): Prognostic value of flow cytometric deoxyribonucleic acid index in endometrial carcinoma: comparison with other clinical-pathological parameters. Am J Obstet Gynecol 170: 527-534.

Suomi R, Hakala-ala-pietila T, Leminen A, Mecklin J-P, Lehtovirta P (1995): Heredity aspects of endometrial adenocarcinoma. Int J Cancer 62:132-137.

Suzuki M, Ohwada M, Sato I, Nagatomo M (1995): Serum level of macrophage colony-stimulating factor as a marker for gynecologic malignancies. Oncology 52:128-133.

Tabibzadeh S (1991): Human endometrium: an active site of cytokine production and action. Endocr Rev 12:272-290.

Takeichi M (1991): Cadherin cell adhesion receptors as morphogenetic regulators. Science 251:1451-1455.

Talavera F, Reynolds RK, Roberts JA, Menon KM (1990): Insulin-like growth factor I receptor in normal and neoplastic human endometrium. Cancer Res 50: 3019-3024.

Thibodeau SN, Bren G, Schaid D (1993): Microsatellite instability in cancer of the proximal colon. Science 260:816-819.

Tornos C, Silva EG, El-Naggen A, Burke TW (1992): Aggressive stage I grade 1 endometrial cancer. Cancer 70-: 790-798.

Tsuda H, Hirohashi S (1992): Frequent occurence of p53 gene mutations in uterine cancers at advanced clinical stage and with aggressive histological phenotypes. Japn J Cancer Res 53:1184-1191.

Umar A, Boyer JC , Thomas DC, Nguyen DC, Risinger JI, Boyd J, Ionov Y, Perucho M, Kunkel TA (1994): Defective mismatch repair in extracts of colorectal and endometrial cancer cell lines exhibiting microsatellite instability. J Biol Chem 269:14,367-14,370

Van der Putten HWHM, Baak JPA, Kenders TJA, Kurver HJ, Stolte HG, Stolte LAM (1989): Prognostic value of quantitative pathologic features and DNA content in individuals with stage I endometrial adenocarcinoma. Cancer 63:1378-1387.

Vasen HFA, Watson P, Mecklin JP, Jass JR, Green JS, Nomizu T, Müller H, Lynch HT (1994): Epidemiology of endometrial cancer in hereditary nonpolyposis colorectal cancer. Anticancer Res 14:1675-1678.

Vogelstein B, Fearon ER, Hamilton SR, Kern SE, Preisinger AC, Leppert M, Nakamura Y, White R, Smits AMM, Bos JL (1988): Genetic alterations during colorectal tumor development. N Engl J Med 319:525-532.

Vogelstein B, Kinzler KW (1993). The multistep nature of cancer. Trend Genet 9:138-141.

Watson P, Lynch HT (1993): Extracolonic cancer in hereditary nonpolyposis colorectal cancer. Cancer 71:677-685.

Watson P, Vasen HFA, Mecklin JP, Tarvinen H, Lynch HT (1994): Risk of endometrial cancer in hereditary nonpolyposis colorectal cancer. Am J Med 96:516-520.

Williams NN, Daly JM (1990): Flow cytometry and prognostic implications in patients with solid tumors. Surg Gynecol Obstet 171:257-266.

Xynos FP, Klos DJ, Hamilton PD, Schuette V, Fernandez-Pol A (1992): Expression of transforming growth factor alpha mRNA in benign and malignant tissues derived from gynecologic patients with various proliferative conditions. Anticancer Res 12: 1115-1120.

Yaginuma Y, Ishikawa M (1993): Rasp 21 expression in human endometrial carcinoma. Int J Gynecol Obstet 42: 52-53.

Yamada H, Sasaki M, Honda T, Wake N, Boyd J, Oshimura M, Barrett JC (1995): Suppression of endometrial carcinoma cell tumorigenicity in human chromosome 18. Genes Chromosom Cancer 13:18-24.

Yamada H, Wake N, Fujimoto S-I, Barrett JC, Oshimura M (1990): Multiple chromosomes carrying tumor suppressor activity for a uterine endometrial carcinoma cell line identified by microcell-mediated chromosome transfer. Oncogene 5:1141-1147.

Yoshida MA, Ohyashiki K, Piver SM, Sandberg AA (1986): Recurrent endometrial adenocarcinoma with rearrangement of chromosomes 1 and 11. Cancer Genet Cytogenet 20:159-162.

Zaino RJ (1995): Pathologic indicators of prognosis in endometrial adenocarcinoma. Pathol Annu 30: 1-28.

Zhang L, Rees MCP, Ticknell R (1995): Isolation and longterm culture of normal human endometrial epithelium and stroma. J Cell Sci 108:323-331.

Etiology of Breast and
Gynecological Cancers, pages 205–215
© 1997 Wiley-Liss, Inc.

RODENT MODEL OF REPRODUCTIVE TRACT LEIOMYOMATA: CHARACTERIZATION AND USE IN PRECLINICAL THERAPEUTIC STUDIES

Sue R. Howe, Jeffrey L. Everitt, Marco M. Gottardis, and Cheryl Walker

Department of Carcinogenesis, University of Texas MD Anderson Cancer Center, Smithville, TX 78957 (CW); Department of Biochemistry, University of Texas Southwestern Medical Center, Dallas, TX 75235 (SRH); Department of Experimental Pathology and Toxicology, Chemical Industry Institute of Toxicology, Research Triangle Park, NC 27709 (JLE); Department of Pharmacology, Ligand Pharmaceuticals, La Jolla, CA 92037 (MMG)

INTRODUCTION

Morbidity from uterine leiomyomas affects an estimated four to fifteen million women in the United states. Despite the startling frequency at which these lesions occur, adequate therapeutic intervention strategies have not been developed for this hormonally responsive tumor type. Clinical impressions indicate that leiomyomas proliferate in response to estrogen, suggesting that antiestrogens may be efficacious in their treatment. The efforts to develop new therapeutic regimes for treatment of uterine leiomyoma have been hampered, however, by the lack of a suitable animal model for this condition. This paper summarizes our work on the Eker rat model for uterine leiomyoma in which these tumors arise spontaneously with a high frequency. Our data indicate that leiomyoma cells proliferate in response to estradiol *in vitro,* and in a nude mouse xenograft system *in vivo.* These data demonstrate the usefulness of the Eker rat model for evaluation of efficacy of potential therapeutic agents for leiomyoma.

Uterine Leiomyoma/Leiomyosarcoma

Uterine leiomyomas (fibroids) are found in 20-25% of premenopausal women and arise from the smooth muscle cells of the uterine myometrium (Buttram and Reiter, 1981). While leiomyomas are considered benign, they have a serious impact on the health of women that develop these tumors. Uterine fibroids can be associated with infertility, can induce abortion by interference with placentation, and can result in menorrhagia, dysmenorrhea, and postpartum hemorrhaging (Rubin, 1990). These tumors also contribute to the high hysterectomy rate of women in the United States. Due to the high incidence of this tumor type, detrimental biological effects, and lack of satisfactory treatment regimens without adverse side effects, uterine leiomyomas are receiving attention as a major women's health issue.

In addition to benign leiomyomas, malignant leiomyosarcomas also arise from the myometrium. In contrast to leiomyomas, leiomyosarcomas have a very poor prognosis (Wen et al., 1987). These tumors can metastasize to the lung, kidney, liver, brain and bone. In the case of uterine myometrial tumors, it is not clear if malignant leiomyosarcomas develop independently of myomas, or whether some of the benign tumors progress to malignancy. In general, good progression models for sarcomas have not been described, in contrast to epithelial cancers where stages of progression have been well characterized. Questions therefore remain regarding the potential for progression of leiomyoma to leiomyosarcoma.

Hormonal Responsiveness of Uterine Leiomyomas

Several lines of clinical data exist suggesting that leiomyomas are an estrogen-responsive tumor type. These tumors typically arise during the reproductive years, and may increase in size during pregnancy and diminish in size after menopause (reviewed in Ross et al., 1986). This association between tumor growth and physiological states in which high circulating levels of estrogen exist has been taken as evidence to implicate estrogen as a modulator of the growth of leiomyomas (reviewed in Ross et al., 1986). In addition, investigators have demonstrated an increase in estrogen receptor levels in uterine myomas (Sadan et al., 1987). Lower rates of estrogen metabolism have been noted in the tumors, suggesting that an increase in local levels of estrogen may play a role in the pathogenesis of the leiomyoma formation (Pollow et al., 1978). The risk factors for leiomyoma development are consistent with "unopposed" estrogen stimulation (Ross et al., 1986), and leiomyoma primary cultures have been reported to have elevated transcriptional responses to estrogen when compared with cultures derived from surrounding normal myometrium (Andersen et al., 1995). This large body of work implicating estrogen in the genesis or progression of uterine myometrial tumors suggests that antiestrogenic compounds may prove beneficial in their treatment.

Need for New Therapeutic Approaches

Management of symptomatic uterine leiomyomas is primarily surgical. Either myomectomy or hysterectomy is indicated, depending on the patient's desire to subsequently bear children. Gonadotropin Releasing Hormone (GnRH) agonists create a hypoestrogenic state and have been utilized for treatment of uterine fibroids, but the impact of these compounds on the overall management of this disease is not clear (Adamson, 1992). Although use of GnRH agonists may significantly reduce uterine size and tumor volume (Andreyko et al., 1987; Adamson, 1992), not all tumors respond to this therapy (Maheux et al., 1984). In addition, these compounds must be administered by injection and cannot be taken orally (Friedman et al., 1987). Because long term hypoestrogenic therapies carry risk of significant side effects, continued treatment with these agents is not recommended, and fibroid volume has been shown to return to pretreatment values within two to six months of cessation of therapy (Adamson, 1992). Bone loss, hot flashes, vaginal dryness, and in a small percentage of cases, severe hemorrhage requiring surgical intervention have been reported with the use of GnRH agonists (Healy et al., 1984; Friedman et al., 1989; Adamson, 1992). Because of these complications, several researchers have suggested that these compounds may be best utilized as preoperative or adjunct surgical therapies for leiomyoma, rather than front line treatment strategies for this disease (Friedman et al., 1987; Adamson, 1992).

Because no medicinal therapeutic strategy currently exists to adequately manage uterine leiomyoma, treatment is now primarily surgical (Easterday et al., 1983). Development of new anti-hormonal therapeutic agents for the treatment of leiomyoma would therefore have extraordinary health benefits for large numbers of women. Clinical data indicating that the use of GnRH agonists is beneficial in treating uterine leiomyomas suggests that other antiestrogens may prove beneficial as well, and that development of novel anti-hormones for long term therapy of leiomyoma would have significant clinical application.

The Eker Rat Model of Leiomyoma

High incidence spontaneous tumor models greatly facilitate the study of the biology and responses of individual tumor types. Until recently, no animal model for uterine leiomyoma has been available. We have now reported that in a physiologic model of familial cancer susceptibility, Eker rats that carry a single gene alteration develop multiple primary tumor types with an autosomal dominant pattern of inheritance (Everitt et al., 1992). Carrier animals that are heterozygous for a mutation in the tuberous sclerosis 2 (TSC2) gene (Yeung et al., 1994; Kobayashi et al., 1995) develop spontaneous tumors in the uterus (leiomyoma/leiomyosarcoma), kidney (renal cell carcinoma), and spleen (hemangiosarcoma). Wild-type siblings are completely normal, while animals that inherit two defective copies of the TSC2 gene die *in utero*. The pattern of inheritance of the Eker rat lesions is depicted in Figure 1.

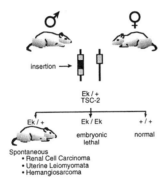

Figure 1: Pattern of Inheritance of the Eker Mutation.
A germline mutation in the TSC2 gene results in the appearance of spontaneous leiomyomas in female rats that carry a defective copy of the gene. Susceptibility to tumor development is transmitted in an autosomal dominant fashion.

The normal allele of the TSC2 gene is lost in leiomyomas that develop in heterozygous animals carrying the mutant allele (Yeung et al., 1995), indicating that inactivation of both alleles plays a role in the pathogenesis of the uterine tumors. The function of the TSC2 protein is not known at this time, and it is unclear whether this gene product plays some critical role in uterine myometrial cell biology. It is possible that loss of function of this tumor susceptibility gene results in a generalized loss of cellular growth control, which sets in motion a cascade of events that ultimately results in tumor development. The diverse nature of the lesions that develop in this animal model would be consistent with this possibility. The mechanism by which alteration of this gene predisposes to uterine leiomyomas has not been determined, nor has the role for this gene in human leiomyoma been elucidated. Both of these questions are being investigated in related studies ongoing in our laboratory.

The clinical aspects and pathological features of the Eker rat reproductive tract tumors have been previously described (Everitt et al., 1995). The spectrum of lesions seen in the rats completely recapitulates the spectrum of lesions seen in the human condition. Early lesions are typified by proliferative changes see histologically within the wall of the myometrium. These foci may progress to form benign leiomyomas, which are usually solitary nodular masses seen at the junction of the uterine body and the cervix. At 14 months of age, 43% of carrier female rats will have grossly visible reproductive tract lesions, while 72% of animals will have lesions that are visible histologically. Anaplastic uterine leiomyosarcomas are seen with a much lesser frequency, just as they are a rare event in the human disease spectrum, and a single incidence of pulmonary metastasis of one of these sarcomatous lesions has been documented in an aged female rat. Both benign and malignant lesions, as well as the pulmonary metastasis, stain positively with smooth muscle markers, confirming their smooth muscle origin (Everitt et al., 1995).

Few clinical signs are associated with the rat leiomyomas unless the tumors are of sufficient size to cause urinary incontinence and constipation (Everitt et al., 1995). Infertility is the primary presenting complaint in women with leiomyomas, however (Rubin, 1990), and the rat tumors appear to be associated with infertility as well. In a pilot study performed to assess the affects of the tumors on fertility, only one viable litter has been produced out of 15 bred tumor-bearing females, as compared with five litters born to 25 non-tumor-bearing littermates (Everitt et al., 1995).

Tumor-derived Cell Lines

We have recently described the isolation of a panel of cell lines derived from Eker rat reproductive tract smooth muscle tumors. Seven cell lines were derived from these tumors and given the designation of ELT (Eker rat Leiomyoma/myosarcoma Tumor-derived (Howe et al., 1995a). Histopathology of the primary tumors from which these lines were derived indicated that five of them were derived from leiomyomas (ELT 3, 4, 6, 9, 10), while two were derived from leiomyosarcomas (ELT 5A, 5B). The characterization of these cell lines has been described (Howe et al., 1995a), and is summarized in Table 1. The smooth muscle origin of the cell lines was confirmed by the presence of the immunoreactive smooth muscle alpha actin isoform. Tumorigenicity of the cell lines was determined by injection subcutaneously in nude mice. Of the seven cell lines, ELT 3 and ELT 5B were tumorigenic. Histologic examination of the nude mouse tumors confirmed that they were of smooth muscle origin, providing further evidence of the smooth muscle nature of the tumors from which the cell lines were derived. Of particular relevance for future therapeutic studies is the presence of estrogen receptor in four out of seven of the cell lines. For hormonally responsive tumor types, estrogen receptor status can affect tumor response to hormonal therapy (Lerner and Jordan, 1990). Northern analysis of poly A+ isolated from the ELT cell lines revealed the presence of a predicted 6.7 kb estrogen receptor transcript in four out of seven of the lines (ELT 3, 4, 9, and 10). In order to confirm the presence of absence of functional receptor, specific binding analysis utilizing 3H-estradiol was performed with ELT 3 and ELT 6. Saturable binding of 3H-estradiol to ELT 3 was readily observed. Scatchard analysis revealed that this cell line had a single class of receptors with a Kd of 0.7nM, binding capacity of 56 fmol/mg total protein, and approximately 14,000 receptor sites/cell. In contrast, ELT 6 did not exhibit specific binding, consistent with the lack of detectable estrogen receptor transcripts on Northern analysis.

Table 1

Cell Line	Histology	α actin	Tumorigenicity	Nude Mouse Tumor Histology	ER
ELT 3	**Leiomyoma**	+	+	**Smooth muscle**	+
ELT 4	Leiomyoma	+	-		+
ELT 5A*	Leiomyosarcoma	+	-		-
ELT 5B*	Leiomyosarcoma	+	+	Smooth muscle	-
ELT 6	**Leiomyoma**	+	-		-
ELT 9	Leiomyoma	+	-		+
ELT 10	Leiomyoma	+	-		+

* Independent tumors isolated from opposite uterine horns of the same animal.
ER = estrogen receptor

Hormonal Responsiveness *In Vitro*

As previously discussed, clinical data indicates that uterine leiomyomas in humans are stimulated to grow by estrogen To examine the estrogen-stimulated growth of leiomyoma cells within the context of a controlled, well-characterized system, the ELT 3 cell line was grown in estrogen-depleted medium supplemented with 0.1 nM to 1.0 μM 17β-estradiol. Data indicate that estrogen was able to stimulate the growth of the cells, and this growth stimulation was significant at each concentration is examined (Howe et al., 1995b). The results of estrogen stimulation experiments are shown in Figure 2.

Interestingly, the estrogen-responsive phenotype characteristic of leiomyomas is not shared by normal myometrial smooth muscle. While estrogen is a proliferative stimulus for leiomyomas, this hormone does not stimulate proliferation in normal and adult uterine myometrial cells. As depicted in Figure 3, in the immature uterus, both endometrial and myometrial cells proliferate in response to estrogen. In the adult animal, however, this proliferative response to circulating estrogen levels is lost in the mature myometrium. During the estrus cycle, in which estrogen levels rise and fall, the myometrium of the uterus does not undergo significant growth or cellular proliferation. This is in contrast to the epithelial cells of the adult uterine endometrium, which retain their ability to proliferate in response to estrogen and differentiate in response to progesterone. In contrast, as discussed above, there is ample evidence that uterine leiomyomas are estrogen responsive, and proliferative in response to this hormone. Elucidation of the molecular mechanism responsible for reversion to an estrogen responsive state may well hold the key to understanding the pathogenesis of these uterine tumors.

The fact that leiomyoma cells are stimulated to proliferate by estradiol suggests that antiestrogens should inhibit the growth of these cells. In order to determine if the Eker rat *in vitro* system was capable of identifying compounds with the potential to inhibit the growth of leiomyoma cells, we chose to examine the effects of the prototypical antiestrogen tamoxifen in this system. While we are not suggesting that

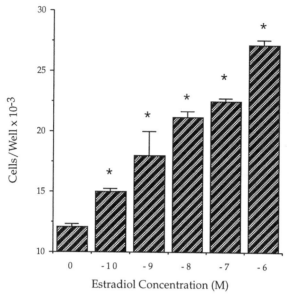

Figure 2: Estrogen Responsiveness in Leiomyoma-derived Call Line ELT 3. ELT 3 cells were grown for 96 hours in estrogen-depleted medium (phenol red-free, stripped serum) supplemented with varying concentrations of 17β-estradiol. Estradiol stimulated proliferation of the leiomyoma cells at all concentrations examined.

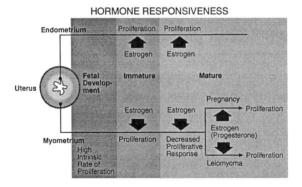

Figure 3: Immature uterine myometrial cells proliferate in response to estrogen, in contrast to adult myometrial cells which do not proliferate in response to this hormone. Leiomyomas appear to have reacquired this estrogen-responsive phenotype.

tamoxifen is an appropriate therapeutic agent for uterine leiomyoma, its use in this system as a well characterized antiestrogen is designed to validate the system. In the rat, as in humans, tamoxifen acts predominantly as an estrogen antagonist. Tamoxifen is well absorbed by rats following oral administration, and metabolism of tamoxifen is similar in both rats and humans; N-desmethyltamoxifen is the major metabolite in both species (Robinson et al., 1991). In treated rats, tamoxifen and its metabolites have been shown to localize to the uterus, and tamoxifen can inhibit the binding of estrogen to its receptor in this tissue (Furr and Jordan, 1984; Pasqualini et al., 1988). Tamoxifen has additional effects on the female rat reproductive tract that are indicative of its action as an estrogen antagonist, including decreased uterine weight, reduced or absent corpora leutea, the presence of follicular cysts, and the disappearance of endometrial glands (Furr and Jordan, 1984; Lyman and Jordan, 1985).

The addition of tamoxifen to cultures of the rat leiomyoma cell line ELT 3 revealed that the antiestrogen was capable of inhibiting the growth of these cells (Howe et al., 1995b). Growth inhibition was seen at concentrations ranging from 0.1 to 10 µM tamoxifen, and was significant at each of these concentrations. Data illustrating the growth inhibitory effects of tamoxifen on leiomyoma cells *in vitro* are shown in Figure 4.

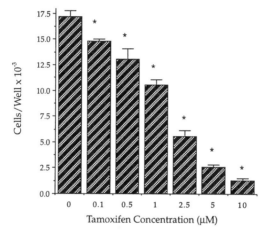

Figure 4: Tamoxifen Inhibition of Leiomyoma Cell Growth *In Vitro.* ELT 3 cells were grown for 96 hours in the presence of varying concentrations of tamoxifen. Inhibition of growth was significant at all concentrations examined.

In Vivo Nude Mouse Xenograft Assay

The ability of ELT 3 cells to produce subcutaneous tumors when injected into athymic nude mice allows us to extend *in vitro* data into a rapid *in vivo* screening assay. We therefore examined the ability of both estrogen and tamoxifen to modify tumor growth in this nude mouse xenograft system (Howe et al., 1995b). ELT 3 cells were injected into female nude mice that had previously been implanted with placebo pellets (Innovative Research), 25 mg tamoxifen pellets (Innovative), or 1.7 mg 17β-estradiol pellets (Innovative). As shown in Figure 5, estradiol stimulated the growth

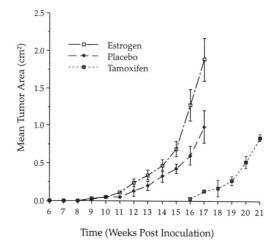

Figure 5: *In Vivo* Modulation of Leiomyoma Growth by Estrogen and Tamoxifen. ELT 3 cells were injected subcutaneously in nude mice that had been implanted with placebo, estradiol, or tamoxifen pellets. Estrogen stimulated the proliferation of these nude mouse tumors, while tamoxifen inhibited their growth.

of leiomyoma cells when compared with placebo-treated controls, while tamoxifen inhibited tumor formation. Such data provides excellent extension of *in vitro* data into this *in vivo* system.

DISCUSSION

This report describes the characterization of a unique animal model for leiomyoma development. Female carriers of the Eker mutation develop reproductive tract smooth muscle tumors with a high spontaneous frequency, and tumor incidence increases with increasing animal age. These tumors demonstrate immunohistochemical staining patterns similar to those found in smooth muscle tumors of women, confirming the smooth muscle origin of the rat tumors.

In order to develop an *in vitro/in vivo* approach to screen for efficacy of potential therapeutic agents, it was necessary to establish a panel of uterine tumor-derived cell lines for use in *in vitro* experiments. Seven cell lines were established from independent benign and malignant smooth muscle tumors, and were characterized for expression of smooth muscle markers and steroid hormone receptors. The cell lines express smooth muscle alpha actin, confirming their smooth muscle origin. Estrogen receptor-positive cell lines proliferate in response to estradiol. In addition, estrogen increases leiomyoma tumor size in a nude mouse xenograft system. The antiestrogen tamoxifen inhibits proliferation of leiomyoma cells both *in vitro* and in nude mice *in vivo*.

Animal models of carcinogenesis have been widely utilized to provide evaluation of cancer chemotherapeutic strategies. The relevance of individual animal models for human cancer, however, varies with the degree of similarity between the animal model and the human disease it is intended to represent. The Eker rat model of human leiomyoma is one in which similarities between the animal and human condition are numerous. The spectrum of lesions seen in the human disease is completely recapitulated in the Eker rat. In addition, just as the ELT cell lines show the same pattern of smooth muscle alpha actin immunofluorescence as that seen in normal rat myometrium in primary culture, smooth muscle cells from human leiomyomas appear to exhibit the same immunofluorescent staining pattern as that seen in normal human myometrial tissue (Eyden et al., 1992). Interestingly, expression of IGF-II by the leiomyosarcoma lines ELT 5A and 5B, but not leiomyoma lines (Howe, unpublished data) is also reflective of what has been seen in human tumors, where overexpression of IGF II in leiomyosarcomas has been observed (Höppener et al., 1988; Gloudemans et al., 1990).

Especially relevant for these studies is that fact that leiomyomas in Eker rats and in humans appear to be estrogen responsive, in contrast to the lack of proliferation that is seen in response to estrogen in the normal adult rat and human myometrium. In Eker rats as well as in humans, the epithelium overlying submucosal leiomyomas appears hyperplastic (Everitt et al., 1995), suggesting that a localized hyperestrogenic environment exists in close proximity to these tumors. These similarities make the Eker rat system an attractive model for studying the molecular and clinical effects of estrogen and antiestrogens on leiomyoma growth and development.

It is important to emphasize that the Eker rat is the only animal model in which these tumors develop spontaneously with a frequency that is significant enough to lend itself to experimental manipulation. In addition, human leiomyomas have been very difficult to culture and there has been no systematic characterization of the few reported successful attempts to culture these cells. Animal tumor models, such as the Eker rat model, offer unique opportunities for the study of molecular mechanisms underlying the development of uterine leiomyomas. Both tumor and normal tissue are readily available, and it is easy to intervene in the whole animal under well-defined experimental conditions with therapeutic approaches at all stages of tumor development. Tumor cells can be established in culture to derive cell lines which can be used in in vitro experiments designed to elucidate mechanisms related to tumor development and to test the efficacy of therapeutic agents. The availability of the Eker rat model makes it possible for the first time to address questions regarding mechanism of tumor development and therapeutic potential of steroid hormone antagonists for uterine leiomyoma in a well-defined experimental model system. The model should therefore prove extremely useful in studies designed to evaluate the biology and responses of these tumors.

As demonstrated and validated with tamoxifen, the Eker rat model allows a rapid system for testing candidate compounds for leiomyoma treatment. The ability of potential therapeutic compounds to modulate the growth of leiomyoma cell lines may be rapidly assessed in vitro. The availability of tumorigenic cell lines makes possible the extension of in vitro data into a rapid nude mouse in vivo screening assay. In addition, Eker rats are available for evaluating efficacy against leiomyomas in situ. The Eker rat system is therefore invaluable for rapid preclinical screening of potential therapeutic agents for what is an extremely important tumor type.

ACKNOWLEDGMENTS

This work was supported in part by the National Institutes of Health grants CA 72253 (CW), HD 33605 (CW and MMG) and CA 66324 (SRH).

REFERENCES

Adamson GD (1992): Treatment of uterine fibroids: current findings with gonadotropin-releasing hormone agonists. Am J Obstet Gynecol 166:746-751.

Andersen J, DyReyes VM, Barbieri RL, Coachman DM, Miksicek RJ (1995): Leiomyoma primary cultures have elevated transcriptional response to estrogen compared with autologous myometrial cultures. J Soc Gynecol Inves. 2:542-551.

Andreyko JL, Marshall LA, Dumesic DA, Jaffe RB (1987): Therapeutic uses of gonadotropin-releasing hormone analogs. Obstet Gynecol Survey 42:1-21.

Buttram VC, Reiter RC (1981): Uterine leiomyomata: etiology, symptomatology, and management. Fertil Steril 36:433-445.

Easterday CL, Grimes DA, Riggs JA (1983): Hysterectomy in the United States. Obstet Gynecol 62:203-212.

Everitt JI, Goldsworthy TL, Wolf DC, Walker C L (1992): Hereditary renal cell carcinoma in the Eker rat: a familial cancer syndrome. J Urol 148:1932-1936.

Everitt JI, Wolf DC, Howe SR, Goldsworthy TL, Walker C (1995): Rodent model of reproductive tract leiomyomata: clinical and pathologic features. Am J Pathol 146:1556-1567.

Eyden BP, Hale RJ, Richmond I, Buckley CH (1992): Cytoskeletal filaments in the smooth muscle cells of uterine leiomyomata and myometrium: an ultrastructural and immunohistochemical analysis. Virchows Archiv A Pathol Anat 420:51-58.

Friedman AJ, Barbieri RL, Benacerraf BR, Schiff I (1987): Treatment of leiomyomata with intranasal or subcutaneous leuprolide, a gonadotropin-releasing hormone agonist. Fertil Steril 48:560-564.

Friedman AJ (1989): Vaginal hemorrhage associated with degenerating submucous leiomyomata during leuprolide acetate treatment. Fertil. Steril. 52, 152-154.

Furr BJA, Jordan VC (1984): The pharmacology and clinical use of tamoxifen. Pharmacol Ther 25:127-205.

Gloudemans T, Prinsen I, Van Unnik JA, Lips CJ, Den Otter W, Sussenbach JS (1990): Insulin-like growth factor gene expression in human smooth muscle tumors. Cancer Res 50:6689-6695.

Healy DL, Fraser HM, Lawson SL (1984): Shrinkage of a uterine fibroid after subcutaneous infusion of a LHRH agonist. Brit. Med. J. Clin. Res. Ed. 289, 1267-1268.

Höppener JWM, Mosselman S, Roholl PJM, Lambrechts C, Slebus RJC, de Pager-Holthuizen P, Lips CJM, Jansz HS, Sussenbach JS (1988): Expression of insulin-like growth factor-I and II genes in human smooth muscle tumors. EMBO J 7:1379-1385.

Howe SR, Gottardis MM, Everitt JI, Walker C (1995b): Estrogen stimulation and tamoxifen inhibition of leiomyoma cell growth *in vitro* and *in vivo*. Endocrinology 136:4996-5003.

Howe SR, Gottardis MM, Everitt JI, Goldsworthy TL, Wolf DC, Walker C (1995a): Rodent model of reproductive tract leiomyomata: establishment and characterization of tumor-derived cell lines. Am J Pathol 146:1568-1579.

Kobayashi T, Hirayama Y, Kobayashi E, Kubo Y, Hino O (1995): A germline insertion in the tuberous sclerosis (Tsc2) gene gives rise to the Eker rat model of dominantly inherited cancer. Natl Genet 9:70-74.

Lerner LJ, Jordan VC (1990): Development of antiestrogens and their use in breast cancer: eighth Cain Memorial Award lecture. Cancer Res 50:4177-4189.

Lyman SD, Jordan VC (1985): Metabolism of tamoxifen and its uterotrophic activity. Biochem Pharm 34:2787-2794.

Maheux R, Guilloteau C, Lemay A, Bastide A, Fazekas AT (1984): Regression of leiomyomata uteri following hypoestrogenism induced by repetitive luteinizing hormone-releasing hormone agonist treatment: preliminary report. Fertil Steril 42:644-646.

Pasqualini JR, Sumida C, Giambiagi N (1988): Pharmacodynamic and biological effects of anti-estrogens in different models. J Steroid Biochem 31:613-643.

Pollow K, Geilfuss J, Boquoi E, Pollow B (1978): Estrogen and progesterone binding proteins in normal human myometrium and leiomyoma tissue. J Clin Chem Clin Biochem 16:503-511.

Robinson SP, Langan-Fahey SM, Johnson DA, Jordan VC (1991): Metabolites, pharmacodynamics, and pharmacokinetics of tamoxifen in rats and mice compared to the breast cancer patient. Drug Metab Disp 36-43.

Ross RK, Pike MC, Vessey MP, Bull D, Yeates D, Casagrande JT (1986): Risk factors for uterine fibroids: reduced risk associated with oral contraceptives. Br Med J 293:359-362.

Rubin A (1990): Uterine fibroids. In ME Rivlin, JC Morrison and GW Bates (eds.): "Manual of Clinical Problems in Obstetrics and Gynecology." Boston, Massachusetts: Little Brown and Co., pp 221-225.

Sadan O, Van Iddekinge B, Van Gelderen CJ, Savage N, Becker PJ, Van Der Walt LA, Robinson M (1987): Oestrogen and progesterone receptor concentrations in leiomyoma and normal myometrium. Ann Clin Biochem 24:263-267.

Wen BC, Tewfik FA, Tewfik HH, Long, JP, Anderson B (1987): Uterine sarcoma: a retrospective study. J Surg Oncol 34:104-108.

Yeung RS, Xiao GH, Jin F, Lee WC, Testa JR, Knudson AG (1994): Predisposition to renal carcinoma in the Eker rat is determined by germ-line mutation of the tuberous sclerosis 2 (TSC2) gene. Proc Natl Acad Sci USA 91:11413-11416.

Yeung RS, Xiao G-H, Everitt JI, Jin F, Walker C (1995): Allelic loss at the tuberous sclerosis 2 locus in spontaneous tumors in the Eker rat. Mol Carcin 14:28-36.

Etiology of Breast and
Gynecological Cancers, pages 217–231
© 1997 Wiley-Liss, Inc.

MECHANISMS OF DES CARCINOGENICITY: EFFECTS OF THE TGFα
TRANSGENE*

Karen Gray, Bill Bullock, Robert Dickson, Kimberly Raszmann, John McLachlan, and
Glenn Merlino

Laboratory of Reproductive and Developmental Toxicology, National Institute of
Environmental Health Science, Research Triangle Park, North Carolina 27709 (KG,KR,JM);
Present Address (KG)-Department of Obstetrics and Gynecology, Uniformed Services
University of Health Sciences, Bethesda, Maryland 20814 [formerly Karen Nelson]; Bowman
Gray School of Medicine (BB), Wake Forest University, Winston-Salem, North Carolina
27709; Department of Anatomy and Cell Biology (RD), Georgetown University Medical
Center, Lombardi Cancer Research Center, Washington, DC 20007 [Supported by DOD
research grant DAMD 17-94-J-4257]; Present Address (JM)-Department of
Pharmacology(JM), Tulane University, Center for Bioenvironmental Research, New Orleans,
Louisiana 70112; to whom correspondence should be sent (GM), Laboratory of Molecular
Biology, National Cancer Institute, National Institutes of Health, Bethesda 20892.
*A portion of this study has been submitted for publication to Molecular Carcinogenesis.

ABSTRACT

Inappropriate estrogen exposure during critical periods of development will cause
numerous abnormalities in the female reproductive tract. Epigenetic effects on the expression
of estrogen-regulated genes is proposed to be one of the mechanisms by which neonatal
estrogen elicits teratogenic and carcinogenic effects. Of note is the existence of an integral
relationship between the regulation of members of the epidermal growth factor (EGF) gene
family and estrogen effects on the growth and differentiation of the reproductive tract. To
determine whether the EGF gene family plays a critical role in mediating the pathogenic
effects of estrogen, we have used transforming growth factor-alpha (TGFα) transgenic mice
to investigate the effects of constitutive TGFα expression in the reproductive tract and whether
TGFα would potentiate carcinogenesis induced by the potent estrogen, diethylstilbestrol
(DES), and by the carcinogen, 7,12-dimethylbenz[a]anthracene (DMBA). The animals were
homozygous TGFα transgenic female mice from the MT42 line and the parental CD-1
outbred mice. Constitutive TGFα expression was found to augment the effects of both DES
and DMBA in eliciting hyperplastic and differentiation changes in the reproductive tract. The
presence of the TGFα transgene significantly increased the incidence of DES-induced vaginal
adenosis, uterine endometrial hyperplasia, hypospadia, and benign ovarian cysts. In addtion,

TGFα potentiated the effects of DMBA in eliciting uterine polyps and benign ovarian cysts, and in the retention of Wolffian Duct remnants. However, the incidence of reproductive tract neoplasia was not promoted by the presence of the TGFα transgene. This study indicates that TGFα plays a role in the developmental and morphogenic events of both the Müllerian duct and urogenital sinus, and that deregulation is associated with pathogenesis of these tissues. Furthermore, the fact that constitutive expression of the TGFα did not substitute for DES as a reproductive tract carcinogen or act as a promoter of DES-induced uterine neoplasia suggest that DES carcinogenesis involves more than aberrant expression of this single growth factor.

INTRODUCTION

Studies have clearly shown that disturbances of reproductive tract growth and differentiation can be elicited by exposure to estrogens during critical developmental stages (Gray, et al., 1994; Iguchi, 1992; McLachlan, et al., 1982; Metzler and Mclachlan, 1977; Noller, et al. 1990). Although the mechanism(s) responsible for the carcinogenic and teratogenic effects of estrogens such as diethylstilbestrol (DES) remains unknown, the premature and permanent induction of genes normally under steroid hormone control has been proposed to contribute to the establishment of the ovarian-independent, "estrogenized" phenotype in the reproductive tracts of exposed animals (Gray, et al., 1994). Substantial evidence points to a critical role of the EGF pathway in the early development of the reproductive tract as well as in mediating steroid hormone effects in the adult (Bossert, et al. 1990; Gardner, et al., 1989; Gray, et al., 1994; Hall and Forsberg, 1993; Nelson-Gray, et al., 1989 and 1992; Pollard, 1990). In fact, exposure to DES during the critical neonatal developmental period in mouse has been shown to result in the persistent induction of EGF in the uterus and vagina. This evidence supports the hypothesis that the developmental toxicity of estrogens is due, in part, to the inappropriate expression of estrogen-regulated genes which may contribute to permanent disruptions in growth and differentiation. Dysregulation of autocrine/paracrine growth pathways due to either elevated expression of growth factors or synthesis, and/or mutation of their receptors is a consistent alteration observed in many neoplastic cells including in reproductive tissues (Gray, et a., 1994).

Studies of transgenic mice expressing growth factor genes have shown direct links between the overexpression or inappropriate expression of a single growth factor and the development of lesions marked by abnormal proliferation and differentiation, and neoplasia (Bockman, et al., 1995; Jhappan, et al., 1990 and 1994; Ma, et al., 1994p; Matsui, et al., 1990; Sharp, et al., 1995; Smith, et al., 1995; Takagi, et al., 1993; Vassar, et al., 1992). In various TGFα transgenic mouse strains, preneoplastic and neoplastic changes have been demonstrated in the mammary gland, salivary gland, stomach mucosa, coagulating gland, liver, and pancreas. Although, in most studies the aberrant expression of a growth factor transgene alone does not result in neoplastic lesions unless long latency periods are accommodated. For example, TGFα overexpression must be combined with wounding, or treatment with either a phorbol ester tumor promoter or an initiator in order to elicit papilloma formation in mouse skin (Jhappan, et al., 1994; Vassar, et al., 1992). Development of mammary gland neoplasia in TGFα transgenic female mice requires exposure to the hormonal milieu of pregnancy (Matsui, et al., 1990; Smith, et al., 1995). Thus, often a proper hormonal or growth promoting environment must be provided before the neoplastic effects of TGFα can be manifested.

In addition to neoplastic lesions, tissues of TGFα transgenic animals exhibit changes that reflect disruption of the mechanisms that regulate tissue homeostasis, involving effects on cell proliferation, cell differentiation, and senescence (Bockman. et al., 1995; Jhappan, et al., 1990; Ma, et al., 1994; Sharp, et al., 1995). This is demonstrated by TGFα stimulating the rediffernetiation of pancreatic acinar cells into simple ductal cells, mucin-producing cells, and occasionally to insulin-producing cells. Disorganization of the gastric mucosa with pathological accumulation of surface mucous cells and depletion in differentiated parietal and chief cells is another characteristic of TGFα mice. Effects of TGFα on the function and response of tissues in the hypothalamic-pituitary-ovarian axis results in alterations of sexual development in the TGFα transgenic animals.

Based on the evidence that TGFα affects reproductive function and that members of the EGF family mediate sex steroid hormone action, we questioned whether the EGF gene family also plays a critical role in pathological changes in the reproductive tract. Here we report the results of our study using TGFα transgenic mice to investigate the effects of constitutive TGFα expression on the induction of reproductive tract alterations by the potent estrogen, diethylstilbestrol (DES), and by the carcinogen, 7,12-dimethylbenz[a]anthracene (DMBA). In comparison to the nontransgenic animals, the presence of the TGFα transgene was found to promote certain reproductive organ-specific pathological abnormalities, but not neoplasia. This supports the hypothesis that deregulation of a single peptide growth factor, like TGFα, can lead to growth and differentiation abnormalities; but, aberrant expression of TGFα alone is clearly not sufficient for carcinogenesis of reproductive tissues.

METHODS

This study was designed to determine whether TGFα expression could modulate DES- and DMBA-induced carcinogenesis of the reproductive tract. The animals were homozygous TGFα transgenic female mice from the MT42 line generated as described previously (Jhappan, et al., 1990) and the parental nontransgenic CD-1 outbred mouse strain. Study duration was 52 weeks with an interim sacrifice at 39 weeks. However, mice that became moribund were sacrificed. After evaluation of the data, there was not a difference between the two major sacrifices and the data were pooled for presentation. Mice were given NIH31 rodent chow (Ziegler Brothers) and water ad libitum. The experimental animal protocol that was followed was in accordance with the NIH approved procedures. At sacrifice, the reproductive tracts were removed, fixed in Bouins' Fixative for 24-48h, washed in water for at least 24h, and stored in 70% ethanol until paraffin embedded. Serial sections (5-7 μM) of the embedded tissues were stained with hematoxylin and eosin and evaluated for histopathological alterations. Unless designated, all chemicals were obtained from Sigma Chemical Company (St. Louis, MO). Data was analyzed by CHI square and observed to significantly different at <0.05 with one degree of freedom.

There were eight experimental groups consisting of the parental CD-1 and TGFα transgenic mice treated with DES (2 ug/pup in sesame oil), DMBA (2mg/20g in peanut oil), both DES and DMBA, or with the vehicles alone using the regimen described below:

Group #1: CD-1 mice, vehicle control, received daily subcutaneous sesame seed oil injections on days 1-5 of age and a single intragastric peanut oil administration at 4 weeks of age.

Group #2: TGFα transgenic mice, vehicle control, treated as described for Group #1.

Group #3: CD-1 mice, neonatal DES treatment, received daily DES treatment by subcutaneous injections from days 1 to 5 of age, and then administered by gavage a single peanut oil vehicle dose at 4 weeks of age.

Group #4: TGFα transgenic mice, neonatal DES treatment, treated as described for Group #4.

Group #5: CD-1 mice, neonatal DES and DMBA treatment, received daily subcutaneous DES treatments on days 1 to 5 of life, then at 4 weeks of age a single intragastric dose of DMBA was administered.

Group #6: TGFα transgenic mice, neonatal DES and DMBA treatment, following the same strategy as performed for Group #5.

Group #7: CD-1 mice, DMBA treatment, received sesame seed oil vehicle subcutaneous injections on days 1 to 5 of age and a single intragastric DMBA treatment at 4 weeks of age.

Group #8: TGFα transgenic mice, DMBA treatment, following the same regimen as Group #7.

RESULTS

Uterine Alterations: A summary of the most distinctive histological changes observed in the uterus of CD-1 and TGFα transgenic mice is shown in Figure 1. Of special note is that the vehicle control TGFα transgenic animals (Group #2) exhibited a significant higher incidence of endometrial hyperplasia (ranging from microcytic to atypical) and of uterine polyps than observed in the vehicle treated nontransgenic CD-1 parental mice.

Similarly, neonatal DES treatment of TGFα transgenic mice (Group #4) resulted in a significantly greater incidence of endometrial hyperplasia than observed in the nontransgenic animals (Group #3), further indicating a propensity of TGFα transgenic mice for the development of hyperplasia. In contrast, the presence of the TGFα transgene did not potentiate the incidence of the uterine adenocarcinomas from that induced by DES in the CD-1 parental strain. Also, DES treatment suppressed the development of uterine polyps in the TGFα animals.

A single DMBA treatment given at four weeks of age did not dramatically modify DES induction of uterine adenocarcinomas in the CD-1 (Group #5) and only slightly decreased the number of tumors in the transgenic (Group #6). In contrast, DMBA exposure significantly reduced cystic endometrial hyperplasia in the CD-1 animals compared to the mice receiving DES treatment only (Group #3). Although not statistically significant, the transgenics also demonstrated a decrease in the incidence of endometrial hyperplasia upon

THE EFFECTS OF THE TGF-ALPHA TRANSGENE ON DES- AND DMBA-INDUCED UTERINE LESIONS

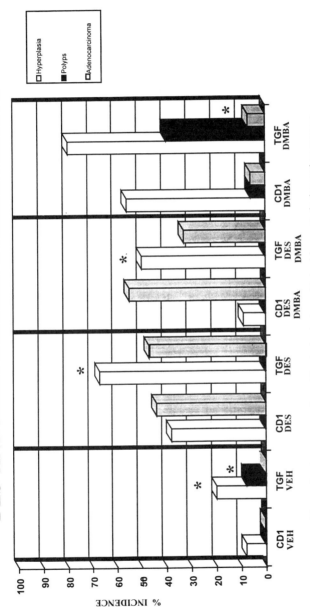

Figure 1: A summary of specific uterine lesions obtained in our study denoted as percent incidence obtained by dividing the number of animals with a lesion by the total number of animals in the treatment group. The asterisk (*) indicates that the TGFα animals exhibit significantly greater number of lesions than observed in the parental CD-1 mice, as determined by CHI square analysis. Note the clear differences in uterine histology between the CD-1 mice and the TGFα transgenic animals.

Abbreviations: CD1=parental mouse strain; TGF=TGFα transgenic mice; VEH=vehicle treated; DES=diethylstilbestrol treated; DES & DMBA=treated with both DES and 7,12-dimethybenz[a]anthracene; DMBA=DMBA treated.

DMBA exposure. Only one animal in Groups #5 and #6, a CD-1 mouse, exhibited a uterine polyp.

Treatment with DMBA alone induced only a low incidence of uterine adenocarcinomas in the CD-1 (Group #7) and the TGFα transgenic (Group #8) animals. In addition, rare tumors, a uterine leiomyosarcoma, a stromal cell sarcoma, and a hemangiosarcoma were found in the DMBA treated CD-1 animals and a single benign leiomyoma was found in a uterus of a TGFα transgenic mouse. Angioecstasis and hemangiomas were commonly found in the uterus of both CD-1 and transgenic mice which are characteristic DMBA-induced lesions. In contrast to the low incidence of adenocarcinomas, a single treatment with DMBA resulted in the greatest induction of endometrial hyperplasia over vehicle controls in both the transgenic and parental mice with the TGFα transgenics demonstrating the greatest response (CD-1 56%; TGFα 80%). Also, DMBA significantly promoted the development of uterine polyps in the TGFα transgenic mice (40%) in comparison to the CD-1 animals (6%).

Of special note is that there did not seem to be a correlation between the incidence of endometrial hyperplasia and the development of adenocarcinoma in animals exposed to the various treatments.

Alterations of Vaginal Histology: A summary of the vaginal abnormalities observed in the CD-1 parental and transgenic animals following DES and/or DMBA treatment in relation to vehicle controls is shown in Figure 2. A striking abnormality exhibited by the TGFα transgenic animals was the retention of the Wolffian duct, also known as Gardner's duct. Wolffian duct remnants, which normally regress during development in females, were consistently found in the TGFα transgenic mice regardless of treatment, but only in the CD-1 parental animals exposed to DMBA with or without DES. In all cases, the presence of the TGFα increased the incidence of Wolffian duct retention over that found in the control animals. Interestingly, retention of the Wolffian duct is documented to be one of the pathological alterations induced by neonatal DES exposure of nontransgenic CD-1, albeit at a very low incidence. This data links abnormal TGFα expression to the pathological occurrence of Wolffian ducts in the female reproductive tract.

Another classical DES-induced vaginal lesions is adenosis which refers to the abnormal appearance of columnar and glandular epithelium within a region of the vagina which is normally lined with squamous epithelium. Vaginal adenosis was consistently observed following neonatal DES exposure in both the CD-1 and TGFα transgenics; however, the presence of the TGFα transgene significantly potentiated the appearance of vaginal adenosis upon exposure to DES with or without subsequent DMBA treatment.

Besides adenosis, TGFα mice also exhibited enhanced sensitivity to DES exposure for the development of vaginal concretions, which are thought to be caused by abnormal urethral development. No concretions were found in the CD-1 mice of this study, but this lesion has been reported to occur in CD-1 mice at a very low incidence as a result of DES exposure. This evidence is the first to suggest that inappropriate expression of TGFα interferes with normal urethral development.

THE INFLUENCE OF THE TGF-ALPHA TRANSGENE ON THE DEVELOPMENT OF ALTERATIONS IN VAGINAL HISTOLOGY UPON TREATMENT WITH DES OR DMBA

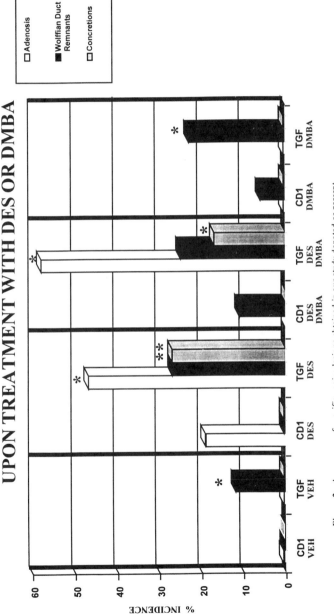

Figure 2: A summary of specific vagina lesions obtained in our study denoted as percent incidence and the asterisk (*) indicates that the TGFα animals exhibit significantly greater number of lesions than observed in the parental CD-1 mice, as determined by CHI square analysis. The presence of the TGFα transgene potentiated DES induction of vaginal adenosis, vaginal concretions caused by abnormal urethral development (hypospadia), and retention of the Wolffian duct.

Abbreviations: CD1=parental mouse strain; TGF=TGFα transgenic mice; VEH=vehicle treated; DES=diethylstilbestrol treated; DES & DMBA=treated with both DES and 7,12-dimethybenz[a]anthracene; DMBA=DMBA treated.

Growth abnormalities in the Oviduct: Exposure to neonatal estrogen induces histological alterations in the oviduct associated with hyperplasia and gland formation (diverticuli) of the oviductal mucosa. The diverticuli extend into the muscle wall, resembling the clinical lesion termed salpingitis isthmica nodosa (SIN). Although there was an elevating trend, the presence of the TGFα transgene did not significantly increase the incidence of SIN-like lesions induced by DES over that observed in the parental CD-1 mice (Figure 3). DMBA treatment did enhance DES-induction of SIN-like oviductal lesions in both transgenic and nontransgenic mice.

Abnormalities of the Ovary: The most notable effect of the TGFα transgene on the ovary was that the transgenic mice treated with vehicle, DES, or DMBA demonstrated significant increases in the incidence of benign ovarian cysts over that found in the parental CD-1 mice (Figure 4). In addition, neonatal exposure to DES was found to significantly promote the development of ovarian granulosa cell tumors upon exposure of both transgenic and nontransgenic animals to DMBA. Although not significant, the presence of TGFα transgene potentiated the development of these ovarian tumors in response to DMBA.

Pathological findings in the Pituitaries: The pituitaries of transgenic animals resembled adenomas with malformed Rathke pouch remnants that formed ductular structures. In contrast, none of the pituitaries obtained from the CD-1 mice exhibited these alterations. Treatment did not influence the histology of the pituitaries (data not shown).

DISCUSSION

Since estrogens are known to regulate the production of members of the EGF family, we have used TGFα transgenic mice as a model system to evaluate the role of TGFα in carcinogenesis of the reproductive tract. Specifically, we wanted to investigate the effects of constitutive expression of this growth factor in the reproductive tract and to determine whether TGFα would potentiate carcinogenesis induced by DES and DMBA. We show here that deregulated TGFα expression augmented the effects of DES and DMBA in eliciting hyperplastic and differentiation changes in the reproductive tract. The presence of the TGFα transgene significantly increased the incidence of DES-induced vaginal adenosis, uterine hyperplasia, uterine polyps, hypospadia, and benign ovarian cysts; however, the incidence of reproductive tract neoplasia was not promoted.

The significant potentiation of DES-induced vaginal adenosis by the TGFα transgene strongly implicates TGFα in pathogenesis of abnormal gland formation that is proposed to be a precursor lesion for the generation of vaginal adenocarcinoma in women (Noller, et al., 1990). Furthermore, the fact that TGFα transgenic animals exhibited a greater incidence of vaginal concretions due to malformation of the urethra and retention of Wolffian ducts suggests that TGFα plays an important role in the regulation of developmental and morphogenic events in both the Mullerian duct and the urogenital sinus of the female animal. Our results are supported by other studies which document that TGFα overexpression alters the growth and differentiation of both glandular and squamous epithelia in several different

INFLUENCE OF THE TGF-ALPHA TRANSGENE ON ABNORMAL GLAND PROLIFERATION IN THE OVIDUCT FOLLOWING DES AND DMBA EXPOSURE

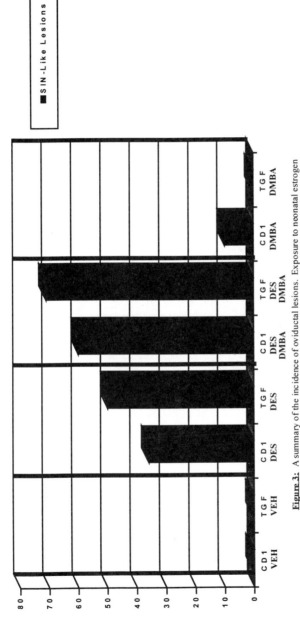

Figure 3: A summary of the incidence of oviductal lesions. Exposure to neonatal estrogen induced histological alterations in the oviduct associated with hyperplasia and gland formation (diverticuli) of the oviductal mucosa which extend into the muscle wall, resembling the clincial lesion, salpingitis isthmica nodosa (SIN). Both CD-1 and TGF α exhibited SIN-like lesions following DES exposure which appeared to be slightly amplified by DMBA treatment. Although, not significant, the percentage of animals with oviductal lesions was consistently higher in the transgenic animals.

Abbreviations: CD1=parental mouse strain; TGF=TGF α transgenic mice; VEH=vehicle treated; DES=diethylstilbestrol treated; DES & DMBA=treated with both DES and 7,12-dimethybenz[a]anthracene; DMBA=DMBA treated.

INFLUENCE OF THE TGF-ALPHA TRANSGENE ON OVARIAN HISTOLOGY FOLLOWING DES AND DMBA EXPOSURE

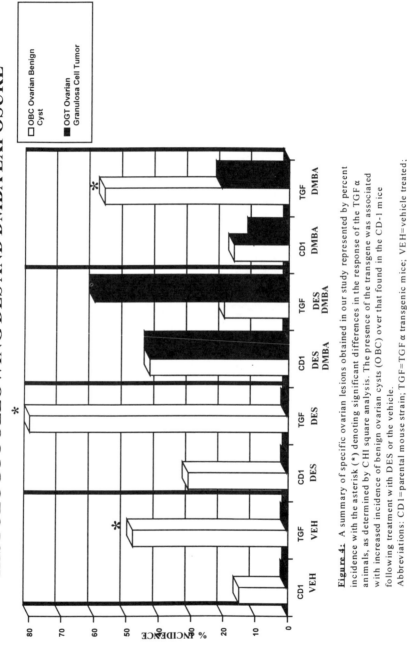

Figure 4: A summary of specific ovarian lesions obtained in our study represented by percent incidence with the asterisk (*) denoting significant differences in the response of the TGF α animals, as determined by CHI square analysis. The presence of the transgene was associated with increased incidence of benign ovarian cysts (OBC) over that found in the CD-1 mice following treatment with DES or the vehicle.

Abbreviations: CD1=parental mouse strain; TGF=TGF α transgenic mice; VEH=vehicle treated; DES=diethylstilbestrol treated; DES & DMBA=treated with both DES and 7,12-dimethybenz[a]anthracene; DMBA=DMBA treated.

organs. As an example, TGFα has been shown to disrupt the normal program of cellular differentiation in the gastric mucosa by interfering with the terminal differentiation of parietal and chief cells while promoting the growth of surface mucous cell progenitors (Bockman, et al., 1995; Sharp, et al., 1995). Zymogen granule-containing cells in the parotid gland have been shown to undergo redifferentiation to form ductular-like structures in transgenic animals. These studies support a morphogenic role for TGFα in that inappropriate expression can redirect epithelia along alternative differentiation pathways.

Interesting, DES- and vehicle-treated TGFα transgenic animals exhibited a significantly greater incidence of benign ovarian cysts than the corresponding nontransgenic mice. Unopposed estrogen in humans is associated with follicular polycystic degeneration of the ovary (Futterweit, 1984). In light of the fact that TGFα is regulated by estrogen in hormonally sensitive tissues and that experimental studies support a role for TGFα in ovarian function, our study provides further support that TGFα has an important role in the development of polycystic ovaries. Also, our data show that neonatal DES treatment promoted the development of ovarian granulosa cell tumors following DMBA treatment which has also been documented by a previous study (Manohara and Rao, 1980). The mechanism of DES action is unknown but it has been proposed that DMBA mediated deletion of oocytes is associated with the development of ovarian tumors in certain strains of mice. The fact that DES also reduces ovarian components (oocytes, follicles, and corpora lutea) and increases the interstitial tissue of the ovary may provide an environment that promotes the development of tumors following DMBA exposure.

Uterine polyps were also another growth abnormality identified in the TGFα transgenic mice. This finding leads to the question of whether up-regulation of TGFα expression may account for polyp development in women, which recently has been found to be a common side-effect of tamoxifen therapy in breast cancer patients (Cohen, 1994).

There is an association between endometrial carcinoma and unopposed estrogen exposure in women. It is proposed that estrogen-related endometrial lesions undergo progression from cystic to adenomatous to atypical hyperplasia to carcinoma (Cohen, 1994; Reinartz, et al., 1994). The observation that TGFα increases the incidence of both cystic endometrial hyperplasia and atypical hyperplasia in mice is of particular importance because there is a strong association between the presence of adenomatous hyperplasia with atypia and the subsequent development of adenocarcinoma. In fact, a role of aberrant growth factor expression such as TGFα has been suggested to be involved in the development of uterine adenocarcinomas in women (Reinartz, et al., 1994). Our results support a role for TGFα as a mediator of events that accompany the development of hyperplastic endometrial lesions; however, whether deregulation of TGFα is involved in the pathogenesis of endometrial cancer is still not clear.

DMBA treatment was found to reduce the incidence of cystic endometrial hyperplasia in both transgenic and nontransgenic although the effect was most significant in the CD1 mice. DMBA treatment has been shown to reduce the mean uterine weight in female rodents which is associated with significant depletion of oocytes, follicles, and corpus lutea (Manoharan and Rao, 1980). The reduction in cystic hyperplasia seen in the uteri of both CD-1 and TGFα transgenic animals upon DMBA treatment may be explained by the depletion of ovarian follicles resulting in decreased ovarian function and less production of the sex steroids in these animals. In fact, it has been shown that combined neonatal estrogen plus DMBA results in a greater depletion of oocytes than in neonatally estrogen treated only. Regardless of the mechanism of DMBA effects, the presence of the TGFα transgene maintained higher levels of cystic endometrial hyperplasia under the influence of DMBA than was seen in the CD-1 nontransgenic mice suggesting that the presence of TGFα may compensates somewhat for reduced ovarian function possibly by mimicking estrogen. However, it is notably that DMBA effects on endometrial hyperplasia was not concordant with the development of uterine adenocarcinomas.

Transgenic studies have clearly demonstrated that the carcinogenic, co-carcinogenic, or promoting effects of TGFα varies depending on the organ, carcinogen, promoter, and hormonal environment. The most impressive characteristic of mammary carcinogenesis in TGFα transgenic mice is that tumor development is clearly dependent on exposure of the mammary gland to multiple rounds of pregnancy involving repeated cycles of lobular-alveolar growth, differentiation, lactation, and involution (Matsui, et al., 1990; Smith, et al., 1995). Inappropriate TGFα expression appears to potentiate the development of preneoplastic hyperplastic alveolar nodules by increasing the proliferative index and enhancing survival during postlactationally-induced apoptosis. These events are proposed to result in the creation of a population of cells that may be more susceptible to additional transforming mutations which ultimately leads to malignant transformation.

We can only provide speculation concerning the mechanism by which TGFα potentiates DES-induced lesions in the reproductive tract. Carcinogenesis of the reproductive tract has several features in common with mammary gland tumorigenesis in that genital tract neoplasia is clearly a multistage process involving pathologically distinct intermediate preneoplastic stages consisting of hyper-proliferative premalignant lesions. Also, long term exposure to endogenous hormones is instrumental to the DES oncogenic process in the reproductive tract. Thus, as found in the mammary gland, we speculate that inappropriate expression of TGFα may contribute to the development of pathological lesions in the reproductive tract by conferring a selective growth advantage and enabling cells to escape from apoptosis.

However, it is clear that the role TGFα plays in hormonal carcinogenesis of the mammary gland is different from that played in the uterus and vagina. Unlike in the mammary gland, TGFα did not significantly increase the development of uterine carcinomas in the transgenic animals compared to the parental mice in the investigated time-frame of 12 months, even though the incidence of various proliferative and differentiation lesions were increased. We raise the question as to why the increase in endometrial hyperplasia seen in the transgenics does not translate into increased tumorigenesis? It is also possible that hyperplastic endometrial lesions may not be precursors to uterine adenocarcinomas so that an increase in hyperplasia will not result in more neoplasias. The role of estrogen in mediating the transition between excessive growth and neoplastic transformation of the endometrium is still unclear. In addition to estrogen-dependent endometrial tumors that progress through distinct precursor stages, it is also proposed that endometrial cancer can arise independent of estrogen without evidence of hyperplastic preneoplastic stages. Consequently, the etiology of these tumors may not involve persistent induction of peptide growth factors such as TGFα. Our study did not show a correlation between the incidence of endometrial hyperplasia and the development of adenocarcinomas which indicates that the mechanism of DES-induced carcinogenesis of the uterus may involve events other than hyperplasia and the overexpression of a single growth factor.

It cannot be ruled out that a general effect of the TGFα transgene on the hypothalamic-pituitary-ovarian axis may be contributing to the development of uterine and vaginal lesions by altering the endocrine environment of the animal. In fact, a recent study by Ma et al (1994) clearly demonstrates that overexpression of the TGFα transgene has disrupting effects on hypothalamic and ovarian function, and that chronic TGFα expression is deleterious to female reproduction. Furthermore, our finding of pituitary adenomas in TGFα female transgenics implicates TGFα in growth regulation of the pituitary (Kudlow, et al., 1989). Clearly further studies are needed to understand the relative contributions of TGFα-induced alterations in the endocrine environment versus direct autocrine/paracrine tissue effects in reproductive tissues; but nonetheless, our study presented here provides further evidence of the importance of TGFα in many aspects of reproductive physiology.

In conclusion, the potentiation of DES and DMBA lesions in TGFα transgenic mice further supports the hypothesis that deregulation of peptide growth factors is involved in the pathogenesis of some reproductive tract diseases. However, the TGFα transgene did not promote DES-induced reproductive tract neoplasia indicating that estrogen carcinogenesis involves more than aberrant expression of this single peptide growth factor.

REFERENCES

Bockman, DE, Sharp, R, Merlino, G (1995): Regulation of terminal differentiation of zymogenic cells by transforming growth factor α in transgenic. Gastroenterol 108:447-454.

Bossert, NL, Nelson Gray, K, Ross, KA, et al. (1990): Epidermal growth factor binding and receptor distribution in the mouse reproductive tract during development. Develop Biol 142:75-85.

Cohen, I (1994): Endometrial changes with tamoxifen: comparison between tamoxifen-treated and non-treated asymptomatic, postmenopausal breast cancer patients. Gynecol Oncol 52:185-195.

Futterweit, W (1984): "Polycystic Ovarian Disease". New York Berlin Heidelberg Tokyo: Springer.

Gardner, RM, Verner, G, Kirkland, JL, et al.(1989): Regulation of uterine epidermal growth factor (EGF) receptors by estrogen in the mature rat during the estrous cycle. J Steroid Biochem 32:339-343.

Gray Nelson, K, Sakai, Y, Eitzman, B, et al. (1994): Exposure to diethylstilbestrol during a critical developmental period of the mouse reproductive tract leads to persistent induction of two estrogen-regulated genes. Cell Growth & Different 5:595-606.

Halling, A, Forsberg, J-G (1993): Acute and permanent growth effects in the mouse uterus after neonatal treatment with estrogens. Reprod Toxicol 7:137-153.

Iguchi, T (1992): Cellular effects of early exposure to sex hormones and antihormones. Intl Rev Cytol 139:1-57.

Jhappan, C, Stable, C, Harkins, RN, et al. (1990): TGFα overexpression in transgenic mice induces liver neoplasia and abnormal development of the mammary gland and pancreas. Cell 61:1137-1146.

Jhappan, C, Takayama, H, Dickson, RB, et al.(1994): Transgenic mice provide genetic evidence that TGFα promotes skin tumorigenesis via H-Ras-dependent and H-Ras independent pathways. Cell Growth Differentiation 5:385-394.

Kudlow JE, Leung, AWC, Kobrin, MS, et al. (1989): Transforming growth factor-α in the mammalian brain. J Biol Chem 264:3880-3883.

Ma, YJ, Dissen, GA, Merlino, G, et al. (1994): Overexpression of a human transforming growth factor-α (TGFα) transgene reveals a dual antagonistic role of TGFα in female sexual development. Endocrinol 135:1392-1400.

Manoharan, K, Rao, AR (1980): Influence of exogenous estrogen on oocyte depletion induced by 7,12-dimethylbenz[a]anthracene in mice. Cancer Letters 10:359-363.

Matsui, Y, Halter, SA, Holt, JT, Hogan, BLM, Coffey, R.J. Development of mammary hyperplasia and neoplasia in MMTV-TGFα transgenic mice. Cell 61:1147-1155,

McLachlan, JA, Wong, A, Degen, GH, Barrett, JC (1982): Morphological and neoplastic transformation of Syrian hamster embryo fibroblasts by diethylstilbestrol and its analogs. Cancer Res 42:3040-3045.

Metzler, M, McLachlan, JA (1977): Oxidative metabolites of diethylstilbestrol in the fetal, neonatal, and adult mouse. Biochem Pharmacol 27:1087-1094.

Pollard, JW (1990): Regulation of polypeptide growth factor synthesis and growth factor-related gene expression in the rat and mouse uterus before and after implantation. J Reprod Fertil 88:721-731.

Nelson Gray, K, Takahashi, T, Bossert, NL, et al. (1989): Epidermal growth factor replaces estrogen in the stimulation of female genital-tract growth and differentiation. Proc Natl Acad Sci USA, 88:21-25.

Nelson Gray, K, Takahashi, T, Lee, DC, et al. (1992): Transforming growth factor-α is a potential mediator of estrogen action in the mouse uterus. Endocrinol 131:1657-1664.

Noller, KL, O'Brien, PC, Colton, T, et al (1990): Medical and surgical diseases associated with in utero exposure to diethylstilbestrol. In Noller LL (ed): "Clinical Practice of Gynecology." New York: Elsevier Science Publishing Co. Inc., pp 1-7.

Reinartz, JJ, George, E, Lindgren, BR, et al. (1994): Expression of transforming growth factor alpha, epidermal growth factor receptor, and erbB-2 in endometrial carcinoma and correlation with survival and known predictors of survival. Hum Pathol25:1075-1083.

Sharp, R, Babyatsky, MW, Takagi, H, et al. (1995): Transforming growth factor α disrupts the normal program of cellular differentiation in the gastric mucosa of transgenic mice. Development 121:149-161.

Smith, GH, Sharp, R, Kordon, EC, et al. (1995): Transforming growth factor-α promotes mammary tumorigenesis through selective survival and growth of secretory epithelial cells. Am J Pathol 147:1081-1096.

Takagi, H, Sharp, R, Taklayama, H, et al. (1993): Collaboration between growth factors and diverse chemical carcinogens in hepatocarcinogenesis of transforming growth factor α transgenic mice. Cancer Res 53:4339-4336.

Vassar, R, Hutton, ME, Fuchs, E (1992): Transgenic overexpression of transforming growth factor α bypasses the need for c-Ha-ras mutations in mouse skin tumorigenesis. Mol Cell Biol 12:4643-4653.

Etiology of Breast and
Gynecological Cancers, pages 233–243
© 1997 Wiley-Liss, Inc.

ESTROGENS AND THE GENETIC CONTROL OF TUMOR GROWTH

Jack Gorski, Douglas Wendell, David Gregg, and Tae-Yon Chun

Departments of Biochemistry and Meat and Animal Science, University of Wisconsin, Madison, WI 53706

The estrogen-induced pituitary tumor of the Fischer 344 (F344) rat has many important similarities to human breast cancer. These tumors occur in 100% of F344 rats treated with estrogen and are discernible by 3 weeks of treatment. Because of the existence of rat strains that are resistant to these tumors, we can use techniques of genetic analysis on this animal model to gain a better understanding of tumor growth.

It is generally accepted that estrogens play a major role in the development of breast cancer in humans. Evidence supporting this hypothesis includes the correlation of lifetime estrogen exposure with breast cancer incidence, and the estrogen-dependence of breast cancer cells grown *in vitro* or when these cells are transplanted into animal models (Nandi et al., 1995). Despite a great deal of experimental and clinical data, estrogen's exact role in breast cancer is not understood. How and when estrogen promotes cancer and its molecular targets needs to be understood in order to design more effective treatments to cure this second-most lethal cancer in women. Such an endeavor is complicated by the fact that estrogen is also required for normal breast development. Thus, estrogen stimulus of mammary growth and development is normally limited by control mechanisms that fail to function in estrogen-dependent tumors.

Such a balance of stimulation and control of growth can be seen in certain animal models. As shown in Figure 1, when estrogen is continuously administered to a variety of rat strains, DNA synthesis rate and cell proliferation increase in the uterus during a 24 to 48 hour period but then return to prestimulation levels despite the continued presence of estrogen (Wiklund and Gorski, 1982). In other words, a control mechanism exists to limit the extent of stimulation.

The pituitary gland of most rat strains responds to estrogen similarly. However, in F344 rats, DNA synthesis remains elevated and growth proceeds continuously for at least 12 weeks of estrogen treatment. After 8 weeks of exposure to chronic high doses of estrogen, the pituitaries of F344 rats increase in mass 5- to

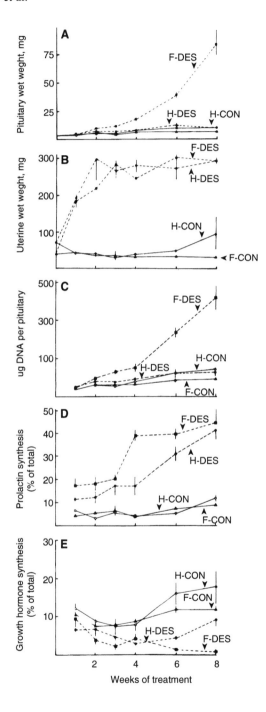

8-fold, from 12 to 15 mg in controls to 80 to 100 mg in the estrogen treated rats, while the pituitaries of Holtzman rats show no significant pituitary mass increase (Wiklund et al., 1981a). The resultant tumor is largely due to an increase in the number of lactotrophs. In control animals, approximately 10 to 15% of the cells are lactotrophs but this increases to 70% after sustained exposure to estrogen in the F344 rats. The uteri of both strains do not show this continuous growth response to estrogen (Wiklund et al., 1981b). Thus, the F344 rat provides an *in vivo*, estrogen-dependent tumor model that has the potential to be manipulated genetically and to reveal the mechanisms of estrogen control of tumor growth.

Early studies in our laboratory showed that the DNA synthesis rate in the pituitaries of Holtzman and F344 rats was similar for 3 to 5 days of estrogen treatment (Wiklund and Gorski, 1982). However, after 7 to 10 days of estrogen treatment, the rate of DNA synthesis drops back to control levels in the Holtzman rats but not in the F344 rats as shown in Figure 2. This decrease in DNA synthesis is not due to a general refractoriness to estrogen since prolactin synthesis continues at a high rate for extended periods of estrogen treatment in the Holtzman rat pituitaries (Wiklund et al., 1981b). That this growth of F344 pituitaries requires continuous exposure to estrogen is shown by the fact that withdrawal of estrogen for 1 week results in a dramatic decrease of pituitary mass (Table 1). These observations suggest that tissue growth and cell replication are normally limited by mechanisms that prevent excessive growth beyond some defined limits. These mechanisms have a genetic basis that can be overcome due to genetic selection or damage. Understanding these growth control mechanisms may provide a basis for understanding other tumors and cancer in humans.

GENETIC ANALYSIS OF ESTROGEN-DEPENDENT PITUITARY TUMORS

The difference between the Holtzman and F344 rat strains in estrogen-induced growth of their pituitaries provides a model for biochemical and genetic dissection. A series of crosses and back-crosses between the two strains provided data for genetic analysis. Wiklund et al. (1981a) suggested that estrogen-dependent pituitary tumor formation in the rat is due to variation at two or three genetic loci. This model viewed estrogen induction of pituitary hyperplasia in terms of a tumor incidence model. Under this model, rats were classified as having developed a pituitary tumor if their pituitary mass exceeded the threshold values of 17.5 mg for males and 19 mg for females. The probability of a given rat developing a pituitary tumor in response to estrogen was hypothesized to be determined by the number of susceptible (F344) alleles at the tumor susceptibility loci. The F344 strain thus had a 100% incidence of pituitary tumor induction due to homozygosity for susceptible alleles at all loci. Wiklund et al. (1981a) measured tumor incidence in F_2 and backcross progeny. They found that the resulting frequency of tumors fit a model of multiple, most likely two or

---

Figure 1. Chronic DES treatment of F344 and Holtzman rats. At zero time, weanling females were ovariectomized and given silastic tubing implants containing 5 mg DES. At the indicated times, animals were sacrificed, and their pituitaries were removed, weighed, and incubated for 1 h in medium containing [^{3}H]leucine. Prolactin and growth hormone syntheses were measured by sodium dodecyl sulfate-polyacrylamide gel electrophoresis. Taken from Wicklund et al. (1981b) with permission of the authors.

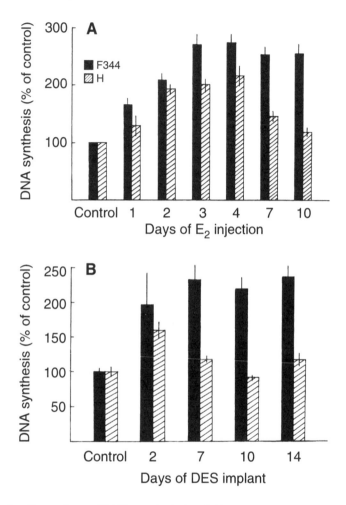

Figure 2. Comparison of DNA synthesis in F344 and strains after daily estrogen treatment. **A.** Male rats (42 to 49 days old) were given daily injections of 10 µg estradiol and DNA synthesis in isolated nuclei was measured 24 h after the last injection. Values are the mean ± SEM of at least five independent groups of animals (three animals per group). **B.** Male rats (42 to 49 days old) were given s.c. silastic tubing implants containing 5 mg DES and were sacrificed at the indicated number of days after implant. Pituitary nuclei were assayed for DNA synthesis. Values are the mean ± SEM of three independent groups of animals (three animals per group). Taken from Wickland and Gorski (1982) with permission of the authors.

three, loci. For example, the three-locus model shown in Figure 3 predicted a tumor incidence of 92% in the progeny of the backcross of F_1 to F344, which the experimental value fit closely at 94% (Wiklund et al., 1981a). This analysis indicated that each locus contributes additively to the overall probability of tumor formation. The data suggest that, although multiple genes are involved, there are probably only a few major loci. Thus, this system is simple enough to be used for finding and characterizing the genes and their products that are involved in estrogen-dependent tumors.

MOLECULAR DISSECTION OF ESTROGEN-DEPENDENT TUMORS

Two approaches have been used to study the molecular basis of pituitary tumor growth. One, the comparison of two-dimensional gel electrophoresis patterns of protein extracts from the two strains, has not revealed any differences (Wiklund, 1980).

Table 1. Average pituitary weights for DES-treated and control animals.

Genotype	Sex	+DES		-DES	
		Pituitary wt (mean ± SD)	No. of animals	Pituitray wt (mean ± SD)	No. of animals
F322	M	47.1 ± 17.5	100	8.5 ± 1.0	12
	F	88.0 ± 27.3	53	11.3 ± 2.0	4
Holtzman	M	12.8 ± 4.7	72	10.0 ± 1.9	23
	F	12.3 ± 4.5	46	12.9 ± 0.1	3
F_1A	M	18.4 ± 4.9	53	10.3 ± 1.2	16
	F	26.8 ± 13.2	59	13.8 ± 1.1	4
F_1B	M	16.1 ± 5.5	29	7.2 ± 1.2	6
	F	18.3 ± 5.2	25	8.4 ± 1.5	4
F_2	M	30.0 ± 17.0	57	9.2 ± 1.0	4
	F	36.4 ± 17.6	67	13.6 ± 1.5	4
Backcross to F344	M	30.6 ± 13.4	47	8.9 ± 0.4	4
	F	43.8 ± 18.5	50	12.4 ± 0.6	4
Backcross to Holtzman	M	18.7 ± 7.8	30	9.2 ± 1.0	4
	F	17.1 ± 6.6	52	13.6 ± 1.3	4

Weanling rats were separated according to sex and given implants containing 5 mg DES. Control animals were left untreated. After 8 weeks, the animals were killed, and their pituitaries were weighed. The number of animals per group is indicated. F_1A and F_1B are reciprocal crosses using Holtzman and F344 dams, respectively Taken from Wiklund et al. (1981a) with permission from the authors.

Three Loci Genetic Model

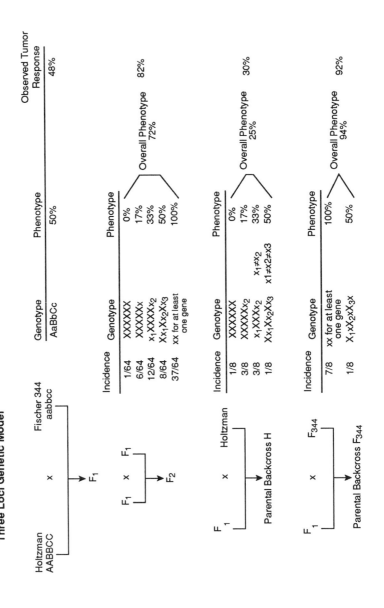

However, this technique shows only those proteins that are present in relatively large quantities. Less abundant proteins that are likely to be involved in regulation will not be detected by this technique. Similarly, subtractive hybridization and differential display electrophoresis of mRNA have been attempted but to date have not revealed any notable difference between the two rat strains in a specific mRNA.

The other approach that has been used to study the molecular difference in the pituitaries of the two rat strains has been the examination of specific genes and their products. We have recently shown that carboxypeptidase E is markedly depleted in F344 pituitaries after continuous estrogen treatment (Gregg et al., 1996). The significance of this observation is not clear but a recent report indicated that carboxypeptidase is found bound to DNA as part of a transcription regulation complex in adipocytes. It was suggested that the peptidase activity might involve modification of transcription factors to more active or less active forms. This enzyme also has a potential role in modifying growth factors or other regulatory proteins removing terminal amino acids. More work is necessary to determine the exact role of this enzyme in pituitary tumor formation.

A number of other proteins and/or their mRNAs have also been examined in this model system. In particular, a variety of oncogene products such as several ras genes, the retinoblastoma gene, cell cycle regulating genes such as cyclin D3 and cyclin dependent kinase 4, etc., have been studied and to date none of these have given any evidence of involvement with the development of estrogen induced tumors (T.-Y. Chun and J. Gorski, unpublished data). This suggests that perhaps a new oncogene or anti-oncogene may be involved. Further analysis is needed, perhaps by using populations comprised of pure or enriched lactotrophs.

ANGIOGENESIS AND TUMOR FORMATION

Angiogenesis is the process by which normal growing tissues as well as tumors achieve neovascularization necessary for their growth. Inhibition of angiogenesis has been shown to stop tumor growth in certain animal models (Millauer et al., 1994;

Figure 3. Genetic model involving three loci. A, B, and C code for three pituitary proteins, each essential for the control of DES-stimulated cell proliferation and resistance to pituitary tumor induction. The Holtzman strain is homozygous normal for all three loci. The F344 strain carries mutant alleles and makes no functional A, B, or C protein. The F_1 generation is heterozygous at all three loci. If the cellular levels of proteins A, B. and C are critical for the control of cell proliferation, then the F_1 heterozygote, which may make half the normal amount of proteins A, B, and C, may have a 50% probability of developing a pituitary tumor. The possible genotypes for the various crosses are listed, with X denoting a gene from the Holtzman strain and x denoting a gene from the F344 strain. The phenotypes are derived by assuming that an F344 allele endows the offspring with 17% (one in six) tumor incidence if accompanied by the corresponding Holtzman allele. the lowercase letters with subscripts (x_1, x_2, and x_3) denote nonallelic F344 genes. If proteins A, B, and C are all essential for cell proliferation control, then genotypes that are homozygous for F344 alleles at any of the loci will yield phenotypes with 100% tumor incidence. The overall tumor incidences predicted by this model are compared to the experimentally observed incidences shown on the far right. Taken from Wicklund et al. (1981a) with permission of the authors.

O'Reilly et al., 1994). In addition to being needed to feed the growing tumor mass, neovascularization provides a route for the spread of metastases and the regulation of their growth (Fidler and Ellis, 1994). Clinical studies have found that increased microvessel density of mammary tumors is correlated with an increased risk of metastatic disease (Weidner et al., 1991).

The estrogen-dependent pituitary tumor of F344 rats also exhibits dramatic vascular changes (Elias and Weiner, 1984). After prolonged estrogen treatment, F344 pituitaries contain hemorrhagic lakes and increased vascular density (Elias and Weiner, 1984; Schechter and Weiner, 1991). Normally, the pituitary receives its blood supply via the hypothalamus. However, Elias and Weiner (1984) demonstrated that in response to estrogen, new arteries invade the pituitary of the F344 rat to provide it with a systemic blood supply. Such drastic changes are not observed in the pituitaries of estrogen-treated rats of tumor-resistant strains. Therefore, as with growth, the F344 pituitary tumor is a model system in which genetic techniques can be used to study tumor angiogenesis.

The relationship between estrogen and mammary tumor angiogenesis is not well defined. Estrogen is known to stimulate normal angiogenesis of other tissues, such as the endometrium of the uterus (Findlay, 1986) and umbilical vein endothelial cells (Morales et al., 1995). Evidence of estrogen's role in the angiogenesis of estrogen-dependent mammary tumors is very limited. Haran et al. (1994) showed that administration of tamoxifen produced a decrease in capillary endothelial density in MCF-7 cell tumors transplanted into mice. A direct effect by estradiol has not been proven, however. This problem is inherent in such experiments because altering the estrogen present in a cultured or transplanted tissue affects growth in general. Is the effect on angiogenesis due to a direct requirement of estrogen by endothelial cells invading the tumor or is it due to the effect of estrogen on tumor cell growth, which in turn regulates angiogenesis?

We have examined the mRNA content for several angiogenic factors in F344 rat pituitaries as compared with Holtzman controls (D. Gregg, E. Goedken, and J. Gorski, unpublished data). Thus far we have not seen any notable differences between the strains in vascular endothelial growth factor, angiogenin, β-fibroblast growth factor, and thrombospondin 1 mRNAs. It is possibile that new angiogenic factors or regulation of the activity of known angiogenic factors by mechanisms were not revealed by our studies of mRNA content. For example, modification of an angiogenic factor protein by carboxypeptidase E might cause a marked effect on tumor vascularization but would not be detected by the screening we have done to date.

GENETIC TOOLS FOR TUMOR BIOLOGY

Estrogen-induced pituitary tumors of F344 rats have been the object of research for many years (Dunning et al., 1947; Kaplan and DeNicola, 1976; Wiklund et al., 1981a; Elias and Weiner, 1984). Unfortunately, the molecular targets of the estrogen-estrogen receptor complex in the estrogen-dependent rat pituitary tumor are still not known. Another approach, gene mapping, can lead to the identification and experimental manipulation of estrogen's target genes that would not be possible through other means. Methods developed in recent years have made it possible to use this system to make new contributions to tumor biology. The genes responsible for this tumor formation can be mapped by detecting the linkage of tumor susceptibility genes to molecular markers (Lander and Botstein, 1989; Lander and Schork, 1994). The advent of simple sequence repeat (SSR) polymorphisms as genetic markers (Litt and Luty, 1989; Weber and May, 1989) and methods for dissecting complex traits by interval mapping (Lander and Botstein, 1989; Zeng, 1994) provide a quantum leap for genetic analysis in mammals. SSRs are abundant, highly polymorphic, phenotypically neutral, and easily scored by polymerase chain reaction (PCR). Powerful statistical software packages such as MAPMAKER/QTL (Paterson et al., 1991) and QTL-Cartographer (Zeng, 1994) have been developed that detect the linkage between molecular markers and genes affecting complex traits in crosses between inbred lines. Mapping tumor formation genes not only identifies these genes from the standpoint of transmission genetics, but gives a starting point for molecular cloning as well.

Interval mapping is the most powerful method of quantitative trait locus (QTL) mapping. Basically, a genetic map is constructed based on segregation of the markers. Intervals along this map are then evaluated for their ability to explain the quantitative phenotypic data, given the hypothesis that the genetic interval contains a locus affecting the trait of interest. In addition to mapping loci, MAPMAKER/QTL can be used to perform other analyses important to understanding the transmission of a complex trait. For each locus identified, it calculates the proportion of phenotypic variance explained. This indicates the relative influence of each of the multiple genes responsible for the phenotype and indicates if all the genetic variance, and, hence, all or most of the genes, have been mapped. In an F_2 intercross, MAPMAKER/QTL can also be used to test whether the alleles at the identified locus have a dominant/recessive or additive relationship (Paterson et al., 1991). A difficulty with this approach is the long time necessary to obtain the animal data, which requires breeding animals and long-time exposure to estrogen of the resulting progeny. In addition, the distribution of markers in the genome may not be optimal for a particular trait. Fine mapping the genes responsible for estrogen-induced tumors will be difficult but should provide exciting data.

SUMMARY

Biochemical and genetic studies of the estrogen-induced pituitary tumors of the F344 rat provide a new model for understanding cancer biology. Because a genetic difference in tumor susceptibly already exists in this animal model it is possible to search for the underlying mechanisms. Interestingly, thus far marked changes in expression of known or unknown oncogenes do not appear to be involved in the formation of this tumor. Similarly, known angiogenic factors have not been implicated in this model's dramatic angiogenic response to estrogen. It will be very informative to dissect out the critical genes and the products that are involved in this system and then to determine whether similar genes are involved in human, estrogen-induced cancers.

ACKNOWLEDGMENTS

The authors would like to thank the current members of the Gorski for help with the critical reading of this manuscript, to former members of the lab for the work that has gone before, and to Kathryn Holtgraver for editorial assistance.

This work was sponsored in part by the College of Agricultural and Life Sciences, University of Wisconsin; National Institutes of Health Grants HD08192, HD07259, and CA58013 awarded to J.G.; by NRSA Fellowship CA67422 and a gift of

Mrs. Ida Soreng-Cobb to the University of Wisconsin Comprehensive Cancer Center awarded to D.W.; and by American Cancer Society Fellowship PF-3673 awarded to D.G.

REFERENCES

Dunning WF, Curtis MR, Segaloff A (1947): Strain differences in response to diethylstilbestrol and the induction of mammary gland and bladder cancer in the rat. Cancer Res 7:511-521.

Elias KA, Weiner RI (1984): Direct arterial vascularization of estrogen-induced prolactin-secreting anterior pituitary tumors. Proc Natl Acad Sci USA 81:4549-4553.

Fidler IJ, Ellis LM (1994): The implications of angiogenesis for the biology and therapy of cancer metastasis. Cell 79:185-188.

Findlay JK (1986): Angiogenesis in reproductive tissues. J Endocrinol 111:357-366.

Gregg D, Goedken E, Galkin M, Wendell D, Gorski J (1996): Decreased expression of carboxypeptidase E protein is correlated to estrogen-induction of rat pituitary tumors. Mol Cell Endocrinol In Press.

Haran EF, Maretzek AF, Goldberg I, Horowitx A, Degani H (1994): Tamoxifen inhibits cell death in implanted MCF7 breast cancer by inhibiting endothelium growth. Cancer Res 54:5511-5514.

Kaplan SE, DeNicola AF (1976): Protein and RNA synthesis in pituitary tumors from F344 rats given implants of estrogens. J Natl Cancer Inst 56:37-.

Lander ES, Botstein D (1989): Mapping Mendelian factors underlying quantitative traits using RFLP linkage maps. Genetics 121:185-199.

Lander ES, Schork NJ (1994): Genetic dissection of complex traits. Science 265:2037-2048.

Litt M, Luty JA (1989): A hypervariable microsatellite revealed by *in vitro* amplificaation of a dinucleotide repeat within the cardiac muscle actin gene. Am J Hum Genet 44:397-401.

Millauer B, Shawver LK, Plate KH, Risau W, Ullrich A (1994): Glioblastoma growth inhibited *in vivo* by a dominant-negative Flk-1 mutant. Nature 367:576-579.

Morales DE, McGowan KA, Grant DS, Maheshwari S, Bhartiya D, Cid MC, Kleinman HK, Schnaper HW (1995): Estrogen promotes angiogenic activity in human umbilical vein endothelial cells in vitro and in a murine model. Circulation 91:755-763.

Nandi S, Guzman RC, Yang J (1995): Hormones and mammary carcinogenesis in mice, rats, and humans: A unifying hypothesis. Proc Natl Acad Sci USA 92:3650-3657.

O'Reilly MS, Holmgren L, Shing Y, Chen C, Rosenthal RA, Moses M, Lane WS, Cao Y, Sage EH, Folkman J (1994): Angiostatin: a novel angiogenesis inhibitor that mediates the suppression of metastases by a Lewis lung carcinoma. Cell 79:315-328.

Paterson AH, Damon S, Hewitt JD, Zamir D, Rabinowitch HD, S.E. L, Lander ES, Tanksley SD (1991): Mendelian factors underlying quantitative traits in tomato: comparison across species, generations, and environments. Genetics 127:181-197.

Schechter J , Weiner R (1991): Changes in basic fibroblast growth factor coincident with estradiol-induced hyperplasia of the anterior pituitaries of Fischer 344 and Sprague-Dawley rats. Endocrinology 129:2400-2408.

Weber JL, May PE (1989): Abundant class of human DNA polymorphisms which can be typed using the polymerase chain reaction. Am J Hum Genet 44:388-396.

Weidner N, Semple JP, Welch WR, Folkman J (1991): Tumor angiogenesis and metastasis: correlation in invasive breast carcinoma. New Engl J Med Wiklund 324:1-8.

JA (1980): Estrogen induced pituitary growth and DNA synthesis: genetic differences in response to chronic treatment in the rat. Ph.D. Thesis. University of Wisconsin-Madison. 185.

Wiklund J, Gorski J (1982): Genetic differences in estrogen-induced deoxyribonucleic acid synthesis in the rat pituitary: correlations with pituitary tumor susceptability. Endocrinology 111:1140-1149.

Wiklund J, Rutledge J, Gorski J (1981a): A genetic model for the inheritance of pituitary tumor susceptibility in F344 rats. Endocrinology 109:1708-1714.

Wiklund J, Wertz N, Gorski J (1981b): A comparison of estrogen effects on uterine and pituitary growth and prolactin synthesis in F344 and Holtzman rats. Endocrinology 109:1700-1707.

Zeng Z-B (1994): Precision mapping of quantitative trait loci. Genetics 136:1457-1468.

Etiology of Breast and
Gynecological Cancers, pages 245–255
© 1997 Wiley-Liss, Inc.

TARGETED ANTIESTROGENS

Debra A. Tonetti and V. Craig Jordan

Robert H. Lurie Cancer Center
Northwestern University Medical School
Chicago, Illinois 60611

TAMOXIFEN THERAPY FOR BREAST CANCER

Tamoxifen, a non-steroidal antiestrogen, was clinically tested as a treatment for advanced breast cancer in 1971, and in the past 25 years has become the endocrine treatment of choice for all stages of breast cancer (Jordan, 1994). The initial observation that estrogen may stimulate the growth of some breast cancers was made by Beatson in 1896. Over a half century later, the estrogen receptor (ER) was identified (Jensen and Jacobson, 1962). Of the 50-80% of all breast cancers that are ER-positive (ER+), 70-80% of these patients with both ER+ and progesterone receptor-positive (PR+) tumors will respond to endocrine therapy. Tamoxifen which is classified as a partial antiestrogen competes with estrogen for the ligand binding site on the ER, and blocks its action. It has also been demonstrated that just 2-5 years of tamoxifen therapy will reduce the risk of contralateral breast cancer by 39% and enhance patient survival by preventing recurrence (Early Breast Cancer Trialists' Group, 1992). In addition to relatively few undesirable side effects, tamoxifen therapy produces several beneficial side effects including the maintainance of bone density and reduced risk of coronary heart disease.

TARGET SITE-SPECIFICITY OF ANTIESTROGENS

Breast

Tamoxifen is a partial agonist/antagonist and therefore may act as an estrogen or an antiestrogen, depending on the tissue and species examined. In the breast, tamoxifen acts as a potent antiestrogen. The tamoxifen metabolite, 4-hydroxytamoxifen (4-OHT) competes with estradiol at the ligand binding domain of the ER. Even though the 4-OHT/ER homodimer binds to the estrogen response element (ERE), transcriptional activation is prevented (Pham et al., 1991), whereas the mechanism of inhibition by pure antiestrogens such as ICI 182,780 is reported to involve degradation of the ER. Unfortunately, often with time, the therapeutic benefit of tamoxifen therapy declines resulting in disease recurrence. The exact mechanism of acquired tamoxifen resistance is at the present time unknown, although due to the complex nature of the ER-mediated signal transduction pathway, the etiology is likely to be multifactorial (Tonetti and Jordan, 1995).

Bone

Since estrogen contributes to the maintainance of bone density, postmenopausal women are at increased risk of developing osteoporosis. Therefore it was initially of concern that the antiestrogenic effects of tamoxifen therapy may promote accelerated bone loss. That this was not the case was first demonstrated in the laboratory where tamoxifen was shown to prevent bone loss in the ovariectomized rat (Jordan et al., 1987). Since these initial observations in the laboratory, numerous clinical studies have demonstrated estrogenic effects of tamoxifen on bone (reviewed in Wright and Compston, 1995). One of the most definitive studies showed that in a randomized double-blind placebo-controlled trial following at least 2 years of tamoxifen therapy in postmenopausal women, bone mineral density was maintained in the lumbar spine compared to bone loss in untreated women (Love et al., 1992). In addition, measurement of biochemical markers of bone metabolism including serum osteocalcin and alkaline phosphatase were consistent with the preservation of bone mass in these women. The current trials of tamoxifen as a preventive for breast cancer ongoing in the UK, Italy and the US (Jordan, 1993) will provide us with further data to ascertain the extent of the bone preserving effects of tamoxifen.

Liver

Tamoxifen exhibits estrogen-like effects on circulating cholesterol levels, another clear beneficial side effect. Specifically, there is a reduction in low-density lipoprotein (LDL) cholesterol, without affecting high-density lipoprotein (HDL) (Love et al., 1994, 1991). These data may have physiological significance because a reduction in the incidence of fatal myocardial infarction was reported following 5 years of adjuvant tamoxifen therapy (McDonald and Stewart., 1991). The lipid lowering properties of tamoxifen may involve an ER-independent mechanism. Possible mechanisms may include inhibition of cholesterol synthesis (Gylling et al., 1992) and prevention of oxidative damage to LDLs (Wiseman et al., 1993), a process known to contribute to atherosclerosis.

Numerous reports in the literature describe tamoxifen's ability to produce liver tumors in rats and induce DNA adducts both *in vivo* and *in vitro* (Williams et al., 1993; Hard et al., 1993). Of concern is the potential risk of inducing hepatocellular carcinoma in patients receiving tamoxifen therapy. Several lines of evidence have now accumulated to allay these concerns. The first is to realize that the relative daily dose used in treatment are far below the levels used to initiate carcinogenesis (250 µg/kg versus 5 mg/kg) and the duration of treatment in the rat is from puberty to the remainder of the animal's life while the patient is usually treated for about 6% of her lifetime (Jordan, 1995). Since only 2 cases of hepatocellular carcinoma have been reported during adjuvant tamoxifen therapy (Fornander et al, 1989), the risk of developing such a cancer must be put in perspective compared to the benefit of therapy. No increase in the total number of DNA adducts was found in the livers of patients treated with tamoxifen compared to an untreated group (Martin et al., 1995).

Uterus

In the uterus, tamoxifen exhibits estrogenic effects. The first indication of this was illustrated in the laboratory when an endometrial carcinoma and a breast carcinoma were transplanted on either side of an athymic mouse and following estrogen + tamoxifen treatment, the breast carcinoma was growth inhibited, whereas the endometrial carcinoma was growth stimulated (Gottardis et al., 1988). It has now been well documented that tamoxifen therapy is associated with increased incidence of endometrial carcinoma (Assikis and Jordan, 1995). However it seems that upon closer examination of the clinical data, the majority of cases of endometrial carcinoma are of low-grade and early stage disease, and therefore the benefit derived from tamoxifen therapy of increased survival from breast cancer far outweighs the risk of developing endometrial carcinoma (Jordan and Assikis, 1995). No DNA adducts are found in the uteri of tamoxifen-treated women (Dr. Lewis Smith, personal communication).

POSSIBLE MOLECULAR MECHANISMS OF ANTIESTROGEN TARGET SITE-SPECIFICITY

Due to the agonist/antagonist nature of tamoxifen action, in addition to the demonstrated increased overall and disease-free survival from breast cancer, the patient also benefits from a reduced incidence of fatal myocardial infarction and a reduced risk of osteoporotic bone fractures. It is also because of this partial agonist/antagonist activity of tamoxifen that there is an increase in the detection of endometrial carcinomas. At present, the precise mechanism of this target site-specificity remains unknown, however several hypotheses to explain this phenomenon have been offered.

Cellular Environment

One potential mechanism responsible for the target-site specificity of antiestrogens may involve the particular cellular environment in which the ER signalling pathway is operating. For example, the presence or absence of certain transcription factors, accesory proteins and/or DNA binding proteins may dictate the interpretation of the antiestrogen/ER complex as an estrogenic or an antiestrogenic signal at the estrogen response element (ERE) (Figure 1). Several recent reports have described at least eight human ER-associated proteins, hsp70, hsp90, and 45, 48, 55, 80, 140 and 160 kDa proteins (Landel et al., 1995, 1994; Cavailles et al., 1994; Halachmi et al., 1994), some of which have been shown to contribute to the stability of the ER/ERE complex. Berry et al., 1990 demonstrated the importance of cellular context by showing transactivational activity of a given ERE is dependent upon the cell type examined. Therefore, for example, endometrial cells may contain an accesory protein that is not found in breast cells which allows the tamoxifen/ER complex to assume a tighter association with the ERE, allowing transcriptional activation to occur, thus accounting for the target site-specificity observed in these two cell types.

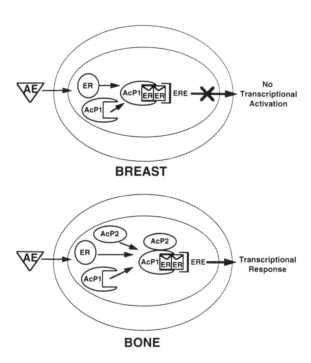

Figure 1. A specific complement of cellular factors that are cell type-specific such as accesory proteins (AcP) may dictate the transcriptional response at the ERE.

Configuration and Placement of the ERE

The configuration, sequence and/or placement of the ERE itself may dictate whether tamoxifen is interpreted as an estrogenic or antiestrogenic signal (Table 1). A plethora of evidence exists in the literature that suggests alterations to the ERE such as sequence variation, placement of multiple EREs and orientation can have a significant impact upon binding affinity of the ligand/ER complex as well as the transcsriptional response to various ligands (Klein-Hitpaß et al, 1988; Tsai et al., 1989, Martinez et al., 1989, Ponglikitmongkol et al., 1990; Naar et al., 1991; Klinge et al., 1992; Dana et al., 1994; Catherino et al., 1995). Tzukerman et al., 1994 reported that promoter context may also play a role in determining the transactivational capacity of liganded ER, specifically their data indicate that tamoxifen is a promoter-specific ER agonist. Alternatively, as a separate entity from the ERE, antiestrogen response elements (AEREs) may be present in certain estrogen responsive genes, such that an antiestrogen/ER homodimer complex may bind with high affinity to such a consensus sequence and regulate transcription. Perhaps minor modifications of the ERE as described occur in a cell-specific manner and may influence the agonist/antagonist nature of tamoxifen.

Design of the Ideal Hormone Replacement Therapy

Tamoxifen is an effective treatment for breast cancer and based upon its ability to reduce the incidence of contralateral breast cancer, three large clinical trials to evaluate its use as a breast cancer preventive agent in a targeted population of high risk women are ongoing. Although tamoxifen has numerous beneficial side effects including the maintainance of bone density and reduced risk of coronary heart disease, the undesirable side effects preclude the use of tamoxifen in women with low risk for developing breast cancer. Therefore it is of great interest to design a targeted antiestrogen to be used as an ideal hormone replacement therapy that would eliminate the concerns associated with the use of tamoxifen in healthy women (Figure 2). Such an agent must not produce liver tumors in rats at any dose and DNA adducts formation should not occur. The ideal targeted antiestrogen should act as an antiestrogen in the breast as well as in the uterus to prevent both breast and endometrial carcinomas. These antiestrogenic effects should be balanced with estrogenic effects to lower circulating cholesterol and to maintain bone density.

Targeted Antiestrogens Currently in Clinical Trial

A number of new antiestrogens have been developed such as droloxifene, raloxifene (initially named keoxifene), idoxifene and toremifene that are currently being tested in the clinic (Jordan, 1995). Two compounds, droloxifene and raloxifene, were developed based on the tamoxifen metabolite, 4-hydroxytamoxifen, that is known to bind

Table 1. Specific Cases of ERE Alterations Affecting Transcriptional Response

ERE CONFIGURATION	ACTIVITY	REFERENCE
Specific base changes within the half-site GGTNA CAG TGACC	Reduced ER binding	Klinge et al., 1992
	Estrogenic activity in response to 4-OHT	Dana et al., 1994
Specific base changes within the spacer GGTCA CNG TGACC	Evidence for a two base preference 3' of the half-site	Dana et al., 1994
Additions to the spacer GGTCA NCAGNNNN TGACC	A negatively regulated ERE contains a 7 base spacer region	Van Dijck et al., 1992
Multimerization of EREs →→ →→ →→ ERE----ERE----ERE	Multimerization of EREs enhance ER binding and estrogenic activity	Ponglikitmongkol et al., 1990; Klinge et al., 1992
Orientation and spacing of EREs →→ →→ ←← ERE-------ERE--/---ERE	Different orientation and spacing of EREs yield distinct transcriptional response	Klein-Hitpa βet al., 1988; Naar et.al, 1991

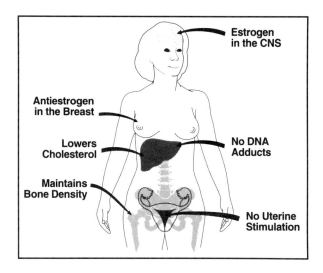

Figure 2. Properties of the ideal targeted antiestrogen

with high affinity to the ER. Droloxifene, or 3-hydroxytamoxifen, has a 10-fold higher binding affinity than tamoxifen for the ER and has a shorter half-life than tamoxifen. In addition, droloxifene exhibits lower estrogenic activity on the immature rat uterus (Hasmann et al., 1994). Based on numerous clinical trials it appears that droloxifene has potential as a treatment for breast cancer (Rauschning and Pritchard, 1994), and may also be tested as a treatment for osteoporosis. Several clinical trials are already evaluating raloxifene as a preventive treatment for osteoporosis. Raloxifene possesses several desirable qualities including preservation of bone density in laboratory animals (Jordan et al., 1987), reduction in circulating cholesterol levels, and lack of estrogenic activity in the uterus (Black et al, 1994). Although raloxifene prevents the development of carcinogen-induced rat mammary tumors, it is not as potent an antitumor agent as tamoxifen (Gottardis and Jordan, 1987).

Future Directions

The development of tamoxifen as a successful breast cancer therapy has laid the foundation for a new strategy of targeted antiestrogens for the prevention of diseases in women. The years of accumulated laboratory and clinical data in the development of tamoxifen will lend insight into the evaluation of the new targeted antiesrogens being developed. In the near future a targeted antiestrogen will be available to be used as a novel hormone replacement therapy to prevent osteoporosis and deaths from coronary heart disease. Furthermore, this new strategy will have the added advantage of reducing the risks of developing breast and endometrial cancer. Through widespread patient acceptance due to the elimination of undesirable side effects, these targeted antiestrogens should have an impressive affect on women's health.

Acknowledgements

The authors would like to acknowledge the generous support of the Lynn Sage Foundation and the Susan G. Komen Breast Cancer Foundation. We also thank Mr. Henry Muenzner for creating the computer generated schematics.

References

Assikis VJ and Jordan VC (1995): Gynecologic effect of tamoxifen and the association with endometrial carcinoma. Int J Gynecol. Obstet 49:241-257.

Black LJ, Sato M, Rowley ER, Magee DE, Bekele A, Willliams DC, Cullinan GL, Bendele R, Kauffman RF, Bensch WR, Frolik CA, Termine JD, Bryant HU (1994): Raloxifene (LY139481HC1) prevents bone loss and reduces serum cholesterol without causing uterine hypertrophy in ovariectomized rats. J Clin Invest 93:63-69.

Catherino WH and Jordan VC (1995): Increasing the number of tandem estrogen response elements increases the estrogenic activity of a tamoxifen analogue. Cancer Lett 92:39-47.

Cavailles V, Dauvois S, Danielian PS, Parker MG (1994): Interaction of proteins with transcriptionally active estrogen receptors. Proc Natl Acad Sci USA 91:10009-10013.

Dana SL, Hoener PA, Wheeler DA, Lawrence CB, McDonnell DP (1994): Novel estrogen response elements identified by genetic selection in yeast are differentially responsive to estrogens and antiestrogens in mammalian cells. Mol Endocrinol 8:1193-1207.

Early Breast Cancer Trialists' Collaborative Group (1992): Systemic treatment of early breast cancer by hormonal, cytotoxic, or immune therapy. Lancet 330:1-15.

Gottardis MM and Jordan VC (1987): Antitumor actions of keoxifene and tamoxifen in the N-nitrosomethylurea-induced rat mammary carcinoma model. Cancer Res 46:4020-4024.

Gottardis MM, Robinson SP, Satyaswaroop PG, Jordan VC (1988): Contrasting actions of tamoxifen on endometrial and breast tumor growth in the athymic mouse. Cancer Res 48:812-815.

Gylling H, Mäntylä E, Miettinen TA (1992): Tamoxifen decreases serum cholesterol by inhibiting cholesterol synthesis. Athero 96:245-247.

Halachmi S, Marden E, Martin G, MacKay H, Abbondanza C, Brown M (1994): Estrogen receptor-associated proteins: possible mediators of hormone-induced transcription. Science 264:1455-1458.

Hard GC, Iatropoulos MJ, Jordan K, Radi L, Kaltenberg OP, Imondi AR, Williams GM (1993): Major differences in the hepatocarcinogenicity and DNA adduct forming ability between toremifene and tamoxifen in female Crl: CD(BR) rats. Cancer Res 53:3919-3924.

Hasmann M, Rattel B, Löser R (1994): Preclinical data for droloxifene. Cancer Lett 84:101-116.

Jensen EV and Jacobson HI (1962): Basic guides to the mechanism of estrogen action. Recent Prog Horm Res 18:387-414.

Jordan VC and Assikis (1995): Endometrial carcinoma and tamoxifen: Clearing up a controversy. Clin Cancer Res 1:467-472.

Jordan VC (1995): What if tamoxifen (ICI 46,474) had been found to produce rat liver tumors in 1973? Annals Oncol 6:29-34.

Jordan VC (1994): The development of tamoxifen for breast cancer therapy. In Jordan VC (ed): "Long-term antiestrogen treatment for breast cancer" Madison: The University of Wisconsin Press, pp 3-26.

Jordan VC (1993): A current view of tamoxifen for the treatment and prevention of breast cancer. Br J Pharmacol 110:507-517.

Jordan VC, Phelps E, Lindgren JU (1987): Effect of antiestrogens on bone in castrated and intact female rats. Breast Cancer Res Treat 10:31-35.

Klein-Hitpaß L, Kaling M, Ryffel GU (1988): Synergism of closely adjacent estrogen-responsive elements increases their regulatory potential. J Mol Biol 201:537-544.

Klinge CM, Peale FV, Hilf R, Bambara RA, Zain S (1992): Cooperative estrogen receptor interaction with consensus or variant estrogen responsive elements *in vitro*. Cancer Res 52:1073-1081.

Landel CC, Kushner PJ, Greene GL (1995): Estrogen receptor accessory proteins: effects on receptor-DNA interactions. Environ Health Perspect 103:(Suppl 7) 23-28.

Landel CC, Kushner PJ, Greene GL (1994): The interaction of human estrogen receptor with DNA is modulated by receptor-associated proteins. Mol Endocrinol 8:1407-1419.

Love RR, Mazess RB, Barden HS, Epstein S, Newcomb PA, Jordan VC, Carbone, PP, DeMets DL (1992): Effects of tamoxifen on bone mineral density in postmenopausal women with breast cancer. N Engl J Med 326:852-856.

Love RR, Wiebe DA, Feyzi JM, Newcomb PA, Chappell RJ (1994): Effects of tamoxifen on cardiovascular risk factors in postmenopausal women after five years of treatment. J Nat Cancer Inst 86:1534-1539.

Love RR, Wiebe DA, Newcomb PA, Cameron 1, Leventhal H, Jordan VC, Feyzi J, DeMets DL (1991): Effects of tamoxifen on cardiovascular risk factors in postmenopausal women. Ann Intern Med 115:860-864.

Martin EA, Rich KJ, White INH, Woods KL, Powles TJ, Smith LL (1995): ^{32}P-Postlabelled DNA adducts in liver obtained from women treated with tamoxifen. Carcinogenesis 16:1651-1654.

Martinez E and Wahli W (1989): Cooperative binding of estrogen receptor to imperfect estrogen-responsive DNA elements correlates with their synergistic hormone-dependent enhancer activity. EMBO J 8:3781-3791.

McDonald CC, Stewart HJ for the Scottish Breast Cancer Committee (1991): Fatal myocardial infarctions in the Scottish adjuvant tamoxifen trial. Br Med J 303:435-437.

Naar AM, Boutin J-M, Lipkin, Yu VC, Holloway JM, Glass CK, Rosenfeld MG (1991): The orientation and spacing of core DNA-binding motifs dictate selective transcriptional responses to three nuclear receptors. Cell 65:1267-1279.

Pham TA, Elliston JF, Nawaz Z, McDonnell DP, Tsai M-J, O'Malley BW (1991): Antiestrogen can establish nonproductive receptor complexes and alter chromatin structure at target enhancers. Proc Natl Acad Sci. USA 88:3125-3129.

Ponglikitmongkol M, White JH, Chambon, P (1990): Synergistic activation of transcription by the human estrogen receptor bound to tandem responsive elements. EMBO J 9:2221-22231.

Rauschning W and Pritchard KI (1994): Droloxifene, a new antiestrogen: Its role in metastatic breast cancer. Breast Cancer Res Treat 31:83-94.

Tonetti DA and Jordan VC (1995): Possible mechanisms in the emergence of tamoxifen-resistant breast cancer. Anti-Cancer Drugs 6:498-507.

Tsai SY, Tsai M-J, O'Malley BW (1989): Cooperative binding of steroid hormone receptors contributes to transcriptional synergism at target enhancer elements. Cell 57:443-448.

Tzukerman MT, Esty A, Santiso-Mere D, Danielian P, Parker MG, Stein RB, Pike JW, McDonnell DP (1994): Human estrogen receptor transactivational capacity is determined by both cellular and promoter context and mediated by two functionally distinct intramolecular regions. Mol Endocrinol 8:21-30.

Van Dijck P and Verhoeven G (1992): Interaction of estrogen receptor complexes with the promoter region of genes that are negatively regulated by estrogens: the $\alpha_{2\mu}$ - globulins. Biochem Biophys Res Commun 182:174-181.

Williams GM, Iatropoulos MJ, Djordjevic MV, et al. (1993): The triphenylethylene drug tamoxifen is a strong liver corcinogen in the rat. Carcinogenesis 14:315-317.

Wiseman H, Paganga G, Rice-Evans C, Halliwell B (1993): Protective actions of tamoxifen and 4-hydroxytamoxifen against oxidative damage to human low-density lipoproteins: a mechanism accounting for the cardioprotective action of tamoxifen? Biochem J 292:635-638.

Wright CDP and Compston JE (1995): Tamoxifen: oestrogen or anti-oestrogen in bone? Q J Med 88:307-310.

Etiology of Breast and
Gynecological Cancers, pages 257–270
© 1997 Wiley-Liss, Inc.

THE METABOLISM AND GENOTOXICITY OF TAMOXIFEN

Ian N.H. White, Elizabeth A. Martin, Jerry Styles, Chang-Kee Lim, Phillip Carthew and Lewis L. Smith

MRC Toxicology Unit, University of Leicester, Lancaster Road, Leicester LE1 9HN UK

Hormones play an important role in the initiation and promotion of certain cancers. About one third of breast tumours grow in response to the hormonal influence of circulating oestrogens. The ability of the antioestrogen tamoxifen (Fig. 1, I) to prevent or delay the recurrence of oestrogen receptor positive breast cancers and its effect on increasing the survival time of treated women has been clearly demonstrated by meta-analysis of trials involving 75 000 individuals (Anonymous, 1992). Tamoxifen is now used by more than two million women worldwide. Epidemiological studies showed, however, that in breast cancer patients, tamoxifen treatment can result in endometrial cancers (Rutqvist et al., 1995; Fornander et al., 1989). In the National Surgical Adjuvant Breast and Bowel Project (*NSABP B14*) study (Fisher et al., 1994), the annual average hazard rate of endometrial cancer for women $\geq$ 50 years of age was approximately 6 fold (0.4/1000 patient years in the placebo group compared to 2.3/1000 in the tamoxifen treated group).

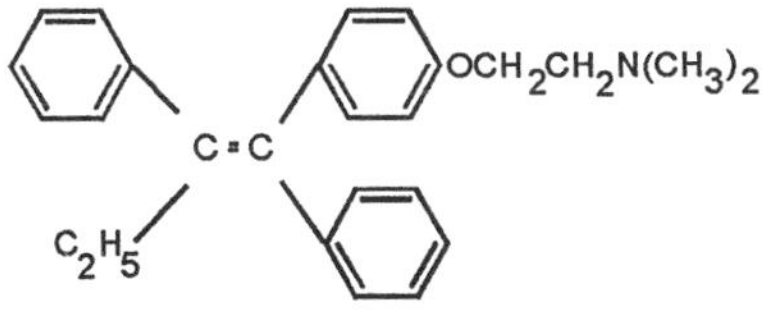

Tamoxifen, I

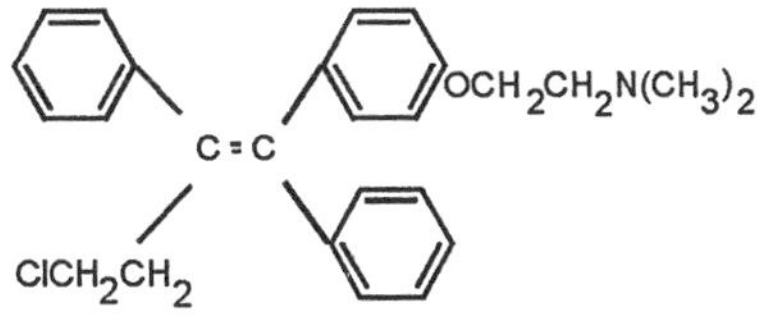

Toremifene, II

Figure 1. Chemical structures of tamoxifen (I) and toremifene (II).

Promotion of endometrial cancers suggests tamoxifen may be having an oestrogen agonist effect on the endometrium, encouraging the proliferation of oestrogen receptor positive cells and promoting endogenous DNA lesions. It has been shown experimentally that the oestrogenic/antioestrogenic properties of tamoxifen are both organ and species specific. In humans and in rats, tamoxifen has both oestrogen and antioestrogenic properties while in the dog and mouse it acts as an oestrogen agonist (Jordan & Robinson, 1987).

It has also been suggested by Rutqvist et al. (1995) that tamoxifen treatment may increase the incidence of GI cancers. It is known that hormones are important to the normal function of this organ but the mechanism by which tamoxifen might exert its carcinogenic effects in this tissue remains to be established. In the future, epidemiological studies comparing tamoxifen and toremifene, since both have such similar oestrogenic/antioestrogenic properties, should be able to show if the carcinogenic side effects of tamoxifen on the endometrium or the GI tract are due to their hormonal effects alone.

EVIDENCE OF HEPATOCARCINOGENICITY OF TAMOXIFEN IN RATS.

Even after two weeks administration of tamoxifen (40 mg/kg) to rats, the induction of γ-glutamyltranspeptidase enzymes activitiy can be demonstrated in isolated hepatocytes, suggesting oxidative stress (White et al., 1996). With longer term exposure (three months) altered hepatic foci and foci expressing glutathione S-transferase P can be demonstrated immunohistochemically (Carthew et al., 1995). In male and female rats, life time exposure to tamoxifen leads to the development of hepatocellular carcinomas (Hard et al., 1993; Greaves et al., 1993). The incidence of such tumours was dependent on the dose of drug administered and even with the lowest dose tested (5 mg/kg/day) there was a significant increase relative to controls. These effects were believed by some to be due to the hormonal actions of the drug acting by an epigenetic mechanism, promoting endogenous hepatocellular lesions as has been described for human endometrial tissues. Support for this view came from the observation that virtually all of the *in vitro* tests for the genotoxicity of tamoxifen, including the Ames *Salmonella* assay and the induction of unscheduled DNA in isolated rat hepatocytes, gave negative results (Tucker et al.,1984).

However, in 1992, work initiated by the MRC Toxicology Unit (White et al., 1992) and at the same time by Han & Liehr (1992) at the University of Texas showed that when tamoxifen was given to rats, even as a single dose, DNA damage could be detected in the liver. This damage was detected using the very sensitive technique of ^{32}P-postlabelling. More recently, the greater sensitivity of accelerator mass spectrometry, has demonstrated the irreversible binding of [^{14}C]tamoxifen, to cellular DNA and the association of the [^{14}C]label with that ^{32}P-postlabelled adduct spots. This conclusively demonstrated binding of an active tamoxifen metabolite with nucleotides of DNA (Martin et al., 1995). The chemical nature of such adducts have not yet been elucidated.

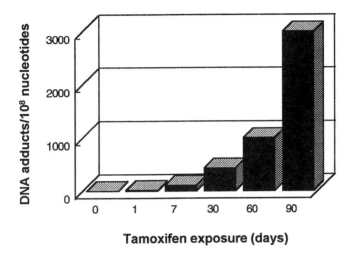

Figure 2. Dependence on time of exposure of female Fischer rats to tamoxifen (~ 40 mg/kg daily) on hepatic DNA damage, determined by ^{32}P-postlabelling. Data taken from White et al., (1992) and Carthew et al., (1995).

The extent of hepatic DNA damage, determined by ^{32}P-postlabelling, following six days dosing with tamoxifen, was dose dependent over the range of 5 - 45 mg/kg. At doses < 5 mg/kg, adducts that could be specifically attributed to tamoxifen treatment, could not be distinguished. This dose in rats is well above that of 20 mg/day (~ 0.3 mg/kg) used therapeutically in women.

It is well known that initiation of DNA damage is only the first step of a multifactorial process which in some instances leads to cancer. With tamoxifen in rats, however, there is now strong evidence that there is a causal relationship between the presence of hepatic ^{32}P-postlabelled DNA adducts and the subsequent development of liver tumours. Results strongly suggest that the hepatocarcinogenic actions of tamoxifen are **not** related to the oestrogenic/antioestrogenic effects of this drug. One powerful piece of evidence which supports this view comes from the studies of Williams et al., (1993) who showed that toremifene (Fig. 1, II), a very closely related triphenylethylenic analogue of tamoxifen, did not cause liver tumours in rats following long term dosing. A similar lack of hepatocarcinogenic action has been reported for 3-hydroxytamoxifen (droloxifene) (Dahme, Rattel,.1994). Both toremifene and droloxifene give little or no DNA damage, as determined by ^{32}P-postlabelling (Williams et al., 1993; White et al., 1992) but pharmacologically, both have similar antioestrogenic properties to tamoxifen in rats and in women.

So far rats are the only species where tamoxifen has been shown to cause liver tumours. One possible reason for this potency is that unlike certain other hepatocarcinogens such as N-nitrosodimethylamine or aflatoxin, where the majority of the

DNA damage is repaired within the first few days, with tamoxifen, the ^{32}P-postlabelled DNA adducts appear to be remarkably stable. With repeated exposure to tamoxifen (~40 mg/kg/day) in female Fischer rats, lesions increase with continued exposure from around 20 adducts/10^8 nucleotides after a single dose to around 3000 adducts/10^8 nucleotides after six months (Fig. 2). After withdrawal of tamoxifen these adducts appear to have a half life of around three months (Carthew et al., 1995; White et al., 1992). Mice given a similar dosing regime for a somewhat shorter length of time do not get liver tumours (Tucker et al., 1984). Both C57Bl/6 and DBA/2 strains of mice when dosed for six days with tamoxifen show the presence of ^{32}P-postlabelled adducts in their liver, but at a level of about one quarter that seen in rats (White et al., 1992). In contrast to rats, with longer exposure, the level of adducts does not increase in the liver (Martin et al., 1994) lending further support to the idea that initiation of DNA damage is an essential component of tamoxifen hepatocarcinogenesis. There is no evidence that tamoxifen causes liver tumours in women. In the study of Rutqvist et al., (1995), in a nine year follow up period, only three cases were found amongst 1372 women taking this drug against one case in 1357 controls. No tests were carried out such as for the presence of α-foetoprotein to establish if the liver tumours were primaries.

PROMOTION OF DNA DAMAGE CAUSED BY TAMOXIFEN

As mentioned above, DNA damage alone is not sufficient to give rise to liver tumours. Promotion and progression involving cell division and changes (mutations) being passed on to daughter cells has to occur. In one study involving three strains of rats (Fischer, Wistar and Lewis) it was found that although the extent of DNA damage was similar in all three strains, the time to tumours in the liver was very much longer in the Fischer animals (Carthew et al., 1995). The extent of parenchymal cell division, relative to controls was shown to be significantly higher after six months tamoxifen exposure in the susceptible Wistar and Lewis strains that in the 'resistant' Fischer animals. It is thought, therefore, as well as initiating DNA damage, tamoxifen can act as a promoter, inducing cell division in the liver. It has in fact been shown by Dragan et al., (1995) that such promoting effects are not confined to tamoxifen. Following initiation of liver tumours by N-nitrosodimethylamine, toremifene can also act as a promoter, although at somewhat lower efficiency than tamoxifen.

It is not known if there is a lower limit for DNA damage caused by tamoxifen which will lead eventually to liver tumours. It was found that after three months tamoxifen treatment in female Wistar rats which gave ^{32}P-postlabelled DNA damage in the liver of around 700 adducts/ 10^8 nucleotides, liver tumours were only found in about one third of the animals in a lifetime study (Carthew et al., 1995). However, if after a three month initiation period with tamoxifen, the classical promoter phenobarbital was included in the drinking water, hepatocellular carcinomas appeared more quickly and at the end of the lifetime study, about 85% of the animals had liver tumours. The results of this study are consistent with the hypothesis that phenobarbital promotes at least some of the same foci that tamoxifen itself is capable of promoting after initiation, and that liver cell proliferation is a major factor in converting DNA adducts to heritable genetic alterations, some of which eventually result in liver tumour formation.

Similar mechanisms of tumour initiation - promotion - progression might be expected to occur in women taking tamoxifen therapeutically. It was therefore of paramount importance to establish if routes of activation of tamoxifen and hepatic DNA damage occurred in human liver and if so, the extent of this damage relative to the susceptible rat species.

^{32}P-POSTLABELLED ADDUCTS IN LIVER OBTAINED FROM WOMEN TREATED WITH TAMOXIFEN.

Following tamoxifen treatment of women ~ 0.3 mg/kg (20 mg daily) serum levels of this drug show a wide range of values but are around 300 ng/ml (Furr, Jordan,.1984; Adam et al., 1980). Because of the more rapid metabolism of tamoxifen in rats compared to women (Robinson et al., 1991), a similar steady state serum level (244 ng/ml) is seen in female rats given 23 mg/kg daily (Hard et al., 1993). In both rats and humans, tamoxifen and its major (detoxication) metabolites N-desmethyltamoxifen and 4-hydroxytamoxifen (Fig. 3) accumulate in the liver to at least an order of magnitude higher concentration than that seen in serum. In rats given 20 mg/kg/day tamoxifen, liver concentrations of this drug were about 9 μg/ g tissue (Carthew et al., 1995). HPLC of liver extracts from a small number of women given tamoxifen, qualitatively showed a pattern of metabolites similar to those of rats and showed a range of liver concentrations between 0.01 to 1.2 μg/g (Lein et al., 1991; Martin et al., 1995). Following ^{32}P-postlablelling and TLC of DNA extracted from the livers of six women taking tamoxifen (20 or 40 mg/kg daily) a variable number of weakly labelled adducts were visualised but none had R_f values typical of those seen in the DNA extracted from tamoxifen treated rats (Martin et al., 1995). Similar low levels of DNA damage were seen in the DNA from the livers of women not taking this drug. Such results posed the question as to whether human liver could activate tamoxifen and if so what was the potential to activate this drug compared to that seen in rats.

ENZYMES INVOLVED IN THE ACTIVATION OF TAMOXIFEN: EVIDENCE FROM CELLS AND MICROSOMAL FRACTIONS.

With respect to hepatocarcinogenesis in the rat, it is clear that it is not tamoxifen itself which is initiating DNA damage but an active metabolite. Initial studies by Mani & Kupfer,. (1991) showed that only after incubation with rat liver microsomal fractions in the presence of NADPH were active metabolites of [14C]tamoxifen produced which bound irreversibly to protein. The enzyme carrying out this reaction had characteristics typical of the cytochrome P450 mixed function oxidases. In rats and humans, N-demethylation of tamoxifen (Fig. 3) is catalysed by the dexamethasone inducible CYP3A

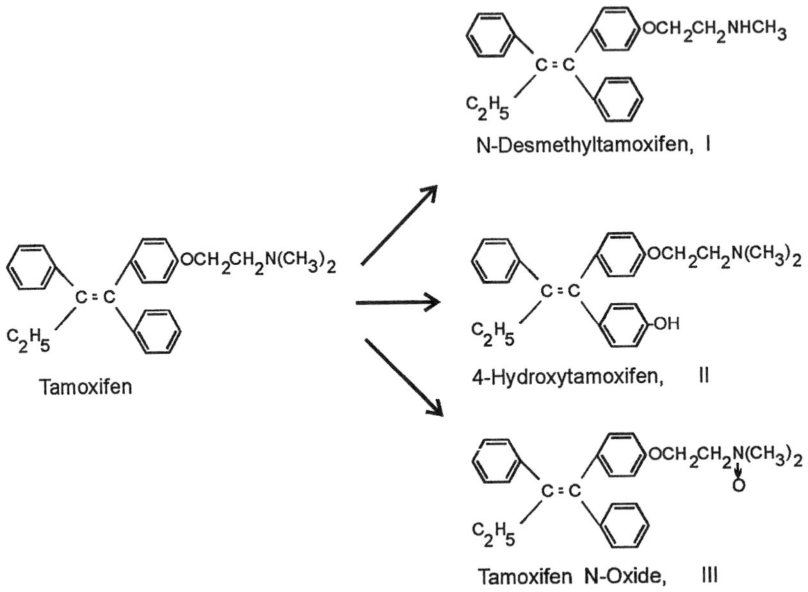

Figure 3. Major liver metabolites of tamoxifen in rats and humans.

family (Jacolot et al., 1991; Mani et al., 1994), while the flavin-containing monooxygenases mediated N-oxidation (Han & Liehr, 1992). In contrast, the N-hydroxylation reaction is catalysed by a constitutive CYP2C8, CYP2C9 family (Daniels et al., 1992). Subsequent studies using covalent binding of [^{14}C]tamoxifen to microsomal protein as a surrogate for DNA binding demonstrated the involvement of CYP3A in activation and covalent binding to rat and human liver microsomes (White et al., 1995; Mani et al., 1994). While phenobarbital pretreatment of rats induces CYP2B/B2 and also increases covalent binding, the involvement of these cytochromes is not so clear cut. Phenobarbital pretreatment of rats also induces CYP3A to a lesser extent. Antibodies directed against CYP2B1/2B2 appear not to inhibit covalent binding of tamoxifen (Mani et al., 1994). In contrast using a series of twelve human liver microsomal preparations which had been characterised for different CYP isoenzymes, a positive correlation was found between the presence of the human ortholog, CYP2B6 in addition to CYP3A4 and covalent binding (White et al., 1995).

GENOTOXICITY OF TAMOXIFEN IN CELL LINES EXPRESSING CYTOCHROME P450s:
a, Crespi cells

The activation of tamoxifen and toremifene has been tested in human lymphoblastoid derived cell lines in which the human cytochrome P450s CYP1A1, CYP1A2, CYP2D6, CYP2E1 and CYP3A4 have been transfected and are functionally expressed (Crespi MCL5 cells). Initial studies showed a dose dependent increase in micronucleus formation with tamoxifen, such increases were significant down to concentrations of 300 ng/ml which is equivalent to the serum levels of tamoxifen in women taking this drug therapeutically (White et al., 1992). In this assay toremifene also gave a positive result, although the extent of activation was less than that seen with tamoxifen. With the availability of cell lines expressing individual CYP isoenzymes, the work of Styles et al., (1994), confirmed that CYP3A4 was the major isoenzymic form involved in the genotoxic effects of tamoxifen. In this study, CYP2E1 and to a lesser extent, CYP2D6, also gave positive dose dependent micronucleus results with tamoxifen. The involvement of these latter isoenzymic forms has not been substantiated by any other tests *in vivo* or *in vitro*.

b, Rat hepatocytes *in vivo*.

Tamoxifen causes no induction of unscheduled DNA synthesis in hepatocytes from untreated rats. However, if the animals are pretreated with this drug to induce CYP2B1/2B2 and CYP3A4, low levels of unscheduled DNA synthesis can be detected following the addition of tamoxifen to the cultured hepatocytes (White et al., 1993). Even after a single dose, tamoxifen can induce both aneuploidy and chromosomal structural aberrations such as mitotic spindle disruption in hepatocytes (Sargent et al., 1994). The hepatocytes were isolated after dosing and stimulated to divide in culture by the addition of epidermal growth factor. Toremifene only caused aneuploidy and droloxifene had no effect (Styles et al., 1995). Aneuploidy is considered to be important in the progression of tumours. Although both tamoxifen and toremifene cause aneuploidy in rat liver cells following EGF stimulation, only tamoxifen is capable of inducing cell division in rats *in vivo* with the resulting formation of aneuploid hepatocytes.

ISOENZYMIC FORMS OF CYTOCHROME P450 INVOLVED IN TAMOXIFEN ACTIVATION

Results from liver microsomal studies suggest that human cytochrome P450's do not show any fundamental difference in specificity from those of rat liver. Comparisons between rat and human detoxication reactions (N-demethylation, N-oxidation and 4-hydroxylation) show qualitatively similar patterns of metabolites, although overall, rates of metabolism in human preparations are about one third those of rats (Robinson et al., 1991; Lim et al., 1993; Lim et al., 1994). With regard to tamoxifen activation, it seems clear that the major isoenzymic forms involved are CYP3A1/3A2 (rat) or CYP3A4 (human). This result with respect to CYP3A4 is confirmed by the micronucleus (Crespi cell) assay described above.

Using irreversible binding to microsomal protein as the index of activation, activities in human liver microsomes are about one third those of rats (White et al., 1995).

It is interesting to note in this respect that microsomal systems show only the *potential* for activation and are poor indicators of the *actual* extent of activation that will occur *in vivo*. This is well exemplified by the mouse DNA damage in the liver following tamoxifen administration which is only about one quarter that seen in rats (White et al., 1992). In contrast, activation of [^{14}C]tamoxifen by microsomal preparations *in vitro* was seven fold greater than seen using the rat liver microsomes (White et al., 1995). A microsomal system with the high tamoxifen concentrations and the absence of many of the Phase II drug metabolising enzyme systems, does not really mimic the situation in the liver. In addition, as with many carcinogens, binding to protein is greater than to DNA when compared on a *per mg* basis. Pathak & Bodell, (1994) demonstrated DNA damage caued by tamoxifen *in vitro*, to be greater using a human liver microsomal activating system than a rat one.

PEROXIDASE MEDIATED ACTIVATION OF TAMOXIFEN AND 4-HYDROXYTAMOXIFEN

Cytochrome P450 is the major enzyme involved in the hepatic activation of tamoxifen. It has recently been demonstrated that a number of different peroxidases, horseradish, lactoperoxidase and prostaglandin H synthase are able to metabolise tamoxifen (Pathak et al., 1995; Davies et al., 1995). The reaction products, N-desmethyltamoxifen and tamoxifen N-oxide are the same as those catalysed by CYP-isoenzymes. In addition, by using radiolabelled tamoxifen, horseradish peroxidase has been shown to catalyse the irreversible binding to added bovine serum albumin or cause damage to added calf thymus DNA. In such peroxidase catalysed reactions, there seems to be little difference between tamoxifen and toremifene in the extent to which activation occurs (Davies et al., 1995). Peroxidases showed very much higher levels of activity towards hydroxylated tamoxifen metabolites, such as 4-hydroxytamoxifen. EPR studies suggest that oxidation of the hydroxy function may give rise to phenoxy radical intermediates (Davies et al., 1995). It is known that peroxidases are widely distributed in the body, but the role that they play in the activation of tamoxifen at extra hepatic sites is not yet clear. It has recently been reported by Hemminki et al., (1995) that DNA damage can be detected in human lymphocytes incubated with relatively high concentrations of tamoxifen *in vitro* and it has been suggested that this may be due to the presence of peroxidases. In addition, high levels of prostaglandin synthase are known to occur in the reproductive tract (Holinka, Gurpide,.1980) but no DNA damage, such as that found in the livers of tamoxifen dosed rats, has been reported in this organ. The presence of 4-hydroxytamoxifen in liver, serum and reproductive tract in women taking this drug therapeutically suggests that peroxidases do not play any major role in the overall metabolism of this drug. This does not exclude the possibility that in certain cell populations, peroxidases or prostaglandin synthase could be involved in selective activation.

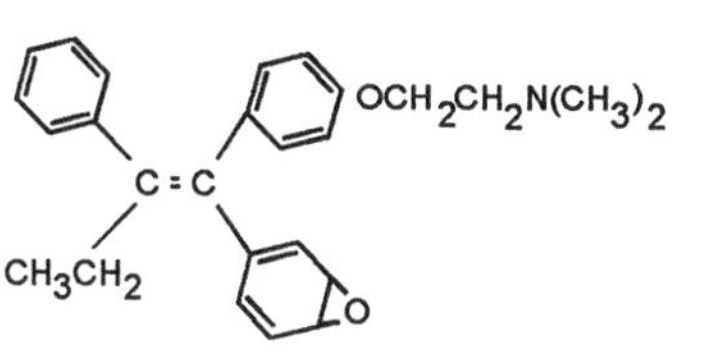

3,4-Epoxytamoxifen

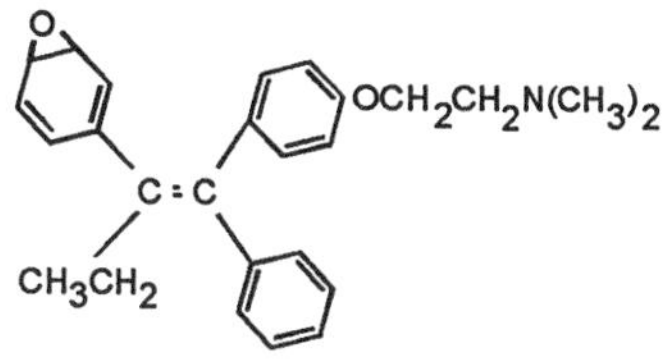

3',4'-Epoxytamoxifen

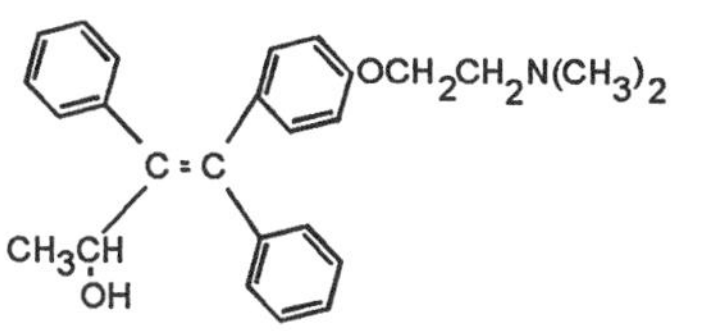

α-Hydroxyethyltamoxifen

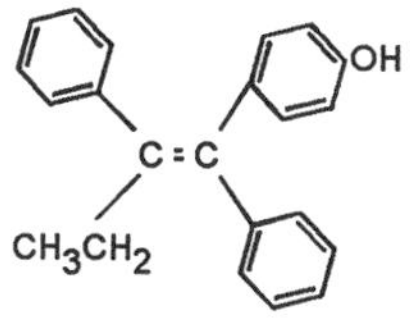

Metabolite E

Figure 4. Chemical structures of proposed active metabolites of tamoxifen.

NATURE OF THE ACTIVE METABOLITE RESPONSIBLE FOR TAMOXIFEN GENOTOXICITY.

Detailed analysis of the tamoxifen metabolites formed following incubation of tamoxifen with female rat liver microsomes by an optimized on-line HPLC-electrospray ionization mass spectrometric (HPLC-ESI MS) method revealed the formation of arene oxides (3,4-epoxytamoxifen and 3',4'-epoxytamoxifen) as potential reactive metabolites (Fig. 4). Arene oxides were hardly detectable in mouse and human liver microsomal incubation mixtures (Lim et al., 1994). Such arene oxides are also formed as putative active metabolites following peroxidase activation of tamoxifen (Davies et al., 1995). Due to their chemical instability, so far such products have not been synthesised and tested.

Using similar HPLC-ESI MS techniques, Phillips et al. (1995), suggested that α-hydroxyethyltamoxifen may be a reactive intermediate. The extent of DNA damage observed when this compound was added to rat hepatocytes, as determined by ^{32}P-postlabelling, was 50 fold higher than tamoxifen itself. By analogy with safrole activation, it has been suggested that an active sulphate ester is formed in the liver from this compound. It was found experimentally that in mice given pentachlorophenol to block sulphotransferase activity just prior to tamoxifen treatment, the extent of the hepatic DNA damage was 8 fold greater than caused by tamoxifen alone. For such a reactive metabolite it is somewhat unexpected to find that α-hydroxyethyltamoxifen, could be detected by HPLC-ESI MS in extracts of Hep G2 cells, liver homogenates and in the plasma of patients following dosing with tamoxifen (Poon et al., 1995).

Not only does α-hydroxyethyltamoxifen give rise to more DNA damage in test systems *in vitro* than tamoxifen but under similar conditions, ring hydroxylated analogues also give rise to a greater level of ^{32}P-postlabelled DNA adducts. The metabolites, which are formed from tamoxifen following administration to rats or to humans, include 4-hydroxytamoxifen (Randerath et al., 1994; Pathak et al., 1995) and (Z)-1.2-diphenyl-1-(4-hydroxyphenyl)but-1-ene (metabolite E, Fig. 4)) (Pongracz et al., 1995).

Evidence for the chemical identification of tamoxifen-DNA adducts have come from the studies of Osborne et al., (1995). This group found an adduct of tamoxifen and deoxyguanosine in which the alpha position of tamoxifen is linked covalently wto the exocyclic amino group of deoxyguanosine. At the same time, Moorthy et al., (1995) found evidence for two active metabolites, one an α-hydroxyethyl derivative as described above the other 4-hydroxytamoxifen.

CONCLUSIONS: POTENTIAL HAZARD OF LIVER CANCER FOR WOMEN TAKING TAMOXIFEN.

For the treatment of women with primary breast cancers, the reduction in the risk of relapse and of contralateral breast cancer makes a clear case for the continued use of tamoxifen (Powles et al.,1995). The principal objective of animal studies on the mechanism of tamoxifen hepatocarcinogenicity is to use our understanding of tits mechanism to define the likely risks to women taking this drug. In order to cause 100 %

Table 1. Relative Risk of Liver DNA Adducts in Rats and Humans

	Safety Factor
Metabolism of tamoxifen:rats greater than women	X 3

Dose of tamoxifen: Rat   40 mg/kg
            Women 20 mg/adult
     (assumes 60 kg body weight)
	X 120

Total	X 360

Rats after six months dosing of 40 mg/kg tamoxifen produce 3000 adducts/10^8 nucleotides. Assume a X 360 safety factor

Therefore women given 20 mg/adult will produce 8 adducts/10^8 nucleotides.

incidence of liver tumours in rats, a daily tamoxifen dose of about 40 mg/kg has to be given. This causes cumulative DNA damage which becomes maximal at about 3000 adducts/10^8 nucleotides. Since, as outlined before, metabolic activation of tamoxifen in humans is about one third of that in rats, this gives an approximate three fold safety factor. In addition, the dose given to humans (0.3 mg/kg daily) is about 120 fold lower than that given to rats. Assuming that the extent of DNA repair and the detoxication of tamoxifen in the two species is similar, there will be an apparent 360 fold safety factor for women taking this drug (Table 1). Martin et al., (1995) showed that in a small population of tamoxifen treated women, there was no evidence of an increase in ^{32}P-postlabelled adducts in the liver. However, given our current understanding of the mechanism of toxicity of tamoxifen, if women were comparable to rats, it would be expected that only 8 adducts/10^8 nucleotides would be present in liver DNA. This is well within the standard deviation of the experimental results. Thus in women treated with tamoxifen, no measurable increase in 32P-postlabelled adducts was expected or found Martin et al., (1995). More importantly, if rats had been given a dose of only 0.3 mg/kg, it is highly unlikely from our knowledge of the liver tumour dose response curve (Greaves et al., 1992) that liver tumours would have been produced. However, it is known that there is a high degree of polymorphism in the drug metabolising enzymes int he human population and this may mean that in a very small number of women, tamoxifen can be metabolised to induce liver DNA lesions which are of biological significance. While the risks of tamoxifen therapy appear to be positively acceptable for women with breast cancer, the risk in normal healthy women given a drug which is a rat genotoxic carcinogen for chemopreventative purposes is less well defined.

REFERENCES

Adam HK, Patterson JS, Kemp JV (1980): Studies on the metabolism and pharmacokinetics of tamoxifen in mormal volunteers. Cancer Treat Rep 64: 761-764

Anonymous. (1992): Systemic treatment of early breast cancer by hormonal, cytotoxic, or immune therapy. 133 randomised trials involving 31000 recurrences and 24000 deaths among 75000 women. Lancet 339: 1-15.

Carthew P, Martin EA, White INH, De Matteis F, Edwards RE, Dorman BM, Heydon RT, Smith LL (1995): Tamoxifen induces short-term cumulative DNA damage and liver tumors in rats: Promotion by phenobarbital. Cancer Res 55: 544-547.

Carthew P, Rich KJ, Martin EA, De Matteis F, Lim CK, Manson MM, Festing M, White INH, Smith LL (1995): DNA damage as assessed by ^{32}P-postlabelling in three rat stains exposed to dietary tamoxifen: the relationship between cell proliferation and liver tumour formation. Carcinogenesis 16: 1299-1304.

Dahme E, Rattel B (1994): Unlike tamoxifen, droloxifene produces no hepatic tumors in the rat. Onkologie 17: 6-16.

Daniels L, Blankson EA, Henderson CJ, Harris AH, Wolf CR, Lennard MS, Tucker GT (1992): Delineation of human cytochromes P450 involved in the metabolism of tamoxifen. Proc Br Pharmacol Soc 153P-154P: -154P.

Davies AM, Malone ME, White INH (1995): Peroxidase activation of 4-hydroxytamoxifen to cause DNA damage in vitro. Biochemical Society Transactions 23: 439S

Davies AM, Martin EA, Jones RM, Lim CK, Smith LL, White INH (1995): Peroxidase activation of tamoxifen and toremifene to cause DNA damage and covalently bound protein adducts. Carcinogenesis 16: 539-545.

Dragan YP, Vaughan J, Jordan VC, Pitot HC (1995): Comparison of the effects of tamoxifen and toremifene on liver and kidney tumor promotion in female rats. Carcinogenesis 16: 2733-2741.

Fisher B, Costantino JP, Redmond CK, Fisher ER, Wickerham DL, Cronin WM, NSABP Contributors (1994): Endometrial cancer in tamoxifen-treated breast cancer patients: Findings from the National Surgical Adjuvant Breast and Bowel Project (NSABP) B-14. J Natl Cancer Inst 86: 527-537.

Fornander T, Cedermark B, Mattsson A, Skoog L, Theve T, Askergren J, Rutqvist LE, Glas U, Silfversward C, Somell, Wilking N, Hjalmar M (1989): Adjuvant tamoxifen in early breast cancer: occurrence of new primary cancers. Lancet 1: 117-119.

Furr BJA, Jordan VC (1984): The pharmacology and clinical uses of tamoxifen. Pharmacol Ther 25: 127-205.

Greaves P, Goonetilleke R, Nunn G, Topham J, Orton T (1993): Two-year carcinogenicity study of tamoxifen in Alderly Park Wistar-derived rats. Cancer Res 53: 3919-3924.

Han X, Liehr JG (1992): Induction of covalent DNA adducts in rodents by tamoxifen. Cancer Res 52: 1360-1363.

Hard GC, Iatropoulos MJ, Jordan K, Radi L, Kaltenberg OP, Imondi AR, Williams GM (1993): Major differences in the hepatocarcinogenicity and DNA adduct forming ability between toremifene and tamoxifen in female Crl: CD(BR) rats. Cancer Res 53: 4534-4541.

Hemminki K, Widlak P, Hou SM (1995): DNA adducts caused by tamoxifen and toremifene in human microsomal system and lymphocytes in vitro. Carcinogenesis 16: 1661-1664.

Holinka CF, Gurpide E (1980): Peroxidase activity in glands and stroma of human endometrium. Am J Obstet Gynecol 138: 599-603.

Jacolot F, Simon I, Dreano Y, Beaune P, Riche C, Berthou F (1991): Identificationof the cytochrome P450 IIIA family as the enzymes involved in the N-demethylation of tamoxifen in human liver microsomes. Biochem Pharmacol 41: 1911-1919.

Jordan VC, Robinson SP (1987): Species-specific pharmacology of antiestrogens:role of metabolism. Fed Proc 46: 1870-1874.

Lein EA, Solheim E, Ueland PM (1991): Distribution of tamoxifen and its metabolites in rat and human tissues during steady-state treatment. Cancer Res 51: 4837-4844.

Lim CK, Chow LCL, Yuan ZX, Smith LL (1993): High performance liquid chromatography of tamoxifen and metabolites in plasma and tissues. Biomed Chromatog 7: 311-314.

Lim CK, Yuan Z, Lamb JH, White INH, De Matteis F, Smith LL (1994): A comparative study of tamoxifen metabolism in female rat, mouse and human liver microsomes. Carcinogenesis 15: 589-593.

Mani C, Kupfer D (1991): Cytochrome P450 mediated action and irreversible binding of the antiestrogen tamoxifen to proteins in rat and human liver: possible involvement of the flavin-containing monooxygenases in tamoxifen activation. Cancer Res 51: 6052-6058.

Mani C, Pearce R, Parkinson A, Kupfer D (1994): Involvement of cytochrome P4503A in catalysis of tamoxifen activation and covalent binding to rat and human liver microsomes. Carcinogenesis 15: 2715-2720.

Martin EA, Rich K, White INH, Woods KL, Powles TJ, Smith LL (1995): ^{32}P-Postlabelled DNA adducts in liver obtained from women treated with tamoxifen. Carcinogenesis 16: 1651-1654.

Martin EA, Rich KJ, Heydon R, White INH, Woods KL, Powles TJ, Smith LL (1994): A comparison of ^{32}P-postlabelled tamoxifen liver DNA adducts in rats, mice and breast cancer patients. The Toxicologist 14: 405 Abstract 1602.

Martin EA, Turteltaub KW, Heydon R, Davies A, White INH, Smith LL (1995): Characterisation of tamoxifen induced-DNA adducts formed in rat liver. The Toxicologist 15: 152 Abstract 811

Moorthy B, Liehr JG, Randerath E, Randerath K (1995) Evidence from 32P-postlabeling and the use of pentachlorophenol for a novel metabolic activation pathway of diethylstilbestrol and its dimethyl ether in mouse liver: Likely alpha-hydroxylation of ethyl group(s) followed by sulfate conjugation Carcinogenesis, 16, 2643-2648.

Osborne MR, Hewer A, Hardcastle IR, Carmichael PL, Phillips DH (1996) Identification of the major tamoxifen-deoxyguanosine adduct formed in the liver DNA of rats treated with tamoxifen Identification of the major tamoxifen-deoxyguanosine adduct formed in the liver DNA of rats treated with tamoxifen. Cancer Res, 56, 66-71.

Pathak DN, Bodell WJ (1994): DNA adduct formation by tamoxifen with rat and human liver microsomal activation systems. Carcinogenesis 15: 529-532.

Pathak DN, Pongracz K, Bodell WJ (1995): Microsomal and peroxidase activation of 4-hydroxytamoxifen to form DNA adducts: comparison with DNA adducts formed in Sprague-Dawley rats treated with tamoxifen. Carcinogenesis 16: 11-15.

Phillips DH, Carmichael PL, Hewer A, Cole KJ, Poon GK (1995): α-Hydroxytamoxifen, a metabolite of tamoxifen with exceptionally high DNA binding activity in rat hepatocytes. Cancer Res 54: 5518-5522.

Pongracz K, Pathak DN, Nakamura T, Burlingame AL, Bodell WJ (1995): Activation of the tamoxifen derivative metabolite E to form DNA adducts: Comparison with the adducts formed by microsomal activation of tamoxifen. Cancer Res 55: 3012-3015.

Poon GK, Walter B, Lonning PE, Horton MN, McCague R (1995): Identification of tamoxifen metabolites in human HEP G2 cell line, human liver homogenate, and patients on long-term therapy for breast cancer. Drug Metabolism and Disposition 23: 377-382.

Powles TJ, Hickish T (1995): Tamoxifen therapy and carcinogenic risk. J Natl Cancer Inst 87: 1343-1345.

Randerath K, Bi J, Mabon N, Sriram P, Moorthy B (1994): Strong intensification of mouse hepatic tamoxifen DNA adduct formation by pretreatment with the sulfotransferase inhibitor and ubiquitous environmental pollutant pentachlorophenol. Carcinogenesis 15: 797-800.

Robinson SP, Langan-Fahey L, Johnson DA, Jordan VC (1991): Metabolites, pharmacodynamics and pharmacokinetics of tamoxifen in rats and mice compared to the breast cancer patient. Drug Metab Dispos 19: 36-43.

Rutqvist LE, Johansson H, Signomklao T, Johansson U, Fornander T, Wilking N (1995): Adjuvant tamoxifen therapy for early stage breast cancer and second primary malignancies. J Natl Cancer Inst 87: 645-651.

Sargent LM, Dragan YP, Bahnub N, Wiley JE, Sattler CA, Schroeder P, Sattler GL, Jordan VC, Pitot HC (1994): Tamoxifen induces hepatic aneuploidy and mitotic spindle disruption after a single in vivo administration to female Sprague-Dawley rats. Cancer Res 54: 3357-3360.

Styles JA, Davies A, Lim CK, De Matteis F, Stanley LA, White INH, Yuan ZX, Smith LL (1994): Genotoxicity of tamoxifen, tamoxifen epoxide and toremifene in human lymphoblastoid cells containing human cytochrome P450s. Carcinogenesis 15: 5-9.

Styles JA, Davies R, Smith LL (1995): Comparison of the clastogenic effects induced in ras by tamoxifen and some of its analogues. The Toxicologist 15: 82

Tucker MJ, Adams HK, Patterson JS (1984) Tamoxifen. In Laurence DR, McLean AEM, Weatherall M (eds): "Safety Testing of New Drugs". Academic Press, New York, pp 125-161

White INH, Davies A, Smith LL, Dawson S, De Matteis F (1993): Induction of CYP2B1 and 3A1, and associated monooxygenase activities by tamoxifen and certain analogues in the livers of female rats and mice. Biochem Pharmacol 45: 21-30.

White INH, De Matteis F, Davies A, Smith LL, Crofton Sleigh C, Venitt S, Hewer A, Phillips DH (1992): Genotoxic potential of tamoxifen and analogues in female Fischer F344/N rats, DBA/2 and C57Bl/6 mice and in human MCL-5 cells. Carcinogenesis 13: 2197-2203.

White INH, De Matteis F, Gibbs AH, Lim CK, Wolf CR, Henderson C, Smith LL (1995): Species differences in the covalent binding of [14C]tamoxifen to liver microsomes and the forms of cytochrome P450 involved. Biochem Pharmacol 49: 1035-1042.

White INH, Razvi N, Lawrence RM, Manson MM (1996): A continuous fluorometric assay for γ-glutamyltranspeptidase. Anal Biochem, in press.

Williams GM, Iatropoulos MJ, Djordjevic MV, Kaltenberg OP (1993): The triphenylethylene drug tamoxifen is a strong liver carcinogen in the rat. Carcinogenesis 14: 315-317.

Etiology of Breast and
Gynecological Cancers, pages 271–282

TAMOXIFEN BREAST CANCER PREVENTION TRIAL - AN UPDATE

Leslie G. Ford, MD
Karen A. Johnson, MD, PhD, MPH

Community Oncology and Rehabilitation Branch
Division of Cancer Prevention and Control
National Cancer Institute
Bethesda, MD 20892

The tamoxifen Breast Cancer Prevention Trial (BCPT) is a randomized, double-blind, placebo-controlled clinical trial to test the effectiveness of 20 mg of tamoxifen versus placebo for preventing the incidence and mortality of breast cancer. In 1996, the incidence of breast cancer is expected to reach a new high of 185,000 cases in the United States (Parker, et al., 1996). Over the span of the next decade, about 2 million women will be newly confronted with this health problem. Although there is now a 4 year trend for decreasing breast cancer mortality in white women (Smigel, 1995), 44,300 deaths from breast cancer are nevertheless expected to occur in 1996 (Parker, et al., 1996), and in the next decade as many as 400,000 women could succumb to this disease unless effective methods of cancer prevention and control are applied. Concern about the magnitude of the incidence and mortality of breast cancer is only accentuated by the reports of newly isolated "breast cancer genes" (Nowack, 1994), that identify carriers as having a relative risk for developing breast cancer that is many times that of the average individual (King, et al., 1993). Trends in incidence and mortality and more specific methods of risk identification have heightened the concern of the average woman, but carry added significance for women of color and members of the so-called breast cancer families, in which generations of women face the consequences of breast cancer in about half the women of their genetic line. In the United States, breast cancer survivors and women at high risk of developing breast cancer are eager to see the development of clinical interventions that prevent the occurrence of breast cancer. An opportunity to develop one such intervention is provided by the evaluation of tamoxifen in the BCPT. This trial is sponsored by the National Cancer Institute (NCI) and is being conducted by the National Surgical Adjuvant Breast and Bowel Project (NSABP) (Redmond, et al., 1993).

Although the primary endpoints of the BCPT are breast cancer incidence and mortality, the trial is not limited to these endpoints. Secondary endpoints for the BCPT include bone fractures and cardiovascular disease incidence and mortality. When compared to breast cancer, the deaths from cardiovascular disease are a large problem with 360,000 female deaths from this cause reported in 1992 (Parker, et al., 1996). Nevertheless, the majority of these deaths occur in women aged 75 and older. Since cardiovascular risk is modifiable and increases once women reach the age of menopause, mortality from cardiovascular disease represents a substantive target for preventive intervention. In postmenopausal women, osteoporosis is also a major health problem leading to over 200,000 hip fractures each year, mostly in women over the age of 70 (Kumanyika, Velez, 1992). The physiologic impact of tamoxifen in women has been found to improve the lipid profile and maintain bone density. These observations and the magnitude of cardiovascular disease and osteoporosis in later years support the collection of data in the BCPT to specifically identify the effects of tamoxifen on bone density and the cardiovascular system.

Tamoxifen is a triphenylethylene derivative that was first synthesized in 1966 and investigated for its potential as an oral contraceptive (Richardson, 1988). Failing in this application, it was subsequently found to have antitumor activity. In the course of preclinical studies, tamoxifen was observed to exhibit a mixed estrogen agonist/antagonist profile (Wakeling, 1994). In a system where estrogen can be virtually eliminated, tamoxifen may function as an agonist with mildly estrogenic effects, but otherwise in the presence of endogenous estrogens, tamoxifen may block the estrogenic effect. A complex mechanism of drug action continues to complicate our understanding of the pharmacologic profile of tamoxifen in humans. Tamoxifen produces an anti-estrogenic effect that suppresses the proliferation of neoplastic breast epithelial cells and exacerbates menopausal symptoms in some women. Estrogenic actions change the lipid profile and bone metabolism, stimulate the endometrium, and alter the levels of coagulation factors in the blood.

The predominant reason for the development of tamoxifen has been its anti-tumor activity. The anti-tumor effect of tamoxifen is accompanied by binding to nuclear estrogen receptors, inhibition of growth factors like TGF-alpha, EGF and IGF-1, stimulation of TGF-beta production, inhibition of protein kinase C, and binding to calmodulin (Nayfield, et al., 1991). In animal model systems, tamoxifen interferes with multiple phases of tumor growth including initiation and promotion (Jordan, 1992). The effect of tamoxifen treatment on the survival of breast cancer patients has been summarized by an ongoing overview analysis (Early Breast Cancer Trialists' Collaborative Group, 1992). In the 1992 overview for 10 years of follow-up, there was a 25 percent reduction in recurrence and a 17 percent decrease in mortality from breast cancer in patients using adjuvant tamoxifen in randomized clinical trials. These reductions have been accomplished with a risk benefit profile that is overwhelmingly positive. An excellent safety profile and a substantial core of data from 42,000 person years of tamoxifen use in randomized clinical trials for breast cancer patients are central to the rationale for the BCPT.

The major justification for investigating tamoxifen as a preventive agent has been the observation in the setting of randomized trials that the occurrence of second primary breast cancers was reduced in about 40 percent of breast cancer patients who used adjuvant tamoxifen (Early Breast Cancer Trialists' Collaborative Group, 1992). The occurrence of contralateral breast cancers in clinical trials of adjuvant tamoxifen is summarized in Table 1, using data that was presented by Zeneca Pharmaceuticals at the June 1994, meeting of the Food and Drug Administration's Oncologic Drug Advisory Committee (ODAC).

Consideration of tamoxifen as a chemopreventive agent for breast cancer prevention has produced an extensive and ongoing analysis of tamoxifen risks and benefits (Cusick, 1986). The major factors contributing to the risk-benefit profile have been the reduction of breast cancer incidence, a decrease in bone fractures and cardiovascular mortality, and the occurrence of thromboembolic events and uterine cancers. Each of these items will be described in turn.

The design of the BCPT was based on a capability to detect a minimum reduction in breast cancer incidence of 30 percent in the participants randomized to take tamoxifen compared to those taking placebo. The number of breast cancer events expected in the placebo arm of the trial is based on the breast cancer risk of individuals entering the trial. Breast cancer risk has been estimated using the Gail, et al. model, which takes into account factors such as age at menarche, number of first degree relatives with a breast cancer diagnosis, age of first live birth, number of breast biopsies, and the presence of atypical ductal hyperplasia on biopsy (Gail, et al., 1989). An additional risk consideration for randomization into the BCPT is a diagnosis of lobular carcinoma in situ. Using these factors, a candidate for participation in the BCPT satisfies the eligibility criteria with respect to risk if her estimated probability of developing breast cancer is a succeeding 5 year period is at least 1.7 percent (National Surgical Adjuvant Breast and Bowel Project, 1994). This level of risk is comparable to that for the average 60 year old woman. For the first 12,000 entrants, the level of risk on average has been twice the required minimum.

Table 1. Contralateral Breast Cancers in Clinical Trials of Adjuvant Tamoxifen

Study	Tamoxifen		Controls	
	Patients	Cancers	Patients	Cancers
20 mg Trials				
NSABP B-14	1419	42	1428	73
Scottish	661	13	651	25
NATO	564	20	567	19
ECOG 1178	91	2	90	5
	2735	77	2736	122
30 mg Trials				
Toronto-Edmonton	198	4	202	9
Copenhagen	52	3	52	4
	250	7	254	13
± Chemotherapy				
CRC (20 mg)	947	30	965	28
Stockholm (40 mg)	1372	40	1357	66
	2319	70	2322	94
Total	5304	154 (2.9%)	5312	229 (4.3%)

Data presented by Zeneca Pharmaceuticals, FDA ODAC meeting 6/7/94.

A second consideration in the use of tamoxifen as a chemopreventive agent has been its impact on cardiovascular events. A 20 percent reduction in mortality from cardiovascular events is projected for the BCPT based on a variety of observations, one of which is an alteration of the serum lipid profile (Love, et al., 1994). For women being treated with tamoxifen, serum cholesterol decreases by 10 to 20 percent, mostly in the LDL fraction. Lipoprotein (a) and fibrinogen levels are decreased and triglycerides may decrease slightly. These changes in the serum lipid profile begin during the first weeks of treatment, persist throughout treatment and may help to explain the observation from the overview analysis which reported a 25 percent reduction in vascular deaths. Contributing to this overall result were the observations from component studies such as the Scottish and Stockholm trials. In the Scottish trial there was a statistically significant reduction in myocardial infarctions (McDonald, Stewart, 1991; McDonald, et al., 1995) and the Stockholm group reported a 30 percent reduction in admissions to hospital for cardiovascular diagnoses (Rutqvist, et al, 1993). Compared to the lipid changes associated with estrogen therapy, the changes seen with tamoxifen are quite favorable; for example, with estrogen therapy, the LDL cholesterol fraction decreases 14 percent and lipoprotein (a) is reduced 17 percent on average. Corresponding figures are 20 percent and 47 percent, respectively for tamoxifen (Love, et al., 1994).

An additional factor contributing to benefit from tamoxifen therapy relates to an effect on bone metabolism. In a rat model, tamoxifen suppresses PTH-mediated bone resorption (Stewart, 1986) and inhibits osteoclast activity (Jordan, et al., 1987). These mechanisms may help to explain the differences in bone-mineral density that are observed in post-menopausal women taking tamoxifen. Tamoxifen-treated women have maintained bone density while placebo-treated controls typically lose bone density at a rate of 1 percent per year over 2 years (Love, et al., 1992). A recent report from the British tamoxifen prevention trial suggests that premenopausal women using tamoxifen may not experience bone density stabilization (Powles, et al., 1996). Verification of these results awaits the report of additional observations.

Weighing in against the potential benefits from tamoxifen therapy as enumerated above are several tamoxifen-associated risks. The most significant of these risks are endometrial cancer and thromboembolic events. Endometrial cancers were first reported in association with daily doses of tamoxifen (40 mg/d) that are higher than those usually employed in the United States (Fornander, et al., 1989). From a compilation of data derived from adjuvant tamoxifen trials and presented at the ODAC in June 1994, it can be seen that uterine cancers have occurred in about 1 percent of some 5,000 patients, consistent with an approximate threefold increase in crude risk (without adjustment for survival).

Table 2. Uterine Cancers in Clinical Trials of Adjuvant Tamoxifen

Study	Tamoxifen		Controls	
	Patients	Cancers	Patients	Cancers
20 mg Trials	2735	25	2736	7
30 mg Trials	250	3	254	1
Other	2319	31	2322	8
Total	5304	59 (1.1%)	5312	16 (0.3%)

Data presented by Zeneca Pharmaceuticals at FDA ODAC meeting June 7, 1994.

A relative risk in the range of 2- to 4-fold or less is suggested by several sources (Cook, et al., 1995; van Leeuwen, et al., 1994). In trying to understand the natural history of this problem, several leads have been pursued. In the British prevention trial with tamoxifen, participants were evaluated after they had started protocol therapy. On endometrial biopsy, a higher incidence of endometrial hyperplasia and polyp formation was found in the tamoxifen arm compared to the placebo arm of the trial (Kedar, 1994). Data is limited from women who have had biopsies at the beginning of tamoxifen therapy and again later during therapy (Gal, 1991).

From the NSABP analysis of endometrial cancer in women who participated in the B-14 trial, it was noted that a high percentage of the women who developed endometrial cancer had prior exposure to hormone replacement therapy (Fisher, et al., 1994). Concern about this issue has led to annual endometrial sampling in the BCPT. A substudy comparing uterine sonography with endometrial sampling is also a part of the approach to gynecologic evaluation of participants in the BCPT.

The incidence of thromboembolic events has been reported for several trials. In the NSABP B-14 trial where tamoxifen was tested as an adjuvant therapy, the rate of thromboembolic events in the tamoxifen arm of the trial was about 1 percent. Although the mechanism is not clear, it has been reported that antithrombin III levels decrease as a result of tamoxifen therapy (Enck, Rios, 1984). This kind of change might disrupt the usual mechanisms of control in the clotting system.

Rare complications of tamoxifen therapy include reports of liver and eye toxicity. There have been isolated reports of individuals with fatty liver, elevated transaminases, and rare reports of liver necrosis (Ching, et al., 1992). Although four cases of hepatobiliary carcinoma have been reported among women treated with tamoxifen in 2 randomized clinical trials, there were also 3 cases in the control groups for those two trials, leaving it doubtful that there is any apparent difference with respect to this outcome (Andersson, et al., 1991; Rutqvist, et al., 1995). Clinical observations have stimulated extensive laboratory work looking for an effect of tamoxifen on liver. Rat studies have demonstrated the development of liver cancers and the formation of DNA adducts in liver cells (Carthew, et al., 1995). Interspecies differences in biology and metabolism are likely to account for the much higher degree of liver toxicity in animals (Robinson, et al., 1991). As Jordan and Morrow have pointed out, part of the difference may also arise from dose and schedule of administration to animals (Jordan, Morrow, 1993). In spite of reports of DNA adducts in the livers of animals treated with tamoxifen, a small series of liver biopsies from 7 women who had taken 20 or 40 mg of tamoxifen daily for at least 2 months and as much as 39 months failed to show any increase in DNA adducts compared to adduct levels in biopsies from seven controls.

Like liver toxicity, ocular toxicity associated with tamoxifen use is rarely encountered in clinical practice. Although an increased incidence of cataracts has been observed in a rat model, tamoxifen associated cataracts have not been a problem in humans. Visual problems related to tamoxifen use were first reported in association with massive doses of tamoxifen (60-80 mg/m^2/day) (Kaiser-Kupfer, Lippman, 1978). When impaired visual acuity is associated with tamoxifen therapy, it usually improves after withdrawal of the medication. With tamoxifen-associated visual problems, there have been reports of paramacular retinal deposits, macular edema, keratopathy and optic neuritis (Nayfield et al., 1991). Although ocular toxicity at relatively low doses of tamoxifen (20mg/day) is rare, work is in progress to establish any differences between treated and untreated groups in the BCPT and NSABP B-14.

In summary, tamoxifen is a well tolerated medication with few side effects. Prior experience with tamoxifen has demonstrated that it is eminently suitable for investigational use in a randomized prevention trial. The potential for tamoxifen to prevent breast cancer is based on a demonstrated reduction of contralateral breast cancers in adjuvant tamoxifen trials. Additional benefits may accrue to tamoxifen users in the form of reduced fractures, and decreased cardiovascular disease endpoints. These benefits will need to be weighed against potential risks largely from thromboembolic events and endometrial cancer.

Risk-benefit analyses of tamoxifen for breast cancer prevention have varied widely in their conclusions (Costantino, et al, 1994). It is clear that real results from a clinical trial are needed to bring a new dimension to the understanding of how tamoxifen performs as a preventive agent. Consistent with this purpose, the BCPT continues to randomize patients. Since starting randomization in June 1992, accrual has reached a level of 12,000 at the time of this writing. The average relative risk for BCPT participants without an LCIS diagnosis is 5.46 times the risk for a group of women of the same age with no risk factors, and for most age categories, twice the minimum risk that is required for entry. At randomization, one-third of the non-LCIS study population is aged 35 to 49, a little over one-fourth are 50 to 59, and about 40 percent are aged 60 or more. This age distribution is very close to the estimated age distribution that was used for designing the trial. The BCPT has been remarkable for establishing exceptionally large groups of women in certain risk categories. At this time, the trial includes about 650 women with a diagnosis of LCIS and over 2,000 women with 2 or more first degree relatives who have been diagnosed with breast cancer. Nearly 80 percent of the participants have at least one first degree relative with a history of breast cancer.

Although a temporary interruption in accrual to the BCPT during 1994 might have been expected to alter statistical power, the ability to detect the primary endpoints of breast cancer incidence and mortality has nevertheless been maintained largely due to the high level of breast cancer risk in participants. As the BCPT moves into the final 25 percent of its enrollment, useful data is already beginning to accumulate. Quality of life data is collected regularly and evaluations of endometrial changes, other cancers, bone metabolism and genetic factors are built into the trial. The baseline assessment of the quality of life for participants has recently been published (Ganz, et al., 1995). As breast cancer susceptibility syndromes become more fully characterized, the BCPT will provide data on how a tamoxifen intervention will affect individuals with increased breast cancer risk defined by genetic factors. The BCPT also has the potential to provide new scientific leads on the prevention of cardiovascular disease, osteoporosis and endometrial cancer. Due to the meticulous collection of data about participants and the tissue and serum samples that they are providing, the BCPT is likely to become a unique resource for advancing the scientific understanding of women's health.

REFERENCES

Andersson M, Storm HH, Mouridsen HT (1991): Incidence of new primary cancers after adjuvant tamoxifen therapy and radiotherapy for early breast cancer. J Natl Cancer Inst 83:1013-1017.

Carthew P, Martin EA, White INH, De Matteis F, Edwards RE, Dorman BM, Heydon RT, Smith LL (1995): Tamoxifen induces short-term cumulative DNA damage and liver tumors in rats: promotion by phenobarbital. Cancer Res 55:544-547.

Ching CK, Smith PG, Long RG (1992): Tamoxifen-associated hepatocellular damage and agranulocytosis. Lancet 339:940.

Cook LS, Weiss NS, Schwartz XM, White E, McKnight B, Moore DE, Daling JR (1995): Population-based study of tamoxifen therapy and subsequent ovarian, endometrial, and breast cancers. J Natl Cancer Inst 87:1359-1364.

Costantino JP, Redmond CK, Fisher B (1994): Response; Re: Endometrial cancer in tamoxifen-treated breast cancer patients: findings from the National Surgical Adjuvant Breast and Bowel Project (NSABP) B-14. J Natl Cancer Inst 86:1025-1026.

Cusick J, Wang DY, Bulbrook RD (1986): The prevention of breast cancer. Lancet I:83-86.

Early Breast Cancer Trialists' Collaborative Group (1992): Systemic treatment of early breast cancer by hormonal, cytotoxic, or immune therapy. Lancet 339:1-15.

Enck RE, Rios CN (1984): Tamoxifen treatment of metastatic breast cancer and antithrombin III levels. Cancer 53:2607-2609.

Fisher B, Costantino JP, Redmond CK, Fisher ER, Wickerham DL, Cronin WM, and other NSABP Contributors (1994): Endometrial cancer in tamoxifen-treated breast cancer patients: findings from the National Surgical Adjuvant Breast and Bowel Project (NSABP) B-14. J Natl Cancer Inst 86:527-537.

Fornander T, Rutqvist LE, Cedermark B (1989): Adjuvant tamoxifen in early breast cancer, occurrence of new primary cancers. Lancet I:117-120.

Fornander T, Hellstrom A-C, Moberger B (1993): Descriptive clinicopathologic study of 17 patients with endometrial cancer during or after adjuvant tamoxifen in early breast cancer. J Natl Cancer Inst 85:1850-1855.

Gail MH, Brinton LA, Byar DP, Corle DK, Green SB, Schairer C, Mulvihill J (1989): Projecting individualized probabilities of developing breast cancer for white females who are being examined annually. J Natl Cancer Inst 81:1879-1886.

Gal D, Kopel S, Bashevkin M, Levowicz J, Lev R, Tancer ML (1991): Oncogenic potential of tamoxifen on endometria of postmenopausal women with breast cancer - preliminary report. Gynecol Oncol 42:120-123.

Ganz P, Day R, Ware JE Jr, Redmond CR, Fisher B (1995): Base-line quality-of-life assessment in the National Surgical Adjuvant Breast and Bowel Project Breast Cancer Prevention Trial. Natl Cancer Inst 87:1372-1382.

Jordan VC, Phelps E, Lindgren JU (1987): Effects of anti-estrogens on bone in castrated and intact female rats. Breast Cancer Res Treat 10:31-35.

Jordan VC (1992): The role of tamoxifen in the treatment and prevention of breast cancer. Curr Probl Cancer 16:134-176.

Jordan VC, Morrow M, (1994): Should clinicians be concerned about the carcinogenic potential of tamoxifen? Euro J Cancer 30A:1714-1721.

Kaiser-Kupfer MI, Lippman ME (1978): Tamoxifen retinopathy. Cancer Treat Rep 62:315-320.

Kedar RP, Bourne TH, Powles TJ, Collins WP, Ashley SE, Cosgrove DO, Campbell S (1994): Effects of tamoxifen on uterus and ovaries of postmenopausal women in a randomized breast cancer prevention trial. Lancet 343:1318-1321.

King M-C, Rowell S, Love SM (1993): Inherited breast and ovarian cancer. What are the risks? What are the choices? JAMA 269:1975-1980.

Kumanyika SK, Velez R (1992): Aging Processes, pp 161-170. *In* Report of the National Institutes of Health: Opportunities for Research on Women's Health, U.S. Department of Health and Human Services, NIH Publication No.92-3457.

Love RR, Wiebe DA, Feyzi JM, Newcomb PA, Chappell RJ (1994): Effects of tamoxifen on cardiovascular risk factors in postmenopausal women after 5 years of treatment. J Natl Cancer Inst 86:1534-1539.

Love RR, Mazess RB, Barden HS, Epstein S, Newcomb PA, Jordan VC, Carbone P, DeMets DL (1992): Effects of tamoxifen on bone mineral density in postmenopausal women with breast cancer. N Engl J Med 326:852-856.

McDonald CC, Alexander FE, Whyte BW, Forrest AP, Stewart HJ (1995): Cardiac and vascular morbidity in women receiving adjuvant tamoxifen for breast cancer in a randomized trial. Br Med J 311:977-980

McDonald CC, Stewart HJ (1991): Fatal myocardial infarction in the Scottish adjuvant tamoxifen trial. The Scottish Breast Cancer Committee BMJ 303:435-437.

National Surgical Adjuvant Breast and Bowel Project (NSABP). NSABP Protocol P-1: a clinical trial to determine the worth of tamoxifen for preventing breast cancer. Pittsburgh, PA: National Surgical Adjuvant Breast and Bowel Project, September 23, 1994.

Nayfield SG, Karp JE, Ford LG, Dorr A, Kramer BS (1991): Potential role of tamoxifen in prevention of breast cancer. J Natl Cancer Inst 83:1450-1459.

Nowack R (1994): Breast cancer gene offers surprises. Science 265:1796-1799.

Parker SL, Tong T, Bolden S, Wingo P (1996): Cancer statistics, 1996. CA Cancer J Clin 46:5-27.

Powles TJ, Hickish T, Kanis JA, Tidy A, Ashley S (1996): Effect of tamoxifen on bone mineral density measured by dual-energy x-ray absorptiometry in healthy premenopausal and postmenopausal women. J Clin Oncol 14:78-84.

Redmond CK, Wickerham DL, Cronin W, Fisher B, Costantino JP and NSABP Participants (1993): The NSABP Breast Cancer Prevention Trial (BCPT). Proc ASCO 12:69.

Richardson DN (1988): The history of Nolvadex. Drug Design and Delivery 3:1-14.

Robinson SP, Langan-Fahey SM, Johnson DA (1991): Metabolites, pharmacodynamics, and pharmacokinetics of tamoxifen in rats and mice compared to the breast cancer patient. Drug Metab Dispos 19:36-43.

Rutqvist LE, Mattsson A (1993): Cardiac and thromboembolic morbidity among postmenopausal women with early-stage breast cancer in a randomized trial of adjuvant tamoxifen. J Natl Cancer Inst 85:1398-1406.

Rutqvist LE, Johansson H, Signomklao T, Johansson U, Fornander T, Wilking N for the Stockholm Breast Cancer Study Group (1995): Adjuvant tamoxifen therapy for early stage breast cancer and second primary malignancies. J Natl Cancer Inst 87:645-651.

Smigel K (1995): Breast cancer death rates decline for white women. Natl Cancer Inst 87:173.

Stewart PJ, Stern PH (1986): Effects of the antiestrogens tamoxifen and clomiphene on bone resorption in vitro. Endocrinol 118:125-131.

van Leeuwen FE, Benraadt J, Coebergh JWW, Jiemeney AM, Gimbrere CHF, Otter R, Schouten LJ, Damhuis RAM, Bontenbal M, Deipenhorst FW, van den Belt-Dusebout AW, van Tinteren H (1994): Risk of endometrial cancer after tamoxifen treatment of breast cancer. Lancet 343:448-452.

Wakeling AE (1994): A new approach to breast cancer therapy - total estrogen ablation with pure antiestrogens. *In* Jordan VC (ed): Long-Term Tamoxifen Treatment for Breast Cancer. Madison, WIS, University of Wisconsin Press, pp. 219-234.

Index